Vegetarian Diet and Healing in 10 body system

Scientific healing mechanisim of cancer, metabolic syndrom, diabetes, obesity, depression, autoimmune disease, atopy

Aaron Lee

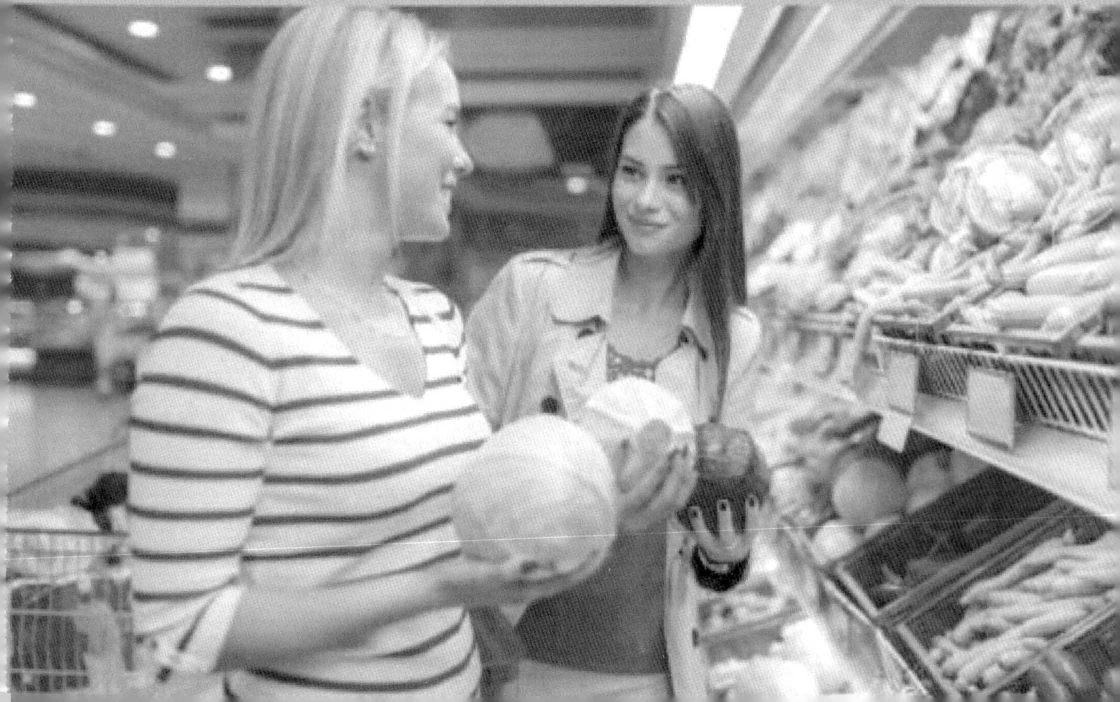

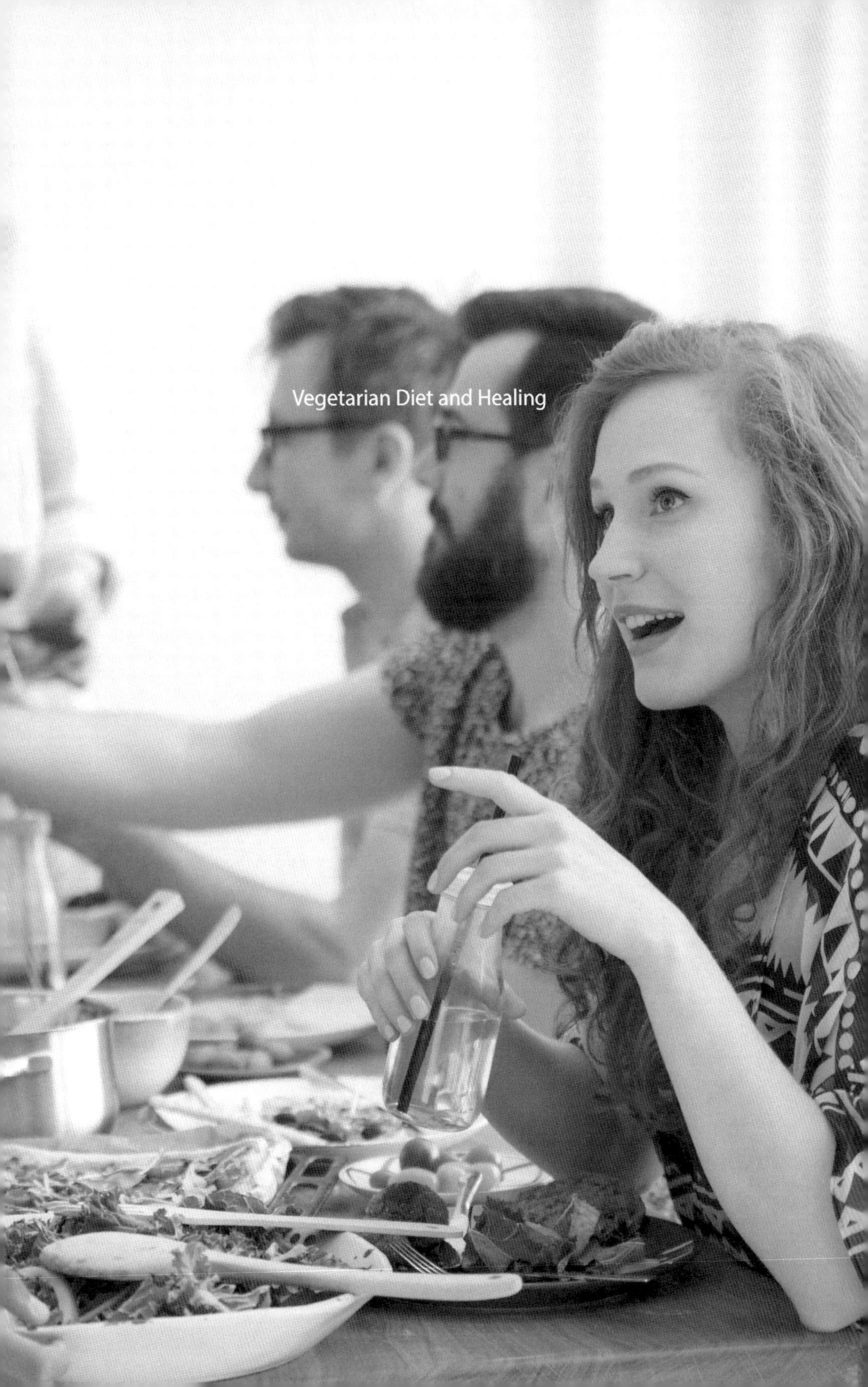

Vegetarian Diet and Healing

Vegetarian diet and Healing. 3rd ed. 2018. 8. 20 (Korean)
Vegetarian diet and Healing. 1st ed. 2019. 5. 27 (English)

Author Ph.D. Aaron KJ Lee
Publisher Soypaper

Telephone 82-2-3789-7891
E-mail soypaper@daum.net
Homepage http://soypaper.co.kr/

Vegetarian Diet and Healing

Ph.D. Aaron KJ Lee

Greetings

Food and nutrition are the components and the energy sources of the human body, and they are essential to the maintenance and health of life. Therefore, it is natural that they depend on what you eat. And, even if you are already sick, you can recover to the original healthy state by eating the right food. This is easy to understand if we accept that the original natural state of our body is healthy.

Life is precious, and people want to live healthily and happily. In the age of living 100 years, health has become more important. Along with this, the information about the useful food became more important. This is because a person behaves as much as he or she knows, and this gets back the result of that act.

The purpose of this study is to provide the systematic and accurate information on nutrition, food, and the health-related scientific research reports on the 10 systems of the human body, including the skeletal system, the nervous system, the endocrine system, the immune system, etc.

The final conclusions of this paper are: First, consume the whole grains, such as brown rice and whole wheat. Second, consume the beans, nuts and seeds. Third, consume the fresh vegetables and the fruits. Just by practicing it, you will see for yourself that the many people who suffer from diabetes, a cardiovascular disease, atopy, obesity, osteoporosis, and depression are restored to their original health states.

In order to consume healthy food, it does not require a doctor's prescription, expensive drugs, complex tools and facilities, and many economic payments. Only the understanding, the belief, and the practice are required. The purpose of this paper is to provide the information on the scientific researches and to help the rational judgments that are based on reason. I hope that you will get a little bit of help regarding the health you need to successfully lead your precious life. I pray for your victory.

This first book of english version was printed by Kim Jin-hwa's donation.

About the author

Aaron K.J. Lee

For the first time in Korea, in 1999, he created a vegetarian club at HiTel Communications(Early forms of internet). In the same year, the first vegetarian campaign in Korea was at Jongno street and at the Maroney Park. During the vegetarian campaign, he felt that he needed an understanding of the nutritional aspects of vegetarianism. In 2004, he entered the Department of Food and Nutrition at the Seoul National University, and he received his doctorate degree in food and nutrition in the year 2014.

As a graduate student at the Seoul National University, He had organized a vegetarian club for the Seoul National University, and he had proposed a vegetarian buffet to the Seoul National University and the Dongguk University.

His books include the effects of the prevention of the metabolic syndrome through the diet, the costs of the national health care, the world's vegetarian diets and the story of vegetarianism. The body wants to have a vegetarian diet. And a vegetarian in history has been promoting the benefits of the vegetarian diet through a number of vegetarian lectures including the temple food conferences. Currently, he is the Director of the Korean Vegetarian and Nutrition Research Institute, and he has been studying the neuroendocrinological effects of nutrition.

0.1. How much meat are we eating?

Along with the increased intake of the animal foods, many chronic diseases, such as cancer, diabetes, cardiovascular disease, osteoporosis, autoimmune disease, atopy, asthma, rheumatoid arthritis, and depression, have been increasing. According to the Korea Food and Drug Administration (KFDA), the amount of the meat consumed per capita per year was only 2.5kg in 1969, and there was a 17-fold increase to 44kg in 2013. Calculated on a daily basis, the average daily intake of the meat in 1969 was only 6.6 grams per day, and it was 120 grams in 2013. This, of course, excludes dog meat, cat meat, and the non-livestock that are not a part of the official count.

Excessive meat consumption can lead to a variety of problems such as excess calories, saturated fats, and cholesterol, thereby, leading to illness. Nevertheless, the fictitious superstitions about eating meat in order to feed the protein have still been circulating, thereby, leading people on the wrong paths. The World Nutrition Society (WNS) allows you to multiply your body weight by 0.8 (g) per day of protein. If you weigh 60 kilograms, you need 60 times 0.8,the 48 grams are enough, and there is no reason to supply the animal food.

0.2. Is it a vegetarian? Is it meat?

The theme of this book is not a debate on whether it is a vegetarian diet or a meat diet, but, rather, a dialogue on the healthy eating for the healthy nations, peoples, and societies. It is because it is food and nutrition that supply our energy to for our body and enable our activities.

In the recent decades, there has been a continuing rise of the dietary patterns in the context of the today's topics– 'vegetarian', 'meat or non–vegetarian', or 'omnivorous'. Therefore, this paper can be said to be very important as a process for identifying what is the first problem, which is an important process for resolving the problem.

Historically, humankind, especially ours, has been living on a vegetarian diet for a long time. This seems to have been an influence of the Buddhism religiously, as well as an influence of the development of rice farming locally.

In Samguk Yusa(Korea ancient history book), the 29th King of Baekje kingdom says that he forbade the all people from killing.

"The name of the 29th King of Baekje kingdom is, also, called "Sun" or "Hyosoon". In the 10th year of the king (A.D. 599), I understood that, in the winter, king dictated that people prohibited the killing in the private households, burning down the fish catching devices, and fishing. "

There is a record that,in the Samguksagi (Korea ancient history book) Silla Kingdom, King Hyeongheung had forbidden all of the people from killing.

"In the 16th year of King Hyeongheung (A.D. 529), the law was banned all live animal from killing."

After the invasion of Mongolia, the consumption of the meat had gradually increased, and, in the Chosun Dynasty, it had not had much meat consumption.

0.3. A vegetarian perspective?

People are vaguely vegetarian and do not lack nutrition. On the contrary, they think that some nutrients will be very scarce. This issue is a personally important information for the ongoing vegetarianism, and it is a key element in the discussions for the provision of the socialized vegetarian foods, such as the school meals. According to the accumulated research results, the degree of the availability of the information about vegetarian nutrition directly affects the view regarding, and behavior of, the vegetarian diet.

In 2004, at the Seoul National University (SNU), about 600 students were surveyed. About 18% of the students said that they did not engage in the vegetarianism due to the 'nutritional imbalance', while 49% of the vegetarian students said that it was 'for health' [1]. The opposite view on, and the subsequent behavior regarding, such vegetarian nutrition are, also, attested to by the dietitians as well as the general public, which is influenced by the amount of the nutritional information on the vegetarian diet.

In 1999, Duncan and Bergman asked 182 registered dietitian in

Washington, Nebraska, and Vermont in the United States about their knowledge and opinions on the vegetarian diet. According to the results of the questionnaire, there was a high correlation between the amount of the knowledge on the vegetarian diet and the attitude [2]. That is, the more the knowledge of the vegetarian diet, the more positive the vegetarian viewpoint (correlation coefficient r = 0.434, p 〈0.01).

The dietitians who were vegetarians at the time of the survey or before the survey had more information about the vegetarian diet than those who did not, and, at the same time, had a more positive view. The dietitians who had a negative view on the vegetarian diet were about one–third of the respondents, and the longer they worked as a dietitian, the more negative the vegetarian diet was. The authors summarize the study with the following phrases: "More and more people are vegetarian than in the past, and the nutritionists have been often asking for the dietary information. Thus, the nutritionists have had more opportunities to have a positive impact on the vegetarian diet, but, one–third of the dietitians who responded to the questionnaire did not adequately respond to the nutritional information questions about the vegetarian diet. "

As can be seen from the study that said that the vegetarians have a higher negative perception during the period of working as a dietitian, the viewpoint on the vegetarian diet of the nutrition experts may be more negative than those of the general public. In 2004, according to a research report by Jin et al., the ratio of the vegetarian diet among the general students and the nutrition students was 10% and 5%, respectively, and the general students were twice as much vegetarians that the

Introduction

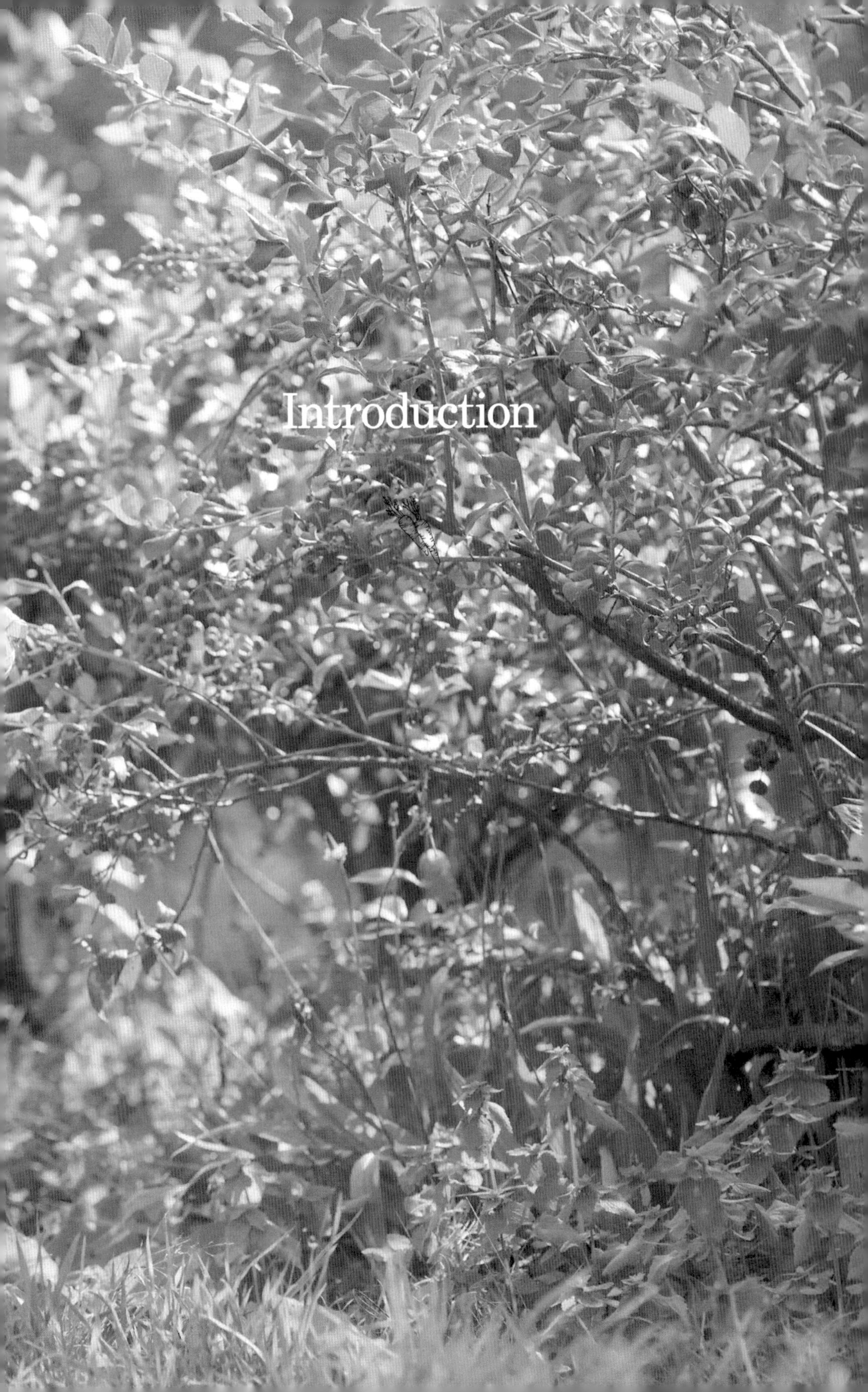

I am writing this letter to the late Miss. Song Sook-ja who has led me to the way of vegetarian nutrition and to the friend of vegetarian club.

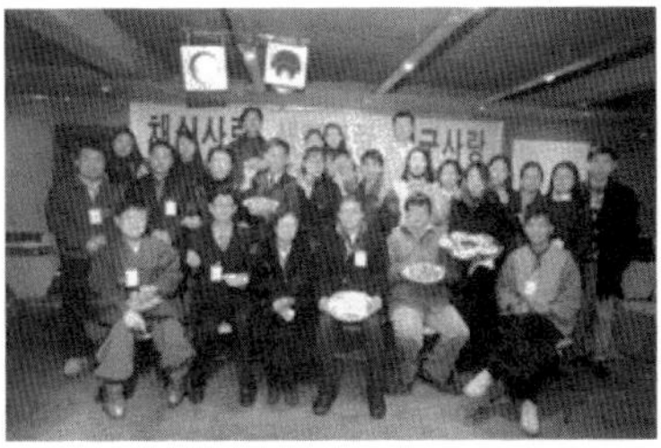

In 1999, the first meeting of the Haitel Vegetarian Society, Insa-dong Zelkova cafe

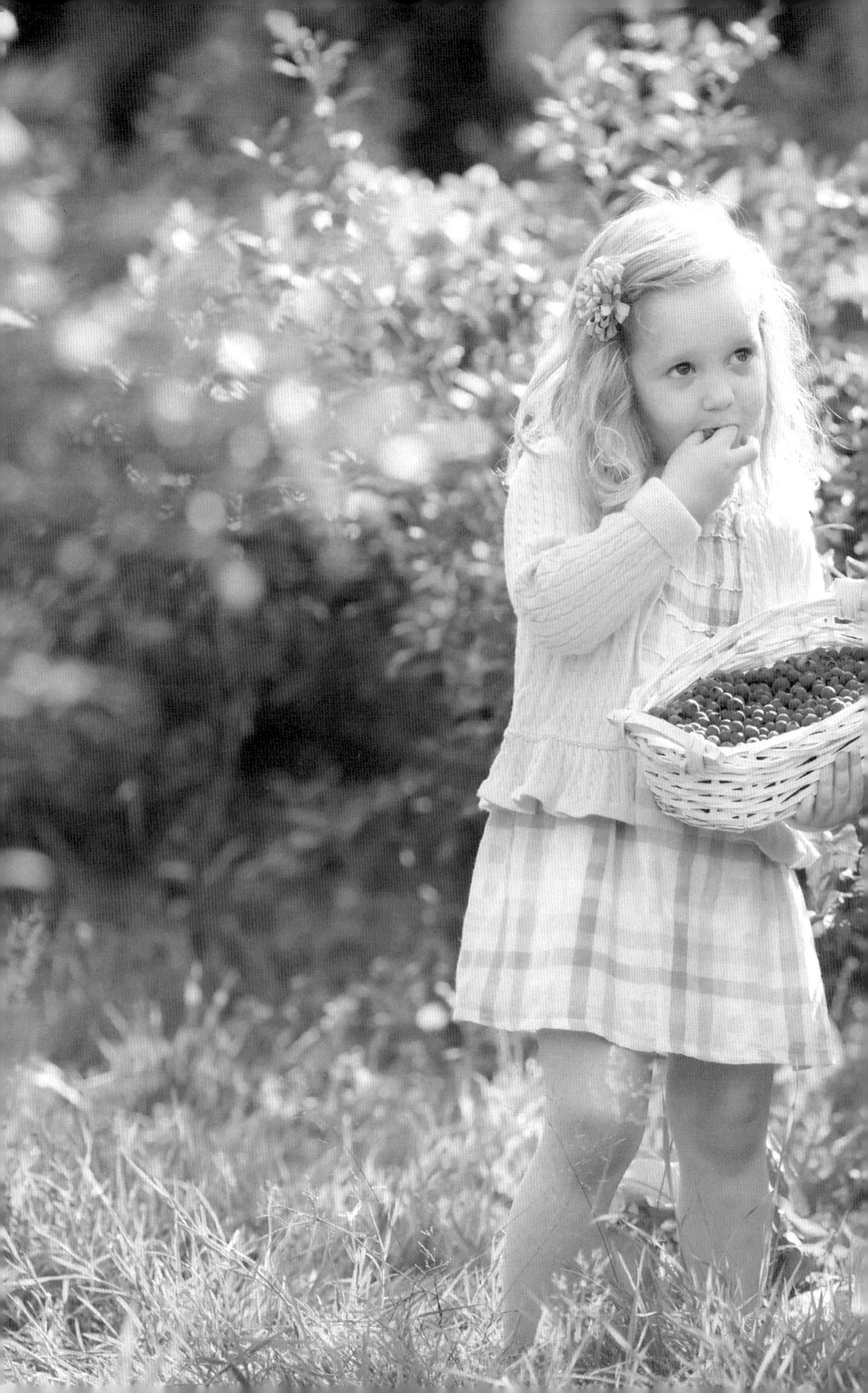

nutrition students [1]. In addition, according to their survey, regarding the introduction of the vegetarian restaurants, the general students showed the favorable rate of 53%, while that of the nutrition students was only 29%. Based on these results, the authors note that the students majoring in nutrition may be a negative factor in the introduction of vegetarianism when they work in the field as the nutritionists.

0.4. Can we provide enough nutrition through the vegetarian diet?

The nutritional safety of vegetarianism has long been recognized in the nutritional world of the advanced countries in the West. In the West, they have been focusing on the rapidly growing vegetarian population since the 1970's, and they have studied whether vegetarianism can supply enough nutrition for the human body through the vegetarian diet. In addition, the positive attitudes toward the vegetarian diet have been formally expressed by the public nutrition and government agencies, beyond the study groups. In 2003, the American Dietetic Association and the Canadian Dietetic Association jointly stated the following in a paper entitled, 'The Stance of the American and Canadian Dietetic Associations on Vegetarianism':

"When we consider the main stages of life as being the infancy, childhood, adolescence, pregnancy, and lactation, the various vegetarian diets can supply the nutrients needed for each cycle and can allow the normal growth. In childhood and adolescence, vegetarianism promotes the healthy eating habits in the long–term, and it has the advantage of lowering the cholesterol, the saturated fatty acid, and the total fat intake in the nutrition and the advantage of increasing the dietary fiber intake through the fruits and the vegetables. The vegetarian children are, also, known to have the lower serum cholesterol levels than the non–vegetarian children [3]. "

Even in the large–scale surveys, such as the National Health and Nutrition Examination Survey (1999–2004), the vegetarian nutrition was not a problem. According to this study of 13,000 people aged 19 and over, the vegetarians were higher than the non–vegetarians with regard to the fibrin, vitamin A, vitamin C, vitamin E, thiamine, riboflavin, folate, calcium, magnesium, and iron [4].

In addition, the US Department of Agriculture (USDA) website kindly introduces how to make a vegetarian diet with the health benefits of vegetarianism.

Fortunately, the social movement on the vegetarian diet has been positive, partly. The most representative example is the school food service site. In October 2010, the University of Seoul hosted a vegetarian buffet at the Dongguk University in June 2011, and the great responses were received from the many students and faculty members. In addition, for the first time in 2011, the Jeonbuk Provincial Office of Education chose dozens of elementary, junior high, and senior high schools in the province for a number of years, and it successfully gave a demonstration on the

Vegetarianism Day with the increasing number of the atopy students and with the increasing environmentally-friendly green-eating habits. However, in spite of the desirable social change of such a vegetarian diet, there is still no information on the vegetarian nutrition in Korea. Therefore, we want to respond to the request for this information.

0.5. Is our body suitable for vegetarianism?

In the fluctuations of the evolution that has been going on for a very long time in comparison with our human history, securing the nutritional sources of the diverse spectrum will be very advantageous for our survival. However, if we look at the basic structure and physiological phenomena of our body, we can estimate the evolution of our body and mind through a long-term view.

Amylase (carbohydrate enzyme of human), which is produced only in the herbivore. And DHA and EPA, which cannot synthesize in the carnivores, are produced by the linolenic acid. The acidity of human stomach, which is only one tenth of the carnivores. The flat nail and tooth structures of human that cannot easily tear, even the thin skin. The broad molars of human with which it is easy to grind the grains or the grass (the molars are not in carnivores). The structure in which the upper jaw and the lower jaw can move left and right in human and herbivore. The carnivorous animals must shake their heads because they cannot move left and right when they feed.

More than anything, the instinctive emotions are involved. As a vegetarian said, "When you bring a little baby with the apples and the rabbits, does he spit on your rabbits and taste them again? When I see the cruelly dying lives, my compassion that turns my head and hurts my heart proves that the human beings instinctively value and care for life.

The ability to eat and digest a broader spectrum of food can be beneficial in the evolutionary process. Especially, at the time of the Ice Age, when food was lacking, there was not enough to worry about whether the food should be the plants or the animals.

However, as can be seen in the case of the cattle rabbits, which do not die right after eating the other animals' flesh, meat cannot be said to be necessary because humans can eat meat. Rather, the vegetable dietary pattern is more suitable for the human body. These claims will be substantiated through the practical evidences that are based on the various scientific experiments and the studies to be presented in this book later on. Originally, we, the humans, had been based on the vegetable diets, so, when we return to the vegetarian diet, we will naturally regain a healthy state. Our body is made in a very sophisticated way, and it is surprising to see the strong resilience if you only fit in a few conditions such as nutrition and air. The healthy body and mind are the precious heritages of our human and vital world that have been refined for a long time, and they can be retrieved if we make the right environment at any time. I hope that this article will help you to be sure of this.

0.6. It should be prepared for the aged-society with vegetarian paradigm.

In the near future, Korea will enter an aging society. According to a report by the US Bureau of Statistics, the proportion of the population over 65 years old in 2050 will be 35.9% already, second only to Japan. Four out of 10 people will be over 65 years old. In 1980, the proportion of the 65-year-old population was only 3.8%, but, in 2000, it entered the aging society with 7%, and, in 2026, it entered the super-aged society with more than 21%. Currently, the medical expenses are 100 trillion won per year. In 2030, the cumulative deficit of the medical expenses will be 400 trillion won. The developed countries in the West are promoting a policy of the vegetarian diet suitable for the human body. There is now the need for a policy to nutritionally prevent the personal and national disasters resulting from bankruptcy.

The purpose of this article is to explain how the body system affects each system in a positive way by constructing 10 human systems of the skeletal system, the urogenital system, the cardiovascular system, the digestive system, the nervous system, the respiratory system, the reproductive system, the immune system, the endocrine system, and the skin system. The results are introduced. This will help you to understand the principles and processes of healing more systematically and synthetically. The content of each chapter consists of its own complete structure, so you can begin reading from any part of your interest.

All the cells in the human body are connected with the blood vessels, and they supply the nutrients and the oxygen through the blood, and they remove the waste products. Therefore, one improvement in many systems of the human body means that the other systems will, also, change in a positive direction. In other words, the fact that the whole body interacts with the whole helps in accepting that the same vegetarian diet is effective, whatever makes the body healthy. This is one of the benefits of nutritional therapy, unlike the drugs with the side effects and the incompletely limited efficacy. Nutritional therapy is safe and complete, and it has been proven in nature for a long time.

0.7. Understanding the system.

The purpose of this study is to understand the health benefits of the vegetarian diet in terms of the system and the perspective of 10 human body systems. Therefore, it is helpful to understand some of the concepts of the system, the cell, the tissue, the organ, and the human system.

In a lexical sense, the 'system' is an aggregation of the complex entities, each component interacting or being interdependent. In general, one system is represented as a closed figure with a circle. The inside of the circle becomes the inside of the system, and the outside of the circle becomes the environment or the outside world. There is an interface between the inside and the outside of the system. The system may often be modeled or visualized as the building blocks with some connection between the members. For example, the sun's radiation between the sun and the earth is represented by a dotted line. The sun and the earth are different in size, composition, and characteristics, but, they are connected by the solar radiations, and they can be regarded as a system of the solar system. In other words, it is arbitrary for the observer to set up a system as a system, but one system has the complex interactions or interdependencies among the elements.

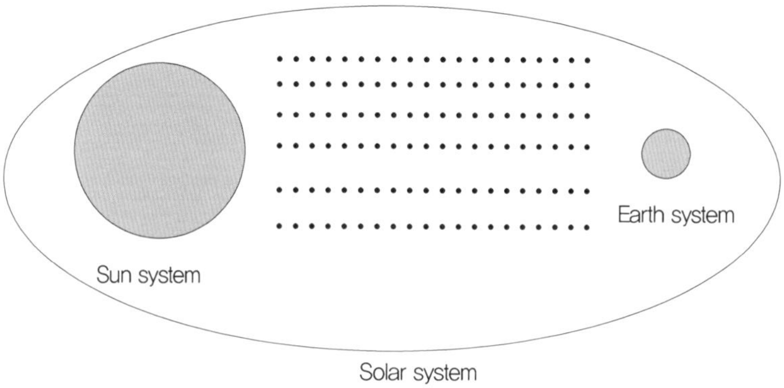

Figure 0–1. Examples of various systems

0.8. The characteristics of the system.

The system has the following, several characteristics: First, the system has the structure that is defined by the parts and the processes. For example, in the solar system, the components are parts of the sun, the earth, and the other planets. And there are the processes of transferring the energy, such as the solar radiation between them. Second, the system is a generalization of the entities. Third, the system tends to function in the same way. This means that the input and the output of the material or the energy and the aspects of the processing change within the system. Fourth, the various parts of the system are structurally related as well as functionally related. Fifth, the relevance of the functions that exist between the parts means the flow and the transfer of some forms of the energy

* Most systems have eight common characteristics.

1. Parts and processes
2. Entities
3. Same function
4. Structural and functional associations of parts
5. Flow and delivery of energy or materials
6. Movement of energy and matter between the external environment
7. Propulsion
8. High level of bonding

or the material. Sixth, one system exchanges the material or the energy with the other systems or environments through the various input and output processes, beyond the boundary with the outside environment. Seventh, the functional relationships can occur due to the presence of the driving force. Eighth, the parts of the system constitute a somewhat well-coupled level, although the levels of the couplings are different. Three characteristics can be found inside the boundary of the system, that is, inside the system.

The first is each of the parts that make up the system as the elements. The part may be as small as an atom or a molecule, depending on the system, or it may be a larger component like the sun or the galaxy. The system of the earth can be regarded as the component of the river, the sea, the continent, the mantle, and the nucleus. In the system, the house,

> Within the system there are three characteristics: components, attributes, and relationships.
> 1. Components –〉 Parts
> 2. Attributes –〉 Measurement or recognizable attributes
> 3. Relationship–〉 Relevance between elements

the room, the kitchen, and the living room become the components. The second are the attributes that are the attributes of the elements that can be recognized or measured, such as the mass, the number, the size, the color, the volume, and so on. The third are the relationships that occur between the elements or the attributes. These relationships are the basis of the cause and effect causation. The state of the system can be expressed through, and determined by, these three characteristics. That is, the state of the system can be defined by the elements, the attributes, and the relationships within the system.

0.9. Three types of systems : The Isolated System, the Closed System, and the Open System.

The 'system', also, refers to an aggregate in which the behaviors of the members in the social system must be controlled or maintained. In the nineteenth century, the French scientist Carnot studied the thermodynamics and introduced the concept of "system" to the natural

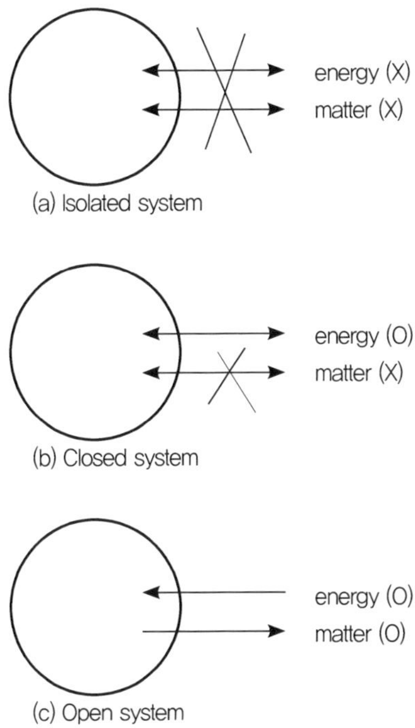

Figure 0-2. Three types of systems, Isolated system (a) closed system (b), open system (c)

Each system unit of living organisms such as cell organelles, cells, tissues, organs, and the human body are all open systems and interact vertically and horizontally between systems.

sciences. Based on the transfer of energy and matter, the scientists have classified the system into three categories: The Isolated System, the Closed System, and the Open System. An isolated system is one in which the system does not interact at all over the interface. That is, there is no material, energy, or information transfer between the inside and the outside of the system beyond the interface.

The Closed Systems have a transfer of energy between the system and the external environment, but, there is no transfer of the material. An Open System is where the materials and the energy are transferred between the external environment and the system. Most ecosystems are the open systems, and they include the human systems. 'Dynamic equilibrium' is an important concept in understanding the characteristics of an Open System. In other words, when the inward flow and outward flow of the system are the same amounts, the inside of the system is kept constant,

Table 0-1. The size of various cells of the human body

Cell type	Average volume (μm^3)
Sperm cell	30
Red blood cells	100
Lymphoid cells	130
Neutrophil	300
Beta cells of the pancreas	1,000
Fibroblast	2,000
Osteoclast	4,000
Macrophages of bronchi	5,000
Heart muscle cells	15,000
Oocyte cell	4,000,000

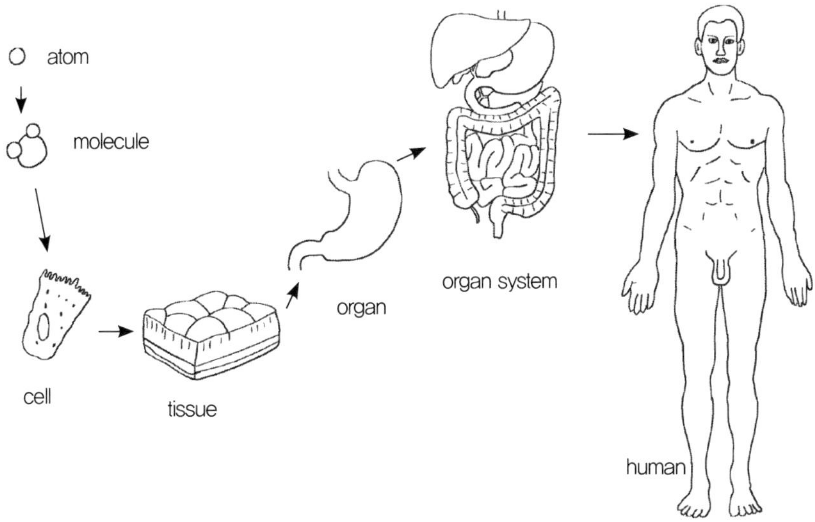

Figure 0–3. Various levels of systems

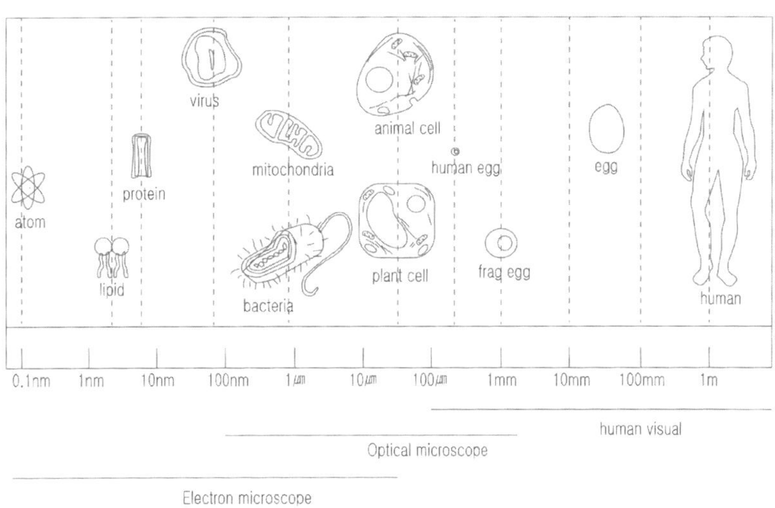

Figure 0–4. Comparison of size of life systems

which is called the "dynamic equilibrium". The opposite of the dynamic equilibrium is the static equilibrium, which is to maintain a constant state inside the system when there is no entry into, or exit from the system, such as an Isolated System. In the case of life, the substances and the energy go in and out constantly, and the adults can maintain a constant weight because of the same dynamic equilibrium between the ingestion and the excretion.

0.10. The characteristics of the biological systems.

The functions that an organism must perform in order to survive include the following:

1. Obtain oxygen to be used for the cell respiration and release the carbon dioxide as a by-product.

2. You must be able to ingest and digest food to obtain the sugars and the other nutrients.

3. It must be able to transport all the necessary materials, such as oxygen and the nutrients, to all the cells.

4. It should be able to remove the toxic wastes generated from the cells and the body.

5. Be responsive to the environment.

6. Be able to fight against invader.

7. For the survival of the species, each individual must be able to

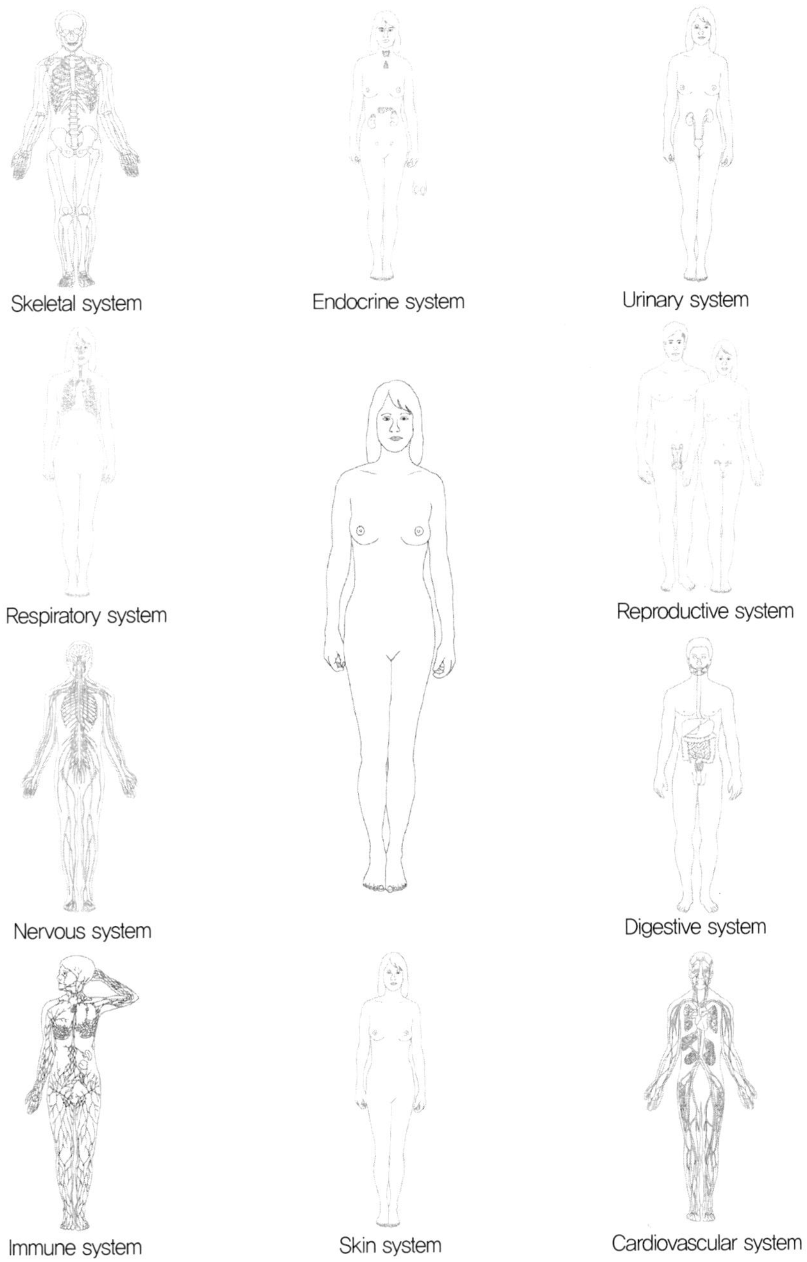

Figure 0–5. Ten systems that make up the human body

reproduce.

0.11. systems of the human body.

The human body can be divided into 10 systems based on the close relationship and function of each component. In this article, we explain the benefits of the vegetarian diet by classifying the 10 systems.

Respiratory System : Allows the gas exchanges between the cells and the environment. Includes the tracheas and the lungs.

Digestive System/Excretory System : Allows the nutrients to be consumed by digesting and decomposing the food. And it discharges the solid wastes. It includes the mouth, the esophagus, the stomach, and the intestines.

Cardiovascular/Circulatory System : Transfers oxygen, nutrients, hormones, and waste products between the body systems. It includes the heart, the arteries, and the veins.

Renal System/Urinary System : The wastes released from the cells are taken from the blood and are cleaned. Includes the kidneys and the bladder.

Endocrine System : The body secretes the chemical signals so that the body system can perform the necessary cooperative actions. Includes the pineal gland, the pituitary gland, the thyroid gland, the adrenal gland, the pancreas, the ovary, and the testes.

Nervous System : Allows rapid response to the cognition, the emotion, the thought, and the environment. The brain and the nerves are involved.

Musculoskeletal System : Allows the body to move according to the commands of the nervous system.

Integral System/Exocrine System : Covers the body and controls the exchanges with the outside. Includes the skin, the hair, the nails, the sweat, and the other glands that secrete the substances from the skin.

Lymphatic System/Immune System : Fights infections. Includes the lymphatic vessels that penetrate the body.

Reproductive System : Allows the production of the offsprings. Includes the ovaries, the mammary glands (the breasts), the penis, and the testes.

References

1. Jang Sang Hyun and Ko Eun Joo: Perceptions of Vegetarians in Nutrition Major and General University Students. Environmental Sociology Research 2004, 7:115–139.

2. Duncan K, Bergman EA: Knowledge and Attitudes of Registered Dietitians Concerning Vegetarian Diets. Nutrition Research, 19:1741–1748.

3. American Dietetic A, Dietitians of C: Position of the American Dietetic Association and Dietitians of Canada: Vegetarian Diets. Can J Diet Pract Res 2003, 64:62–81.

4. Farmer B, Larson BT, Fulgoni VL, III, Rainville AJ, Liepa GU: A Vegetarian Dietary Pattern as a Nutrient-Dense Approach to Weight Management: An Analysis of the National Health and Nutrition Examination Survey 1999–2004. Journal of the American Dietetic Association, 111:819–827.

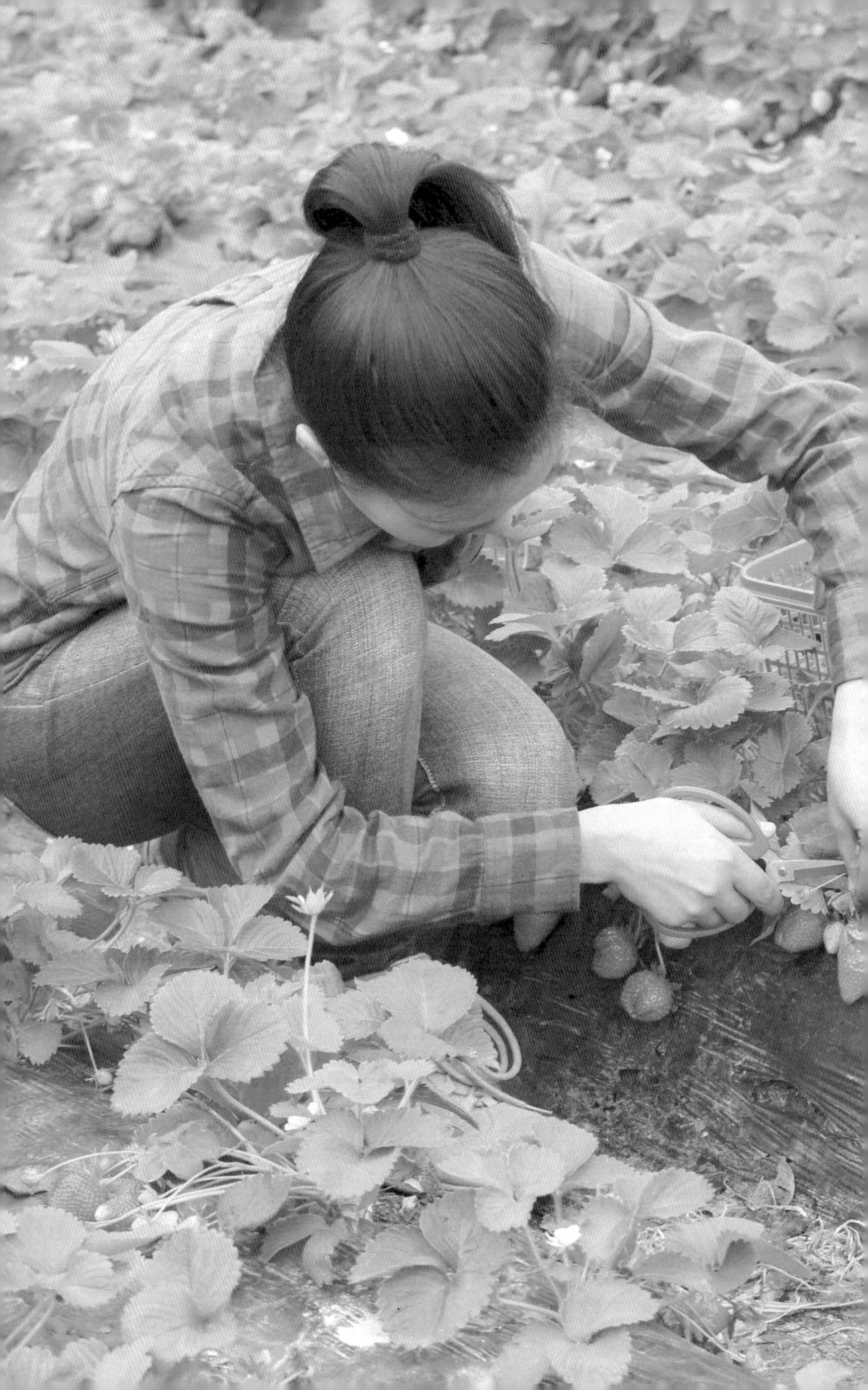

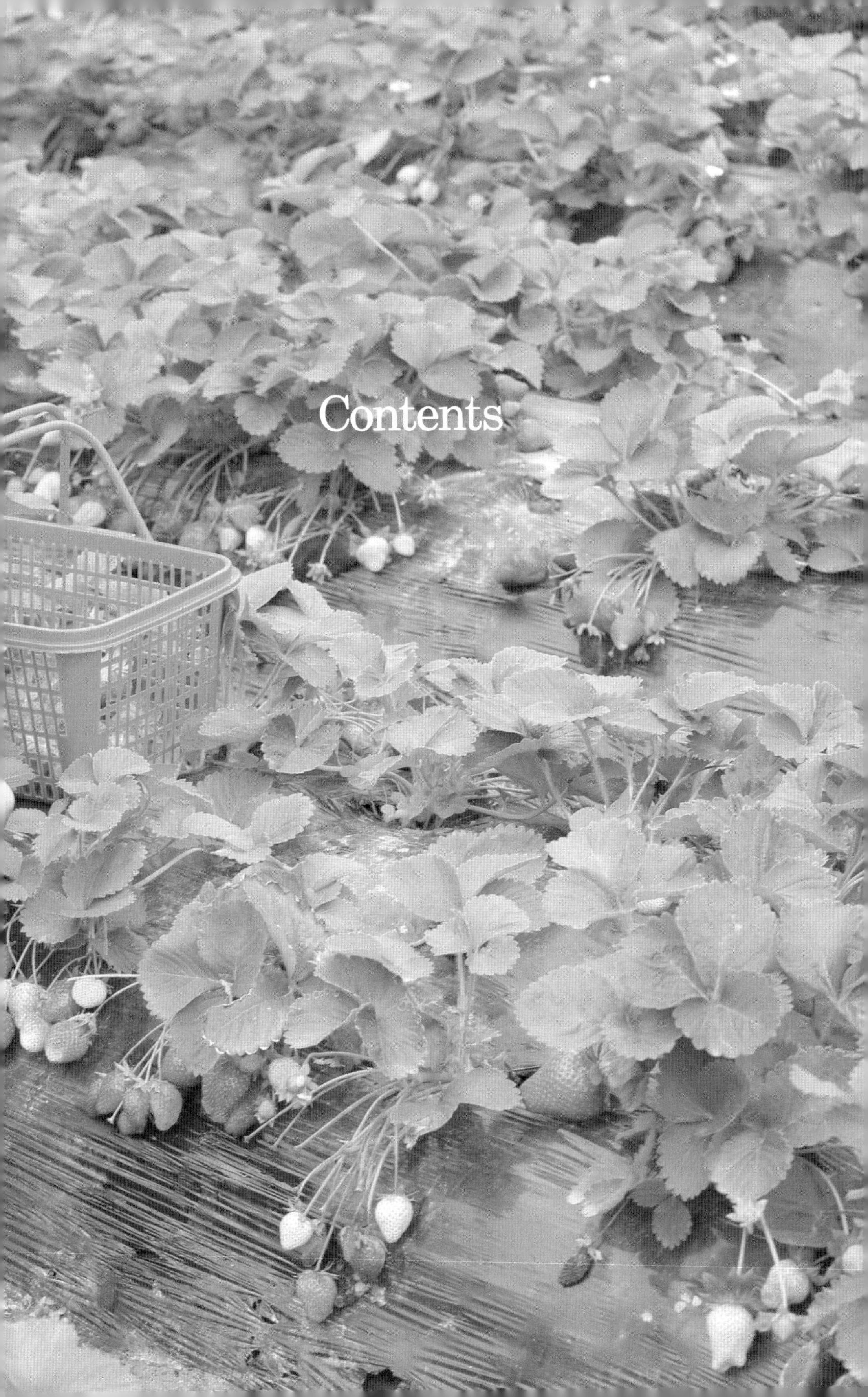

Contents

Vegetarian diet and Healing (3rd ed.)

Chapter1. Skeletal system and vegetarian diet

Chapter 2. Urinary and vegetarian diet

Chapter 3. Cardiovascular and vegetarian diet

Chapter4. Digestive system and vegetarian diet

Chapter5. Nervous system and vegetarian diet

Chapter6. Respiratory system and vegetarian diet

Chapter7. Reproductive system and vegetarian diet

Chapter8. Immune system and vegetarian diet

Chapter9. Endocrine system and vegetarian diet

Chapter10. Skin system and vegetarian diet

Chapter11. Understanding Nutritional Recommendations

Chapter12. Preventive Nutrition and Vegetarianism

Epilogue

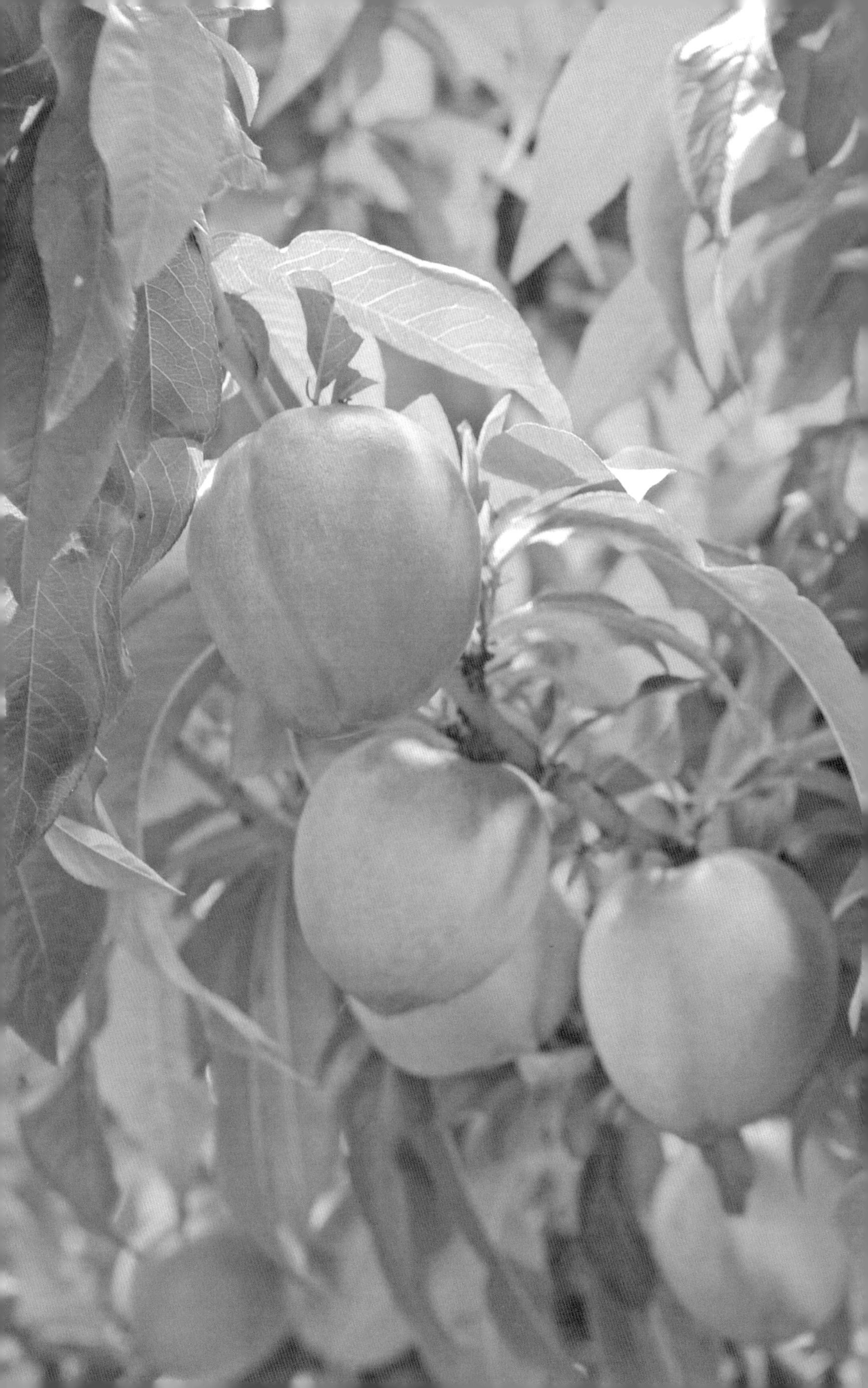

Chapter1. Skeletal System and Vegetarian Diet

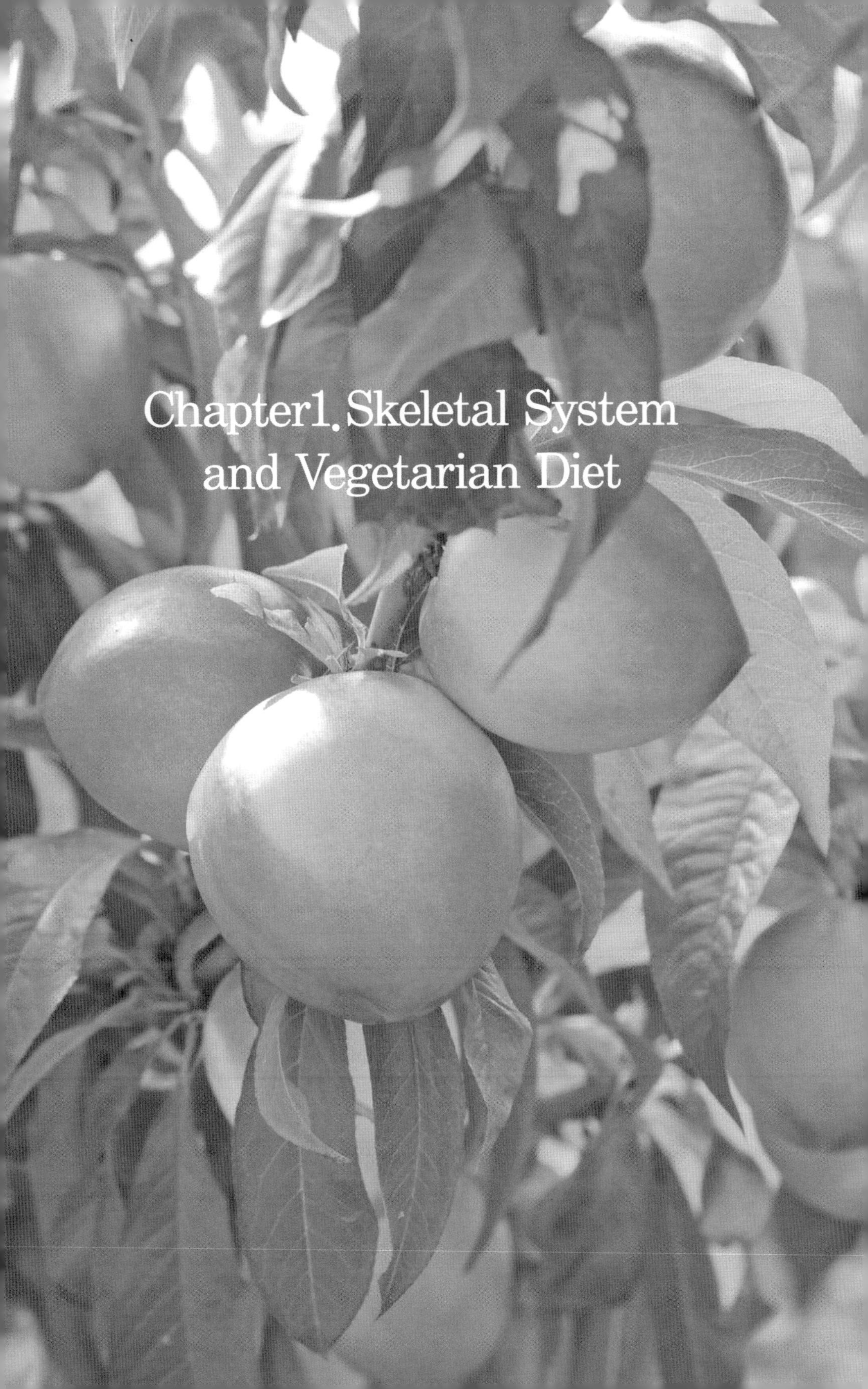

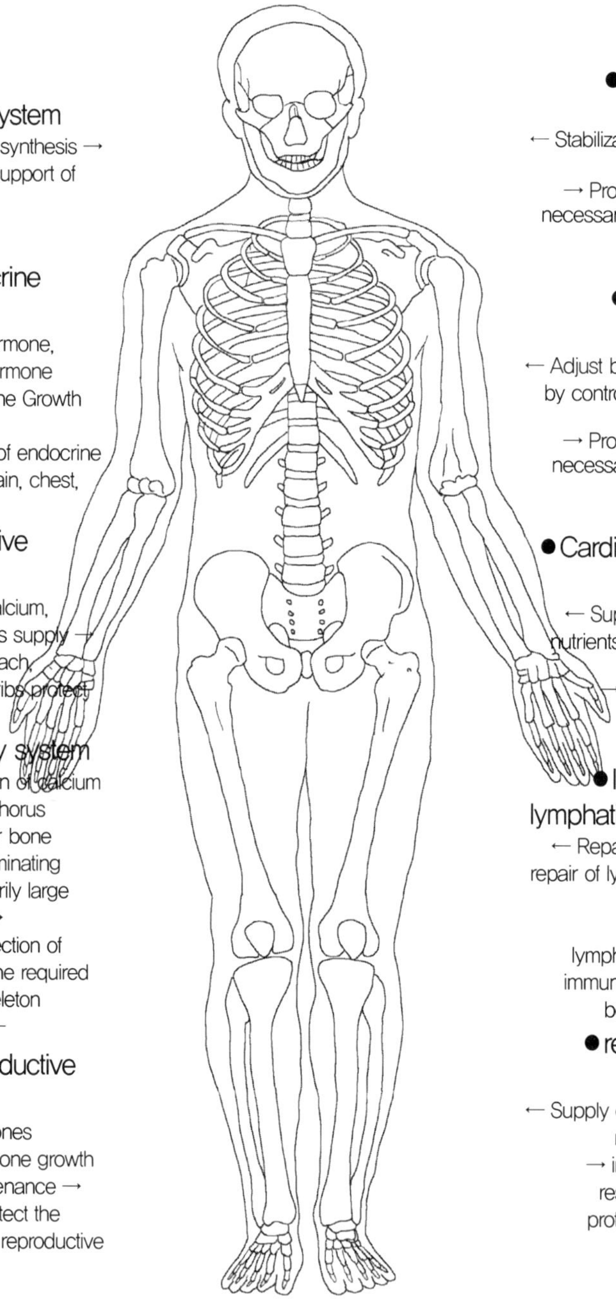
● Skin system
Vitamin D_3 synthesis →
Structural support of skin ←
● Endocrine system
Growth Hormone, Thyroid Hormone Control Bone Growth →
Protection of endocrine system (brain, chest, pelvis) ←
● Digestive system
Nutrient, calcium, phosphorus supply →
Liver, stomach, intestines, ribs protect ←
● Urinary system
Preservation of calcium and phosphorus required for bone growth, eliminating unnecessarily large amounts →
In the protection of kidneys, The required vertical skeleton Provided ←
● Reproductive system
Sex hormones stimulate bone growth and maintenance →
female Protect the pelvis, the reproductive organ ←
● Muscular system
← Stabilization of bone position
→ Provide calcium necessary for muscle contraction
● Nervous system
← Adjust bone position by controlling muscle contraction
→ Provide calcium necessary for nerve function
● Cardiovascular system
← Supply oxygen, nutrients, hormones, blood cells
→ CO_2, Waste removal
● Immune / lymphatic system
← Repair of bones, repair of lymphocytes, defense
→ Produce lymphocytes and immune cells from bone marrow
● respiratory system
← Supply oxygen and remove CO_2
→ important for respiration, rib protection, lung protection

Chapter1. The skeletal system and the vegetarian diet

1.1. The bone function and the remodeling

There are two general misunderstandings about the bones. bones are merely a skeleton that supports the body, and after bone are used once, they are permanently fixed. In addition to the body support function that maintains the basic structure of the human body, the bones, also, protect the brain, the spinal cord, the heart, and the lungs, and they exercise the function of acting as a leverage of the movement by attaching the skeletal muscles and the various minerals, such as calcium phosphate. And they exercise the hematopoietic functions that produce the white blood cells, the red blood cells and the platelets.

In addition, the hard–looking bones seem to have stopped the metabolic activity, but they are, also, the very dynamic structures that are constantly extinguished and generated. These dynamics are made possible by the operations of the osteoclasts and the osteoblasts, which have the many blood vessels and nerves that are

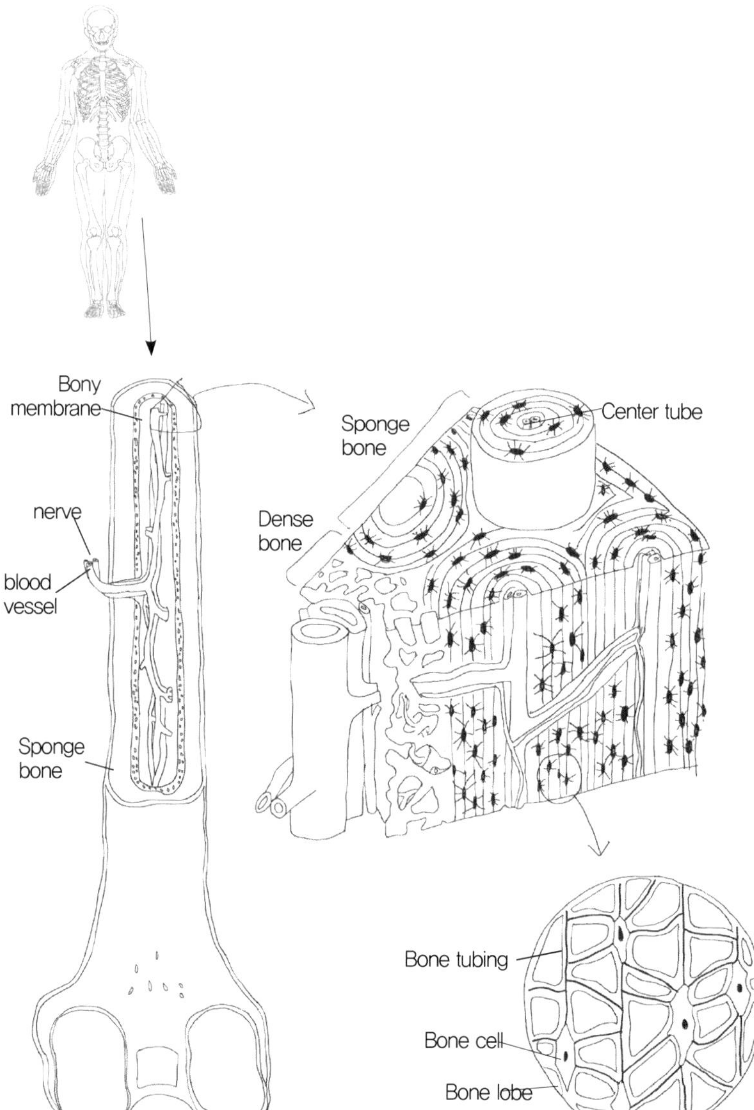

Figure 1-1. Structure of bones

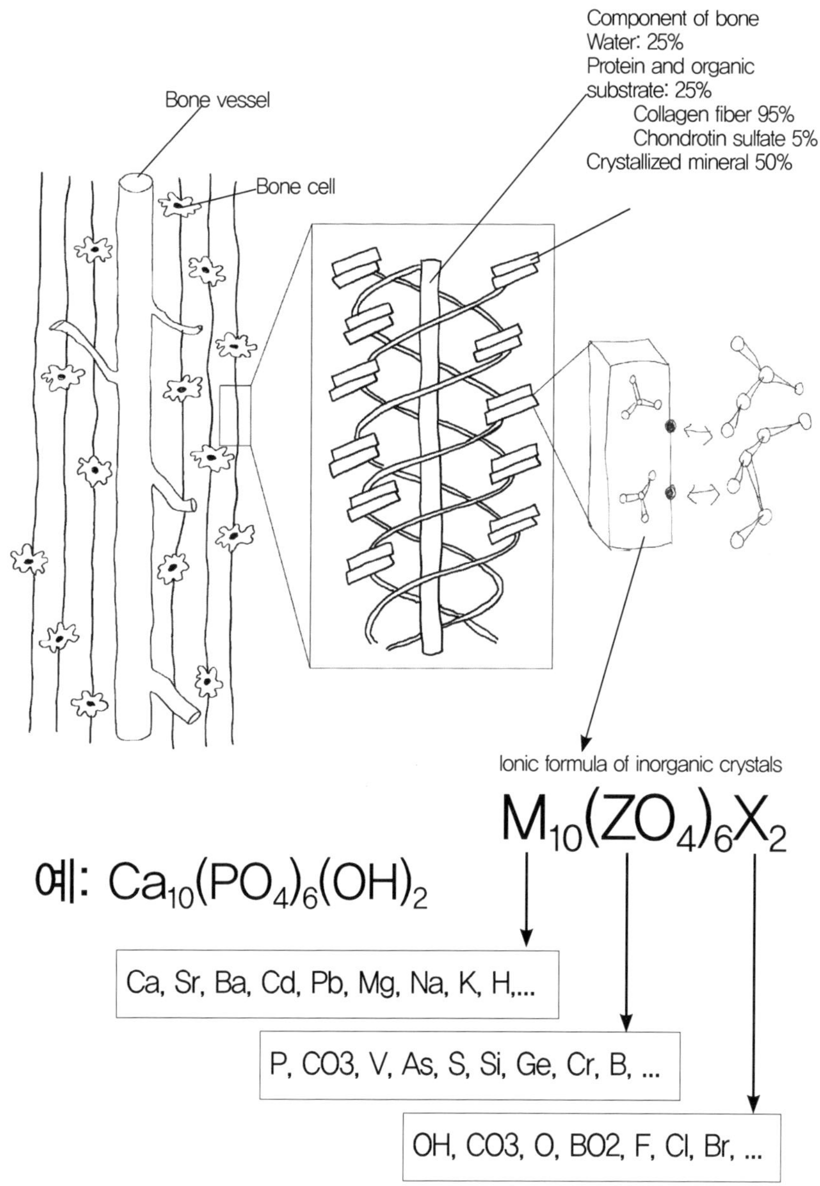

Figure 1–2. Components of bone cells and matrix

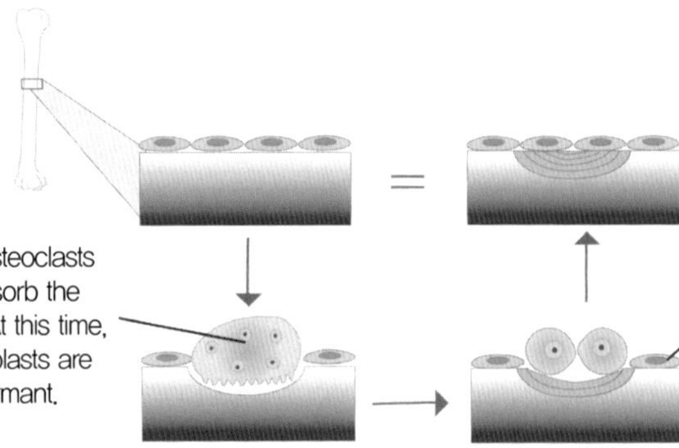

Figure 1–3. Bone remodeling process, a dynamic balance of healthy adults

connected to the inside of the bones, bone cells remove the aged–bone matrix and that make the new ones.

Bones are composed of the bone cells and the bone matrices. The bone cells are, again, divided into the osteoblasts and the osteoclasts. The osteoclast dissolves and resorbs the bone matrix for the continuous growth of the bone. The osteoblast cleaves the protein called the "collagen" in the part that has been degraded by the shape of the osteoclast and attaches the bone, the calcium, the magnesium, the phosphorus, etc., to the bone matrix. For the normal adults, 700 mg of calcium comes out of the bones every day, and this is about from 15% to 20% of the total bone mass from each year. This process is called the "remodeling of the bones".

Osteoporosis is known to be a representative, geriatric disease, and it has, also, been frequently seen in the young people in the recent years. 'Osteoporosis' refers to a state in which the strength of the bone is weakened and the fracture is easily caused by the reduction of the strength of the bone constituents. The constituents of the bone, here, are the minerals, which means the calcium and the other minerals. Osteoporosis is called "a metabolic bone disease", and it is affected by the various factors.

Bone health is influenced by a number of factors, including physical exercise, genetic factors, hormones, and nutritional status. Particularly, the appropriate types of food and the adequate nutrient intake can affect the hormones and the genetic factors, especially the acid–base balance.

1.2. Bone health and the acid–base homeostasis

All activities of the human cells operate normally when the pH of the blood is between 7.35 and 7.45. The human body uses three mechanisms to maintain this range: The buffer system, the CO_2 emission, and the urinary system. The center of the buffer system is the minerals of the bone, and, therefore, the acid–base homeostasis is very important for the health of the bone.

Adults have from 1,000 grams to 1,500 grams of calcium in their bodies, of which 99% are in the bones and the teeth and of which the remaining 1% is in the blood and the soft tissues. If, for some reason, the blood is acidified, the body releases the bone calcium and the other minerals to maintain a pH of between 7.35 and 7.45.

Although the theory that the bone minerals, mainly calcium, will protect against the acidified blood was already there in the late 1880s, the specific experimental evidences began to emerge in the late 1960s and the early 1970s.

In 1969, Barzel and Jowsey had consumed the acid ammonium chloride (NH_4Cl) in the rats, and the bone densities of the rats had gradually decreased and progressed to osteoporosis. Their acid–base equilibrium hypothesis was further confirmed by the addition of the acidic ammonium chloride and the potassium bicarbonate ($KHCO_3$) as the bases, resulting in the bone loss [1,2].

So, through what mechanism does the acid damage the bones in the human body? An important experiment to answer this question was conducted in 1986 by Arnett and Dempster. They had tissue-cultured the mouse bone cells in vitro and had lowered the pH of the culture medium (acidification). The bone resorption rate had increased rapidly as the osteoclast activity had increased [3].

As we have seen, the osteoclasts are the cells that absorb the bone matrix during the remodeling process of the continuous absorption and production of the bone. However, the acidic environment in which the blood is acidified (acidosis) causes an abnormal, bone-mineral re-uptake by the osteoclasts in the body, resulting in the net release of the bone minerals and the osteoporosis.

1.3. Types of food and the acid production

Eating foods makes and also uses the acids in our bodies. Therefore, the daily food intake will affect the body's acid-base homeostasis and will be an important factor regarding the bone health. Therefore, depending on the type of the food, would the level of the acid burden not change? It is natural to ask this.

Remer and Manz investigated the acidities of the various foods in 1995 and investigated the potential kidney burdens. Meat produces about 8mEq per 100g, which is very acidic, while fruits and vegetables showed an increase of the renal, birth-weight value and appeared to be the alkaline foods which are beneficial to the human

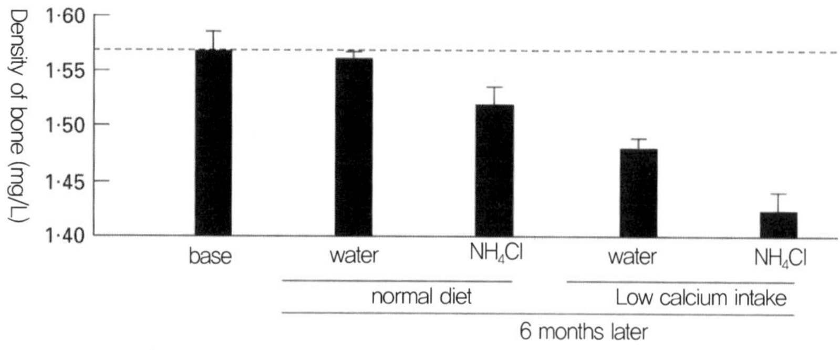

Figure 1–4. Reduction of bone density due to prolonged intake of acid ammonium chloride

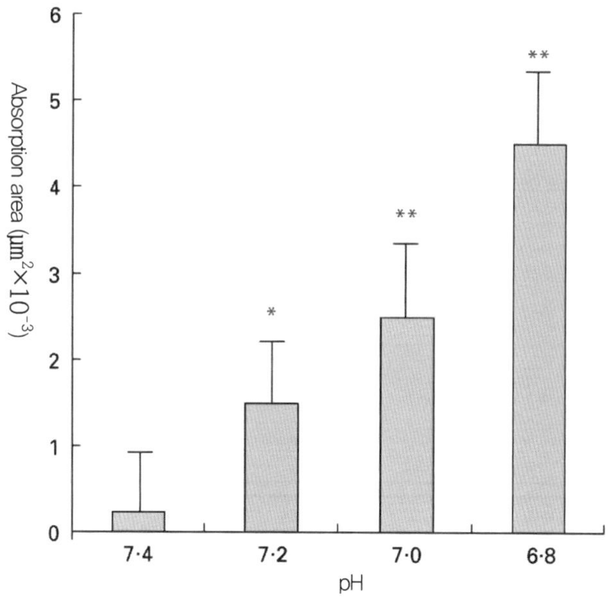

Figure 1–5. Increase of osseointegration area of osteoclast by pH decrease (increase in acidity) of extracellular fluid

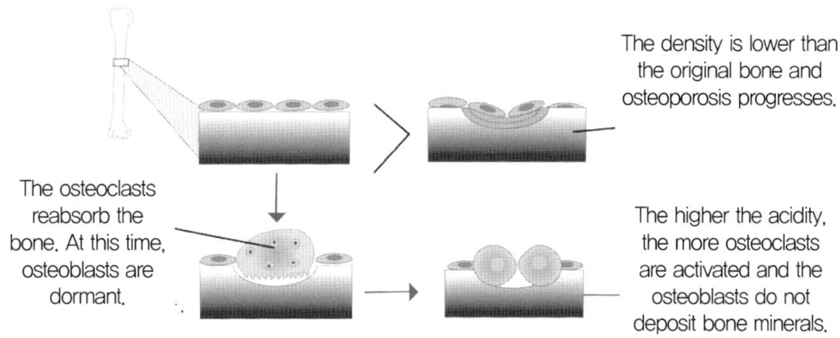

Figure 1–6. Progression of osteoporosis due to ingestion of acid foods

bone health [4].

The notable point is the high burden of the cheeses. Cheddar cheese is 26.4, which is about three times higher than meat. Eggs are, also, very high at 23.4. And these foods are the foods which the lacto–ovo vegetarians enjoy and also intake a lot.

1.4. Animal protein intake and calcium balance.

Is there any evidence that eating meat is bad for the bone health? To understand this, let us, first, look at the concept of balance, which is one of the basics of the nutrient setting in nutrition. The balance is positive and negative. The positive balance is more than the amount that is ingested, as a result of examining the amount consumed and the amount excreted. On the other hand, when the amount discharged is greater than the amount consumed, it

Table 1–1. Potential kidney burden of various foods (Remer & Manz, 1995)

food	Acid load (mEq/100g)	food	Acid load (mEq/100g)
Fruit and juice		Dairy products & eggs	
Apple	−2.2	milk	0.7
raisin	−21.0	yogurt	1.5
Grape juice	−1.0	Cheddar cheese	26.4
Lemon juice	−2.5	Cottage cheese	8.7
Vegetables, grains		Egg (yolk)	23.4
spinach	−14.0	Meat, fish	
broccoli	−1.2	beef	7.8
carrot	−4.9	chicken	8.7
potato	−4.0	Pork	7.9
refine wheat	3.7	Liver sausage	10.6
Brown rice	12.5	salmon	7.1

** The larger the minus value, the less the burden of mountains, and the larger the plus + value, the greater the burden on height*

is called a "negative balance". The intake includes not only the solids but, also, the beverages, and the discharge is the sum of the stool, the urine, the sweat, and the saliva. In other words, even if the intake is low, the positive balance of the human body actually absorbs and stores the calcium, and, even if the intake is high, the balance includes the calcium excretion in the human body (Figure 1–7).

In 1968, Wachman and Bernstein had examined the relationship between animal protein intake and osteoporosis in various parts of the world, and found out that the higher the intake of animal protein, the more hip (femur) fractures were caused by osteoporosis.

In Figure 1–6, the estimated daily intake of calcium in South Africa is less than 200 mg, but the fractures occur in less than 10 per 100,000 people, while in the United States, the United Kingdom, and Finland, which consume more than five times the calcium, the fracture rate exceeds 100 per 100,000 people.(Figure 1–8) [5,6].

This fact was made even clearer in 1981 by a team of researchers. As shown in Figure 1–9, when the patient consumed only 500 mg of calcium with a daily intake of 48 g of protein, the calcium had a positive balance (stored in the human body). However, when the calcium intake was 1,400 mg and when 142 g of protein was ingested, the calcium balance was a negative balance (calcium excreted from the human body). Even if the intake of calcium is only one–third of western diet, it is most likely to absorbed, stored in the body and become healthy with high bone density.

Evidence continues to emerge that the meat–centered, high–protein diets produce many hydrogen ions in the body and, thus,

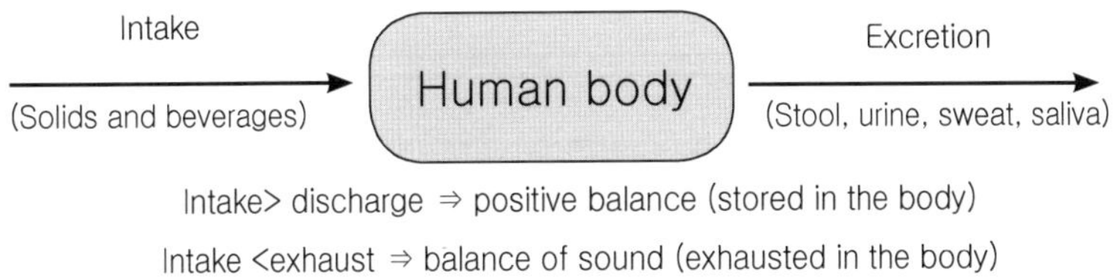

Figure 1–7. Balance between intake and excretion

the body's skeleton continues to release calcium for the acid–base buffering. In 1998, Frassetto and his colleagues had measured the ratio of the protein to the potassium (protein/potassium) and the amount of the acid produced by the kidneys in the 20 non–vegetarian adults, based on the amount of potassium. The higher the protein intake, the higher the concentration of the acid, which burdens the kidneys (Fig. 1–8). This can be interpreted as a high amount of acid production in the body and, therefore, a high possibility of the release of the bone mineral [8]. Amino acids, methionine, and cysteine, which contain a lot of sulfur and animal

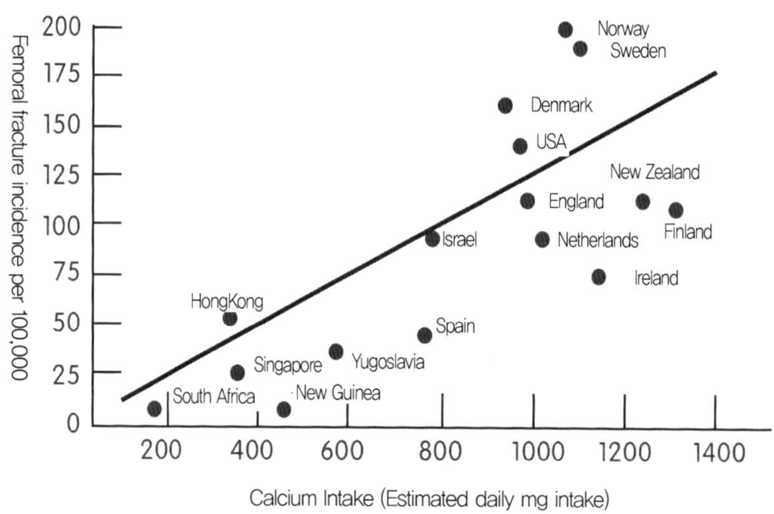

Figure 1–8. Proportion of calcium intake and incidence of femur fracture

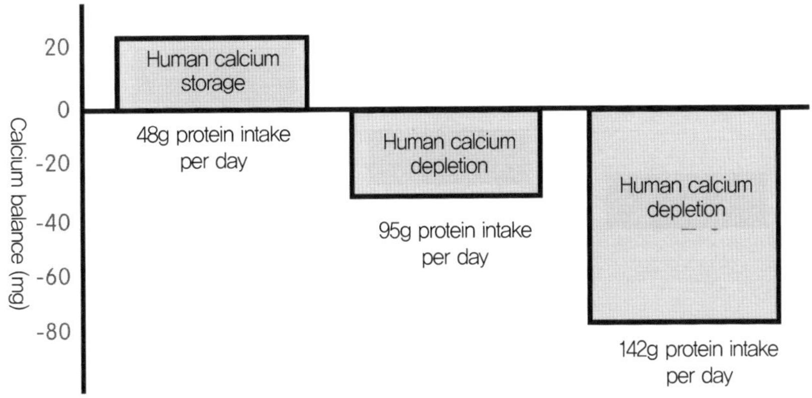

Figure 1–9. Protein intake and calcium balance in the body

As the amount of protein consumed per day increases, calcium excretion increases rather than calcium intake.

proteins, change into sulfuric acid and hydrogen and acidify the blood with the organic acids. Ironically, the prejudice regarding the vegetable proteins is that they have the low quality of protein due to their low content of methionine and cysteine.

Along with the high–sulfur amino acids, many phosphates in the meat protein are also associated with the calcium loss. Calcium is absorbed into the human body at a ratio of 1 : 1 with the phosphoric acid. On the other hand, the soybean–based vegetarian diet has less calcium loss (Table 1–2).

One study in 1998 found out that 150 mg of calcium was excreted when an animal protein was consumed, but only 103 mg of calcium was excreted from the soybean–based vegetarian diet.

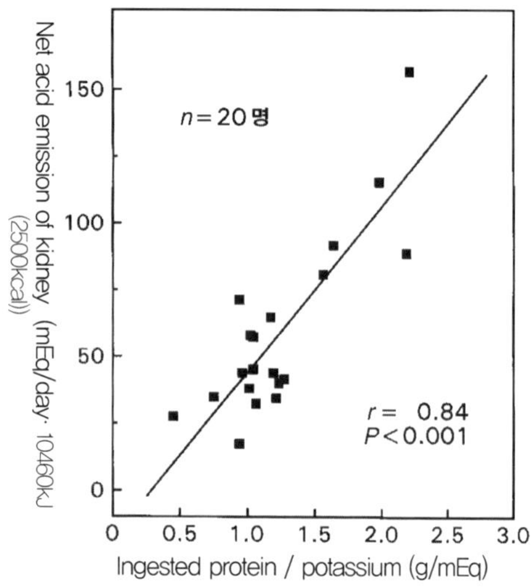

Figure 1–10. The ratio of protein / potassium intake and net acid excretion of kidney (RNAE)

The protein, itself, increases the glomerular filtration rate of the kidneys and promotes the bone loss. The kidneys filter 8,000 mg of calcium daily, and 98% is reabsorbed by the normal people, and the rest is excreted in the urine. However, the high protein diet increases the filtration rate, resulting in the substantial loss. Therefore, doubling the protein intake doubles the calcium excretion.

In 1990, the University of Connecticut researchers found a 60 mg increase in calcium excretion when the protein intake was increased by 50 g, which means that, on the average, 1 mg of calcium is lost per 1 gram of protein. The total amount of the calcium stored in the human body is only from 1,000 g to 1,500 g, which is the sum

Table 1-2. Percentage of calcium and phosphorus in various foods

Food	Calcium (mg)	phosphorus (mg)	Calcium / phosphorus
Diet Coke	0	41	0.1 or less
T-bone steak (90g)	6	198	0.1 or less
salmon (90g)	8	279	0.1 or less
potato (90g)	4	43	0.1
Tofu (half cup)	258	239	1.1
Milk (1 cup)	290	228	1.3
Sesame seed (1 teaspoon)	88	57	1.6
Spinach (half cup)	277	91	3.0
radish slice (half cup)	194	44	4.4
Kale (1 cup)	179	36	4.9

of both the bone and the teeth. Even though the amount of the acidic food is very small, the balance of the calcium throughout life will deplete the bones stored in the human body. The proteins need to be consumed only as needed, and they are safe enough to be supplied with the plant foods.

1.5. . Vegan and calcium balance.

If so, will the vegetarian diet show a positive balance in calcium absorption? In 2003, researchers in Germany studied seven women and one man who were aged from 19 years to 24 years and whose physical growths almost reached the peak. They had been fed a vegan diet for 10 days, they had been fed a turmeric, vegetable diet for 10 days. Afterward their total calcium intakes in the urine excretions were investigated, and the calcium balances were calculated.

The meals supplied were enough to meet the energy required by the individual. As shown in Table 1–3, the average calcium supplied to the vegans was 843 mg, while the amount supplied to the lacto–ovo vegetarians was 1,322 mg. The approximate calcium absorption rate was 26% for the vegans and 24% for the vegetarians. Figure

Table 1–3. Calcium Balance of Vegans and Uranus (± SD per day)

group	Vegan	lacto–ovo vegetarian	P
Number of subjects	8	8	
Calcium intake (mg)	843±140	1322±303	⟨0.01
Calcium stool emission (mg)	637±224	1002±267	⟨0.05
Calcium absorption	205±112	320±135	NS
Calcium absorption (%)	26±15	24±8	NS
Calcium urine output	87±67	110±46	NS
Calcium balance (mg)	119±113	211±136	NS
Calcium balance (%)	15±14	16±9	NS
Deoxypyridinoline (nmol)	105±31	98±23	NS

1–9 shows the balances of the calcium, a vegan balance of from 27 mg/day to 252 mg/day, and a vegetarian balance of from 32 mg to 283 mg, with the average balance of 211 mg [9].

The conclusion is that modern Westerners prefer a low–calorie diet than a high–calorie diet, which can maintain the healthy state, while a nutritionally–harmonized diet meets this need, whether it is vegan or turmeric.

The vegetable foods rich in fruits and vegetables among the plant foods are especially important to prevent osteoporosis and maintain the healthy bones. In 1997, Arpel et al. found that 157 mg of urine had been excreted when 3.6 servings of the fruits and the vegetables had been consumed, but it had decreased by 110 mg when the dose had been increased to 9.5 servings. This was because the fruits and the vegetables produced less acid in the body and, thus, less calcium excretion for the buffering [10].

Regarding the bone mineral health measurements for the bone marrow biomarkers of 200 native vegetarians and non–vegetarians in the 1980s, which were much more prejudiced against the vegetarians than they are now, it was difficult to choose the vegetarian foods. The study was conducted on 200 lacto–ovo vegetarians and 72 non–vegetarians, who were aged from 20 years to 49 years. As shown in Fig. 1–11 and Fig. 1–12, there was no significant difference in the bone mineral masses between the lacto–ovovegetarians and the non–vegetarians until they were about 50 years old.

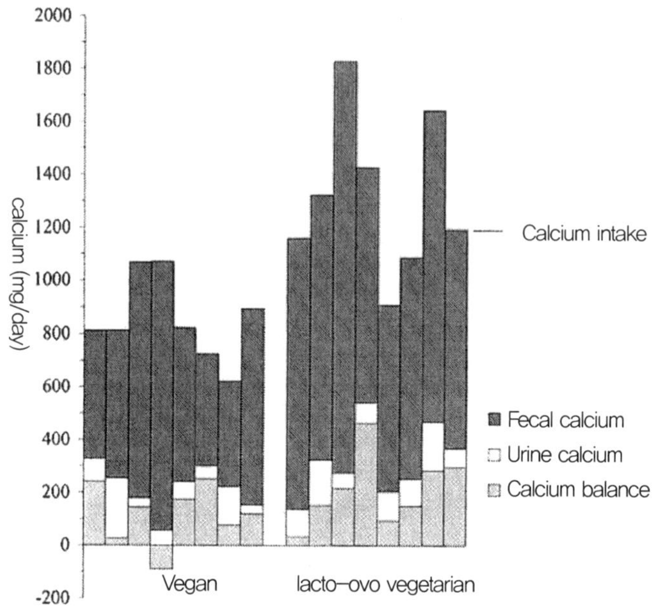

Figure 1-11. Vegetarian Dietary Pattern and Calcium Balance

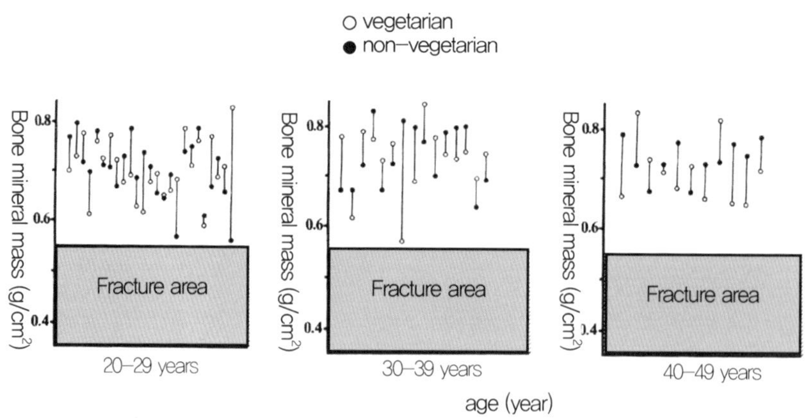

Figure 1-12. Comparison of bone mineral masses between vegetarian and non-vegetarian women. (No statistically significant difference between the two groups of N.S.)

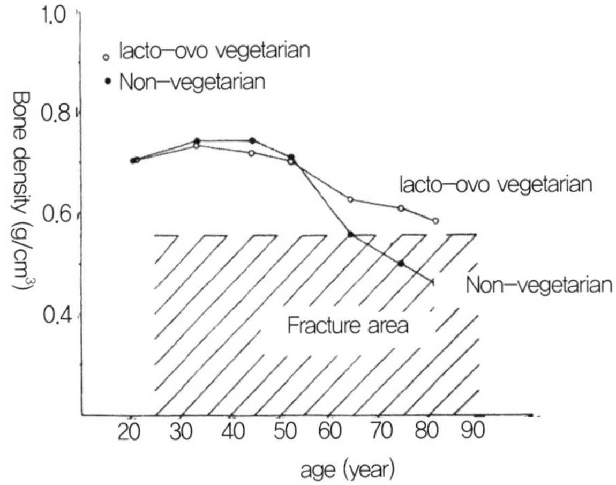

Figure 1–13. Trends in bone density of vegetarians and non–vegetarians by age

Table 1–4. Foods with a particularly high calcium content (per 100g edible portion) [11]

food	black green bean	black bean	Yellow beans	mung beans (green soy)
mg	224	220	246	107
food	tofu	Chestnut	Cone Sushi	Azuki bean
mg	126	239	295	128
food	Perilla	Sesame	Sweet potato stem	Leaf mustard kimchi
mg	351	1,245	1,552	118
food	Sesame	Wasabi	wild chive	Dried radish slice
mg	325	145	124	310
food	Dried leaves	Grapefruit	garland chrysanthemum	Kale
mg	335	236	119	320
food	taro	Pumpkin	fig G N	black sesame
mg	709	165	171	1,237

An edible portion refers to a portion of the food that can be eaten.

(Calcium content per 100g is 6mg of beef, 8mg of pork, 5mg of chicken, the processed meat is not more than 40mg, and the egg does not exceed 100mg.)*

However, after turning 50 years of age, the bone mineral content of the vegetarian diet did not decrease significantly, but it remained healthy because it was still outside the fracture range. However, the bone mineral content of the non-vegetarians had been rapidly lowered, and the bone density had decreased below the fracture area (Figure 1-13). In other words, between 50 and 89 years of age, the bone mass of the vegetarians was healthier than that of the non-vegetarians [10]. This may be the result of a little depletion of the bone that had been stored young by the continued acidic diet with the meat. And the growth hormone weakens the acidic action in the body. According to this, the ingestion of the young meat is presumably due to the growth hormone, which alleviates the acid action, but the acid action due to the meat, which was, again, due to the decreased growth hormone at the age had lowered the bone mineral density.

1.6. The calcium amount and the absorption rate of vegetarian food

In contrast to our general preconceptions, regarding all the items of the beans, seedlings, such as seaweed (224mg / 100g), sesame (1,237), sweet potato stem (1,552), cyanide (145), and tranquilizer (709),the vegetarian foods have the high calcium contents. On the other hand, beef is 6mg per 100g, pork is 8mg per 100g, chicken is 5mg per 100g, and eggs do not exceed 100mg per 100g.

So, is it true that, despite the abundant calcium contents, the vegetable calcium is low in terms of the absorption? Scientific research says that this is a superstition. In normal, vegetarian diets, the calcium absorption is inhibited by the oxalic acid, the fiber, and the phytic acid, which are actually the oxalic acid-rich spinach, which has the constant calcium absorption rate of from 25% to 35%. And, usually, the absorption rate of the calcium in soybean and food is 20%, and the leaf vegetables absorb more than 50%. Therefore, the calcium inhibition due to the vegetable foods is practically unnecessary.

The vegetarians generally consume twice as much fiber and phytic acid than non-vegetarians. However, according to the actual experimental results, the calcium absorption inhibition by these foods can't be observed. Because phytic acid is already bound to calcium, it does not bind to the other calciums. The inhibition of the calcium absorption by the cellulose was known to have taken place in 1942 and has been cited for more than 70 years without any further research.

The insoluble fiber can be an important topic, rather than the total fiber, in relation to the topic of calcium absorption. Therefore, even if the total fiber content is high, the content of the insoluble fiber is small, therefore the calcium absorption is good. The insoluble fiber is mainly a lot of the uncomplexed (refined) grains. However, even though the water absorption rate is low, the total calcium content is high. Therefore, the actual amount absorbed becomes, rather, more than the simple grain (white rice and white wheat).

The conclusion is that vegetarian foods contain a lot of fiber, phytic acid, and oxalic acid, but they do not actually interfere with the calcium absorption. The soybeans have a lot of fiber, phytic acid, and oxalic acid, three of the above, however, the absorption of the calcium is high–up to 20%. It is rare to vegetarians to have

Table 1–5. Proportion of protein intake and urinary calcium excretion

Dietary duration	Protein% of total calorie intake	Urinary calcium excretion (mg / 24 h)		
		Low	Medium	High
15day	1%/12%/25%	51	99	161
4day	8%/12%/25%	108	129	196
15day	8%/16%/24%	168	240	301
15day	8%/16%/24%	217	303	426
15day	8%/16%/24%	168	240	301

Table 1-6. Percentage of lactose degrading enzyme degradation

Ethnic	Lactase degradation rate
Bantu	90%
Filipino	90%
Thais	90%
Japanese	85%
Taiwanese	85%
Arab	78%
Peru	70%
Finnish	18%
Danish	2%

osteoporosis.

Another example is the comparison of the Eskimos and the Caucasians whose diets are completely different. On the traditional diet, the Eskimos have been consuming a lot of meat, and the Caucasians have been both very little vegetarian and almost vegetarian. Caucasian women have the higher bone mass than Eskimo women. However, the young Eskimo women have been similar in terms of the bone mass with the young Caucasian women. Among the Caucasians, the women with the high meat intake had the lower bone mineral mass than the women who were the Caucasian vegetarians.

1.7. calcium intake and the nutritional recommendation fiction

In modern nutrition, the calcium recommendation setting is based on three factors. The first is that the adults usually lose from 200 mg to 250 mg of the calcium daily through the urine and the feces. The second assumption is that only from 30% to 40% of the ingested calcium is absorbed by the human body. Therefore, the amount of the calcium you need to ingest is 800mg a day. Third, the nutritional recommendation targets the upper 97.5% of the intake.

However, these three premises have the contradictions. First, the absorption rate of the calcium varies greatly depending on the intake and the growth period. For example, if you eat a lot of calcium, the absorption rate decreases to 15%. In addition, the absorption rate of the calcium reaches up to 75% in the infants who grow up rapidly and who have a high need for calcium [12].

Second, the Western nutritional recommendation does not allow the consumption of calcium unless it is assumed that a dairy product is consumed. In the United States, 75% of the intake of calcium is provided by the dairy products. Two-thirds of the world's population is estimated to have a difficulty digesting the dairy products, and the remaining one-third had become available for the genetic mutations only ten thousand years ago anthropologically[13].

As can be seen in Table 1-6, 90% of the Thais and 85% of the

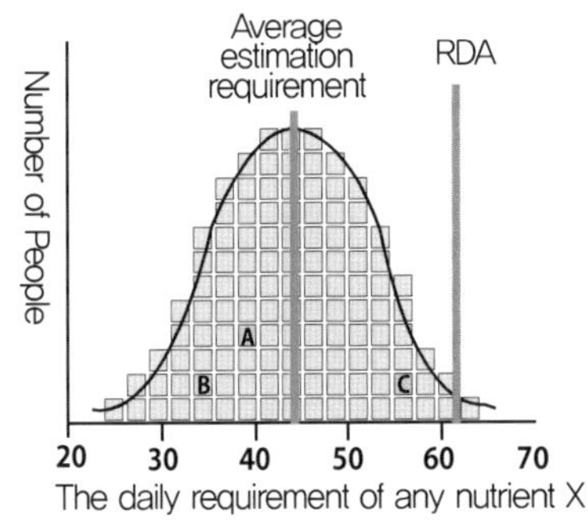

Figure 1-14. Estimated nutrient intake and distribution of normal people

People A, B, and C both consume an amount that is below the recommended intake, but do not say it is not. Other than the lower 2.5% and the upper 2.5%, people interpret that they are nourished within the normal range of intake.

Japanese are the Asians who are similar to the Koreans. The higher the intakes of meat and the dairy products, the higher the calcium excretion from the body, and, thus, the absorption rate of the calcium will be reduced, and the amount required for the ingestion will increase. The diet focused on meat and the dairy products presses the starting button of the vicious cycle of the calcium depletion. In this respect, the current recommendation of the calcium is not at all plausible.

The third is a misconception about the concept of the nutritional recommendation. Nutritional recommendations are not the averages. Rather, the baseline value of the nutrient recommendation is based on the amount that is met by the top 97.5% of the people, assuming the normal distribution of the people's intake needs for the purpose of preventing a deprivation (Fig. 1-12). The average

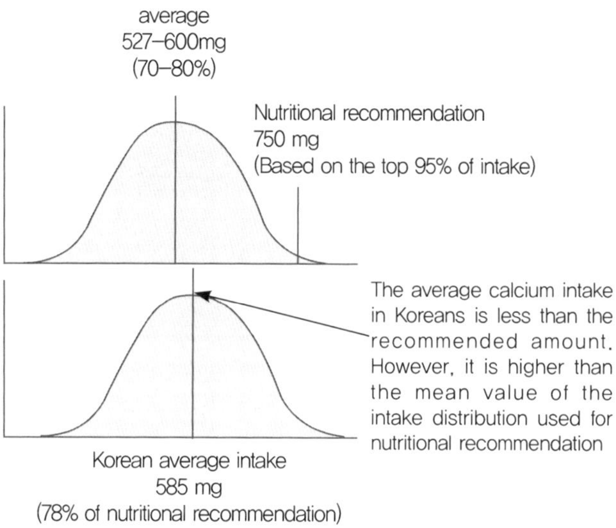

Figure 1–15. Comparison of Calcium Nutrient Intake Level and Korean Average Intake Level Nutritional intake is based on the upper 97.5%. Therefore, the average intake of some groups should be less than the recommended intake

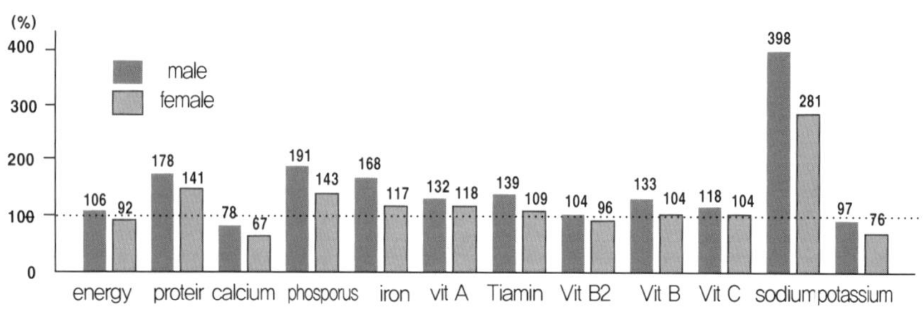

Figure 1–16. Nutritional intake of Koreans (as of 2013)

Percentage of intake based on nutritional standards. The average value of the percentage of individual nutrient intake to nutrition standard. 1 year old or older * Nutrition intake standard: 2010 Korean National Health and Nutrition Standards revised (Korean Nutrition Society 2010) Sodium and potassium are based on adequate intake and others are based on recommended intake. Except for calcium and potassium, all are higher than the recommended intake. Therefore, it can be said that there is a very severe hypertension.

value is obtained by subtracting approximately from 20% to 30% from the nutritional recommendation amount. Therefore, the average intake of a group should be lower than the recommended amount. The average amount of the calcium intakes in Korea is appropriate if the recommended amount of the nutrients is changed to the average of the standard (Fig. 1–13). An excess calcium intake can cause problems, such as cardiovascular deposition and the cataracts. Therefore, it is wiser to eat the calcium–based alkaline foods to increase the actual absorption rate in order to balance the positives in the calcium intake.

1.7. Conclusion

The vegetarian diet reduces osteoporosis. The alkaline vegetarian foods do not put a burden on the human body and, therefore, do not produce the calcium leaks from the bones. On the other hand, the non-vegetarian diet borrows the calcium and the minerals from the bones of the human body as a buffer to neutralize the acids from acidifying the human body due to the excessive protein. Even though their daily amount is small, the result that lasts for life leads to terrible osteoporosis.

In 2010, the number of the osteoporosis patients in Korea already exceeded 2 million, and the rate of the increase has been rising more rapidly. Osteoporosis is associated with back pain, collapse of the kidney, promotion of aging, spine and femoral neck fracture,leading to depression and neuropathy, and calcium is an important substance in the nervous system.

The diet, the lifestyle, the exercise, the sex hormones, and the medication use may be the reasons behind the lowering of the bone mineral density, but the prevention by the vegetarian diet is very important in any situation.

References

1. New SA: Intake of Fruit and Vegetables: Implications for Bone Health. Proc Nutr Soc 2003, 62:889–899.
2. Barzel US, Jowsey J: The Effects of Chronic Acid and Alkali Administration on Bone Turnover in Adult Rats. Clin Sci 1969, 36:517–524.
3. Arnett TR, Dempster DW: Effect of pH on Bone Resorption by Rat Osteoclasts in vitro. Endocrinology 1986, 119:119–124.
4. Remer T, Manz F: Potential Renal Acid Load of Foods and its Influence on Urine pH. Journal of the American Dietetic Association, 95:791–797.
5. Hegsted DM: Calcium and Osteoporosis. J Nutr 1986, 116:2316–2319.
6. Abelow BJ, Holford TR, Insogna KL: Cross-Cultural Association Between Dietary Animal Protein and Hip Fracture: a Hypothesis. Calcif Tissue Int 1992, 50:14–18.
7. Linkswiler HM, Zemel MB, Hegsted M, Schuette S: Protein-Induced Hypercalciuria. Fed Proc 1981, 40:2429–2433.
8. Frassetto LA, Todd KM, Morris RC, Jr., Sebastian A: Estimation of Net Endogenous Noncarbonic Acid Production in Humans from Diet Potassium and Protein Contents. Am J Clin Nutr 1998, 68:576–583.
9. Kohlenberg-Mueller K, Raschka L: Calcium Balance in Young Adults on a Vegan and Lactovegetarian Diet. J Bone Miner Metab 2003, 21:28–33.
10. Marsh AG, Sanchez TV, Midkelsen O, Keiser J, Mayor G: Cortical Bone Density of Adult Lacto-Ovo-Vegetarian and Omnivorous Women. J Am Diet Assoc 1980, 76:148–151.
11. Nutritionists and pre-eaters: Nutrition and cooking. Seoul: Hongik Univ., 1997.
12. Abrams SA: Calcium Absorption in Infants and Small Children: Methods of Determination and Recent Findings. Nutrients 2010, 2:474–480.
13. Bayless TM, Rothfeld B, Massa C, Wise L, Paige D, Bedine MS: Lactose and Milk Intolerance: Clinical Implications. N Engl J Med 1975, 292:1156–1159.
14. Kerstetter JE, Mitnick ME, Gundberg CM, Caseria DM, Ellison AF, Carpenter TO, Insogna KL: Changes in Bone Turnover in Young Women Consuming Different Levels of Dietary Protein. J Clin Endocrinol Metab 1999, 84:1052–1055.
15. Denke MA: Metabolic Effects of High-Protein, Low-Carbohydrate Diets. Am J Cardiol 2001, 88:59–61.

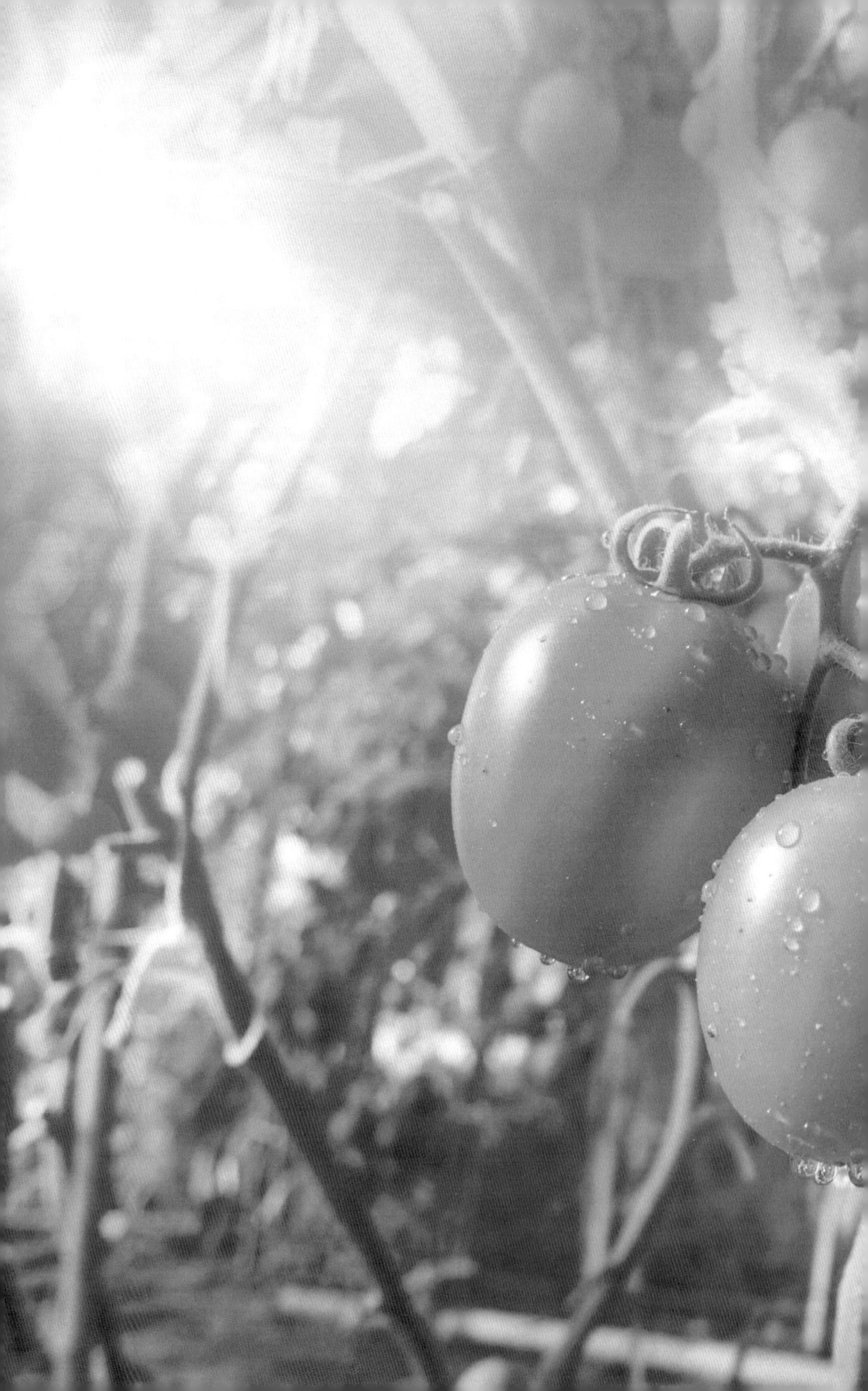

Chapter 2. Urinary System and Vegetarian Diet

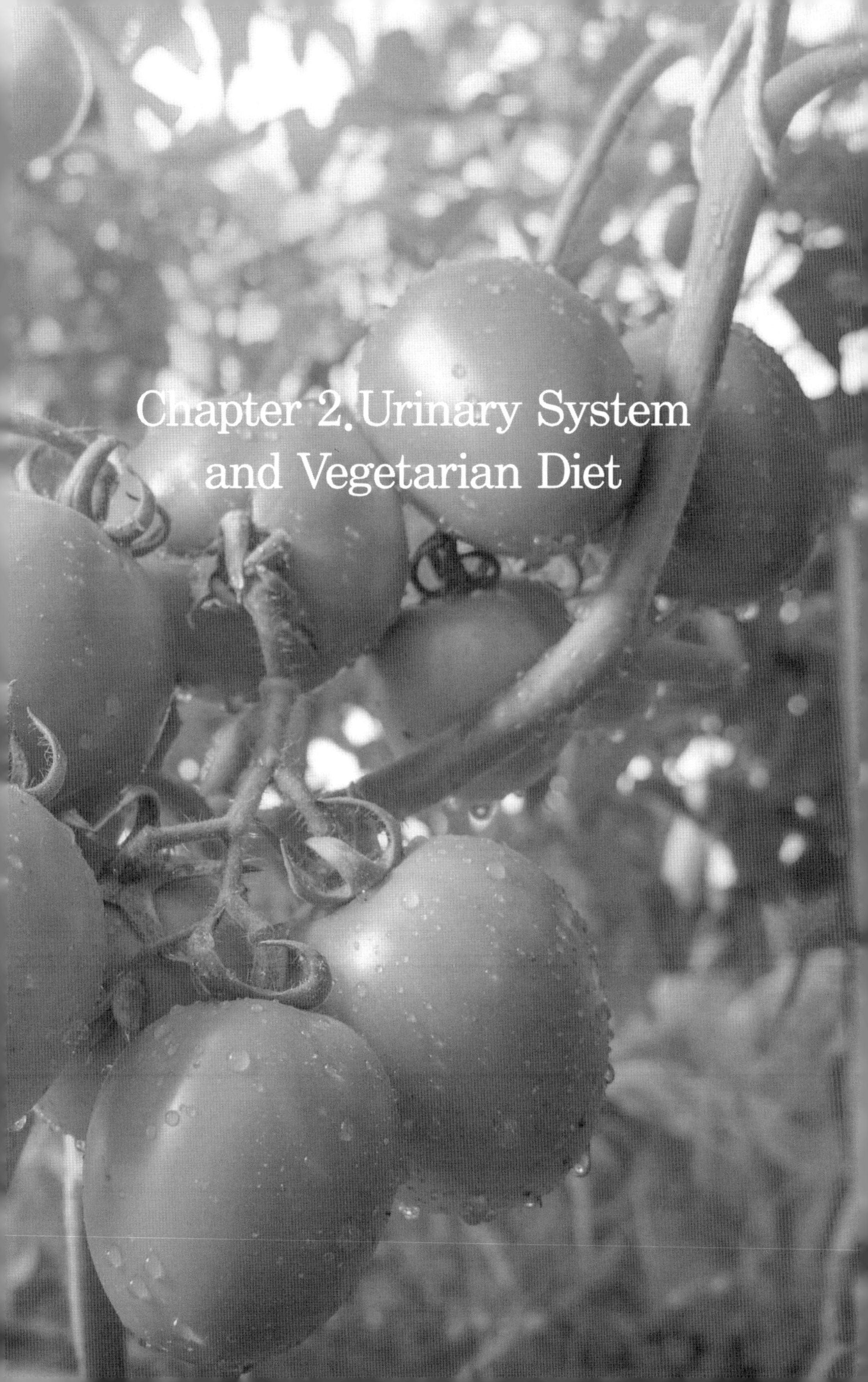

- **Skin system**

The sweat glands are water and moisture.
Elimination of keratinized epidermis prevents excessive liquid loss →

- **Endocrine system**

Aldosterone and ADH regulate blood velocity and electrolyte reabsorption in the kidney →
Renal cells release renin when blood pressure drops ←

- **Digestive system**

Absorbs the water needed to keep the blood concentration constant to remove waste from the kidney →
Emits toxic substances and releases nitrogen waste and bilirubin produced by the liver ←

- **Reproductive system**

Discharge of secretion from adjunct to prevent male urine infection by bacteria →
The male's ureter carries the sperm to the outside ←

- **Skeletal system**

Spine protects kidneys and tubules →
Protect calcium and phosphorus necessary for bone growth ←

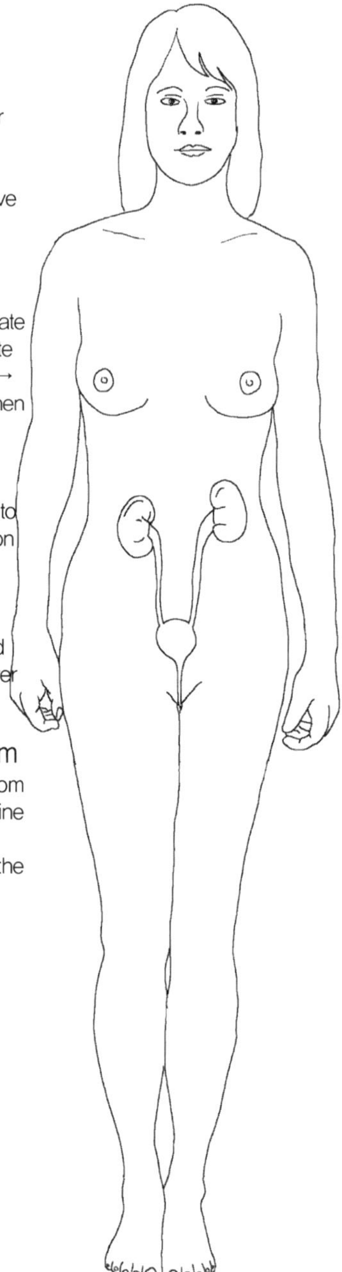

- **Muscular system**

← Sphincter controls the urination by opening and closing the open
→ eliminate noble matter by protein metabolism of muscle

- **Nervous system**

← Adjust the kidney blood pressure
Detect bladder swelling and control urination

- **Cardiovascular system**

← carries blood to the capillary, which acts as a manure, and re–absorbs the electrolyte
→ renin secretion for blood pressure rise

- **Immune / lymphatic system**

← Provides a special defense against ureteral infections
→ eliminate toxins from toxins and cell activity

- **respiratory system**

← Adjust pH by removing CO_2
→ help to remove CO_2

Chapter 2. The urinary system and the vegetarian diet

2.1. The urinary structure and function

The urinary system (the excretory system) is an organ related to the action of sending the waste produced by the metabolism of the body to out of the body. The amount of the tissue fluid in the body should be within a certain range, and the waste produced in the body should be removed. The urinary system is consists of the kidney, the bladder, and the urethra.

The kidney is a bean-shaped organ that is slightly larger than the fist, one part below the diaphragm and one part on each side of the spine. The blood vessels that supply the blood to the lobulated organs are regularly arranged and serve as a standard for distinguishing the area of a lesion. One weighs from 130g to 150g, which is only about 0.5% of the body weight. However, 25% (1.2L per minute ~ 1.3L per minute) of the blood from the heart reaches the kidney through the renal veins. The amount that passes through is 5 tons per day.

The main functions of the normal kidneys are the waste removal, the fluid control and the endocrine function. In other words, the kidneys filter out the body waste, which is represented by the urea, regulates the electrolyte balance and the body fluid, such as the blood at pH 7.3. And it plays an endocrine role related to the red blood cell production, the vitamin D synthesis, etc. in the bone marrow. Kidney, the center of the urinary system, is a purifier that maintains the cleansing and the balancing of the body fluids.

The principle of filtering the waste in the body is like pouring an impure solution into a filter paper. The impurities that are smaller than the fine gaps in the filter paper will pass through the filter paper and not through any larger material. In the body, the blood is a solution containing the impurities, and the glomerulus is the one that plays the role as a filter paper. The fluid that passed through the glomeruli is called the urine, and the water and the minerals in the urine that are necessary for the body are absorbed again, and the remaining solution goes to the bladder and becomes urine.

The kidneys on both sides of the body are composed of one million nephrons, which are the structural, functional units of the kidneys. The nephrons contain a small, structural unit called the "glomerulus", which acts as a kind of filter paper. The glomerulus is a round-shaped filtration unit that has a large surface area due to the depression of the capillary network connected to the imported arterioles. Due to this structure, the blood volume of

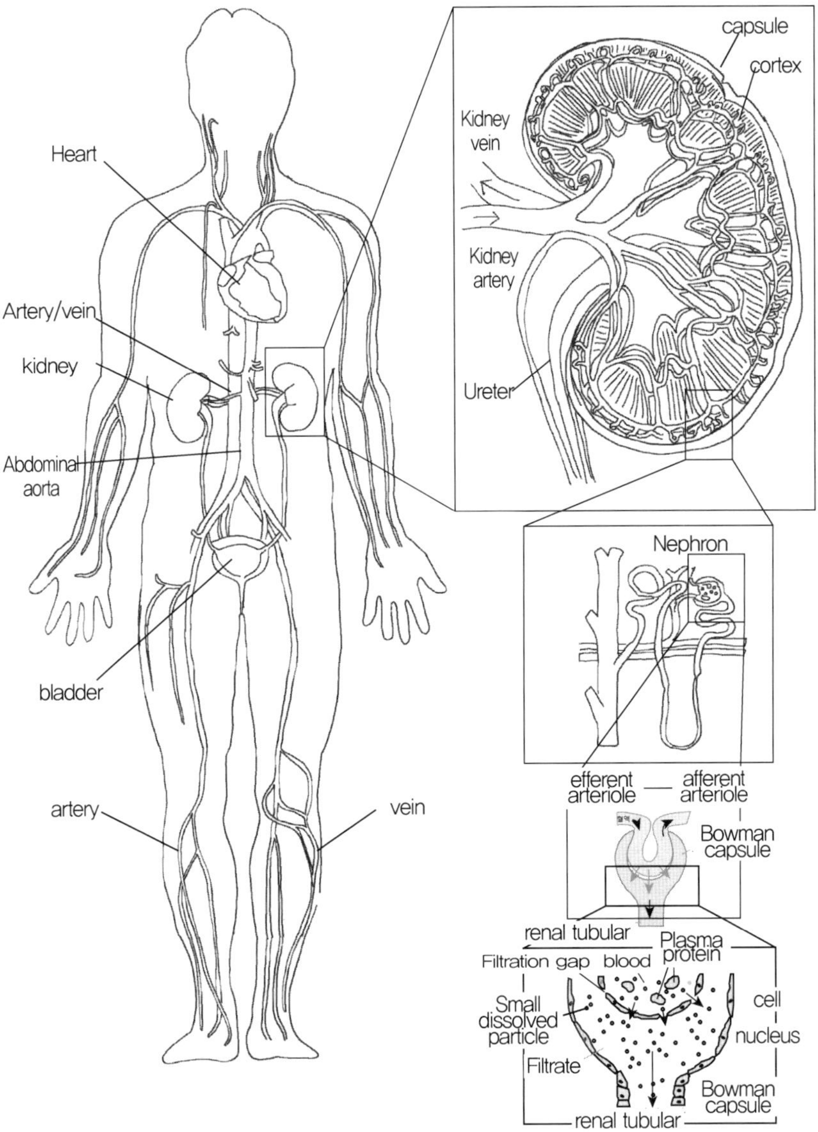

Figure 2-1. Structure of kidney, nephron, bowman's pocket, glomeruli

30ml~40ml contained in the kidney capillary is contacted with the total surface area of the capillary blood vessels of about 12m^2, so that it is efficiently filtered. In men, the glomerular filtration rate (GFR) is 125ml/min/1.73m^2, which is about 10% lower than that of women, which is 17.5L per hour, 180L per day, four times the total body volume, and 60 times the blood plasma.

Adult blood is filtered through the renal glomeruli 400 times per hour to filter out the waste products. The electrically neutral substances with the diameters of less than 4nm(nano meter, 10^{-9}m) are passed through, and no more than 8nm of the charged substances passes through. The red blood cells, the platelets, and the proteins can't pass through the glomerulus. However the salts, the creatinines (the wastes of the muscle energy source), and the uric acid (the cellular, metabolic waste) can pass through glomerulus. When the first 170 liters of the urine are made, the necessary nutrients and the water are reabsorbed into the tubules, and they become only about 1.5 liters of the urine, about 1% of the 170 liters. The urine is 4 times more concentrated than the plasma, and 95% of the components is water.

2.2. The kidney diseases and the low back pain.

The renal diseases include the acute renal failure, the chronic renal failure, and the glomerulonephritis. The acute renal failure cannot supply the blood through the glomeruli due to the severe hemorrhage or the toxic substances, the kidney function is rapidly deteriorated, and the urine cannot be formed. The waste materials stay in the body, and hematuria, pain, and a decrease of the urine appears. The chronic renal failure is caused by two major causes: glomerulonephritis and pyelonephritis. It is caused by hypertension and the urinary stones. The characteristic feature is that the nephronsare destroyed. The nephrons are involved in a kidney function even after 70% of them were destroyed, so one is often unaware of the symptoms in the early days. Therefore, it is common for the complications, such as an infection, to occur later on after the uremia is not treated.

Glomerulonephritis, also known as nephritis, is a type of autoimmune disease in which the antigens and the antibodies accumulate in the glomerular blood vessels and weaken the kidney function. If this condition continues, it may progress to kidney failure.

There are several kidney diseases, but once they are progressed, the function of the kidneys becomes weaker because the wastes that should have been filtered out from the kidneys in the normal state cannot be removed from the damaged kidneys, therefore, circulating in the body and constantly burdening the kidneys. Therefore, slowing the rate of the kidney damage in the treatment of a kidney disease is very important.

However, the protein supply to the patients with a kidney disease is a kind of dilemma. The kidneys of the kidney disease patients are already very much damaged, and the proteins cannot be filtered properly, they leak into the urine, and the kidney cells that were damaged by the disease must be restored to receive a lot of protein. In the normal people, the proteins do not go through the glomerulus, and they go out to the urine. Often, the renal dialysis patients have the protein−calorie malnutrition, which is often associated with a shortage of nutrition. The protein−calorie deficiency becomes more difficult because the protein−calorie deficiency can increase the mortality and worsen the morbidity.

But, the opposite is possible. It is the question of whether a high protein prescription is appropriate for the nitrogen balance. As the protein supply increases, the protein loss in the body increases, and the rate of the nitrogen degradation increases. If there are more elements in the plasma, you need a dialysis. The excessive protein supply can exacerbate the already damaged kidney function. That is, the high−protein diets for the kidney disease patients show a negative balance regarding the protein balance, so that the amount of the elements that are generated in the human body should be minimized to achieve a positive balance. For References, the Food and Agriculture Organization (FAO) sets the minimum daily protein intake of 0.5 grams per kilogram of the body weight. The US nutritional recommendation for the normal people is 0.8 grams per kilogram of the body weight. In this situation, the excessive protein is likely to be a burden on the kidneys. So, what is the actual research result?

The low-protein diet increases the protein content in the serum.

In 1989, the New England Journal of Medicine reported a study of the beneficial effects of the low-protein diet in relation to the kidney diseases. The rate of the removal of the impurities in the body is the glomerular filtration rate, which is about 125ml/min/1.73m^2 for the normal adults. However, when the kidneys are damaged, the essential nutrients are released through the glomeruli. Thus, an increase in the abnormal, glomerular filtration rate is associated with the renal damage.

Figure 2-2 shows that the glomerular filtration rate had been increased to 120ml/min/1.73m^2 when the normal diet had been administered without any restriction regarding the protein intake into the kidney disease patients. After the low-protein diet had been administered, the glomerular filtration rate had decreased. This can be interpreted as a decrease of the nutrients that had been leaked through the glomerulus by improving the kidney function.

If so, could the protein in the body be lacking because the protein intake had been reduced? One of the representative indicators of the protein content in the body is the serum albumin, so, if the serum albumin level is high, the protein is not lacking. After the

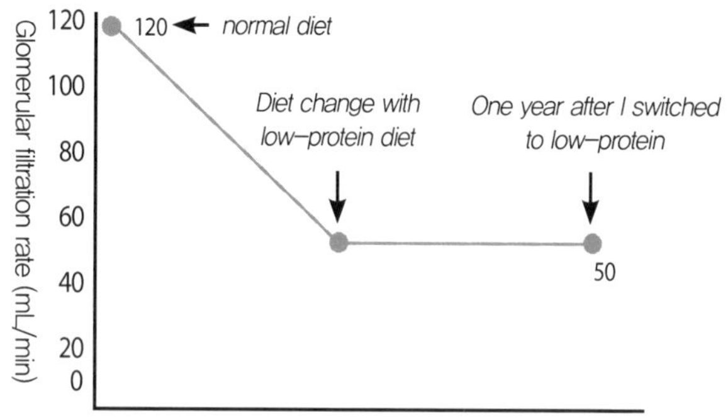

Figure 2-2. Decrease in low-grade lactose and glomerular filtration rate

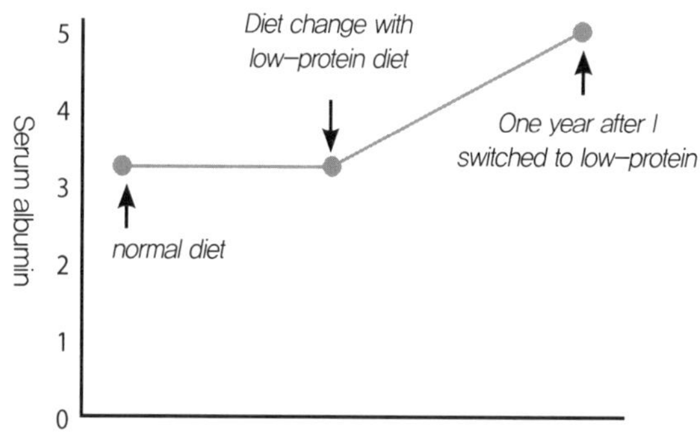

Figure 2-3. Increase of serum albumin by low-back diet

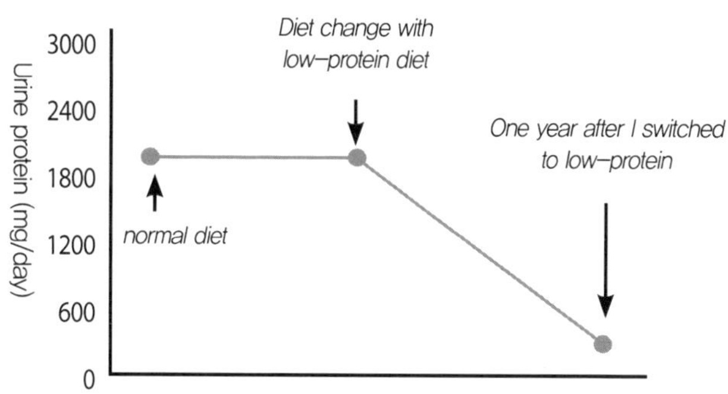

Figure 2-4. Reduction of low protein diet and urinary protein (urine protein)

low–protein diet, the albumin levels in the body were higher than those in the high–protein diet (Fig. 2–3) [1].

This was due to a sharp decrease in the amount of the protein leaking into the urine. That is, 2,000 mg of the urine was excreted per day before the low–protein diet, but it had decreased rapidly to 100 mg after one year of the low–protein diet. In other words, the amount of the protein that had been lost by the damaged kidney had been reduced, and the protein balance was changed to be a positive balance (Fig. 2–4).

The similar results were obtained in a study of the diabetic kidney disease with 82 people with the type 1 diabetes in Denmark in 2002. The typical diets were fed at 1.02 g (1.02 g/kg/day) per kg of the body weight per day and 0.89 g for the low–fat diet. People who died after 4 years or who had been worsened at the end of their kidney were 27% in the general diet and 10% in the low–protein diet [2]. They report that the normal dietary protein restriction has a symptom–improving effect on the type 1 diabetic kidney disease patients and, additionally, has the beneficial effects on hypertension.

2.3. The whole vegans and the low–protein, hypophosphate diet.

Restricting the supply of the protein prevents the residual, renal function from any further damage, and it is, also, effective in preventing the complications due to a kidney disease. However, the protein–restricted diets containing the traditional meat for the therapeutic purposes have some disadvantages. Above all, the low–fat, white meats are tasteless in the long run, they are too expensive, and they are difficult to get when you go out to the market. In view of this problem, Barsotti et al. [3] suggested that the vegan diet could serve as a dietary, protein–free diet without any nutritional deficiencies in the kidney–damaged patients [3].

The whole vegetarian diets are fed from the plants with all the nutrients being lower in the protein–energy ratio and the phosphate–energy ratio than the animal foods. In addition, the essential amino acid feeds in the protein–restricted diets can meet the demand by the mixing legumes (the low valine, the low tryptone, and the high lysine) and the cereals (the methionine rich and the low lysine) (Fig. 2–5).

They calculated the essential amino acid feeds in a traditional, protein–restricted diet and a whole–vegan diet, both of which were the animal foods and both of which were higher than the nutritional requirements regarding the both groups (Table 2–1).

The researchers then divided them into the two groups who were

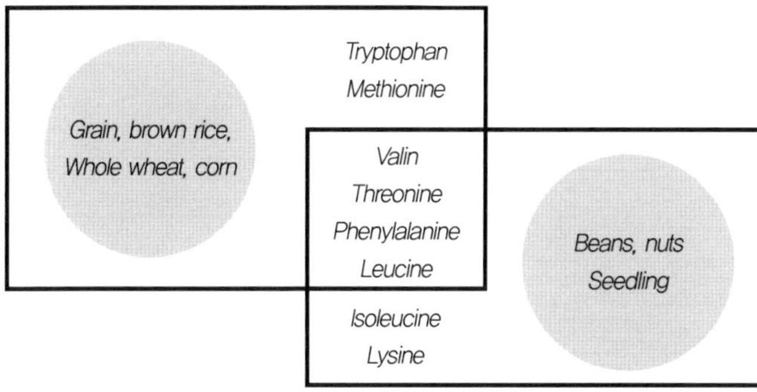

Figure 2–5. Tips for protein intake to balance amino acids when vegetarian

on the 22 protein–free diets– a group that was converted to the vegetarian diet and a group that was converted to the vegetarian diet, both of which were after the animal protein–restricted diet. The vegetarian diets had been from 14.1 months to 12.8 months, respectively, and they had been supplied at a ratio of 1 : 5.6. The protein supply was 0.7 g/kg of the body weight per day. In the case of the 70kg of the body weight, 36.4g of the cereals and 6.5g of the protein in the legumes had been supplied. The total calories were 57% carbohydrate, 34% lipid and 8% protein.

The experimental results showed that the urea concentration of the serum was 60 mg/dl on the average when the protein was not restricted, but it had decreased to 45 mg/dl after 14 months. The concentration of the urea in the urine was 18.4 mg/dl to 10.1 mg/dl. This means that the protein–restricted diet through the whole vegan diet is very effective. Even when converting from an animal

Table 2-1. Average daily intake of essential amino acids (mg, calculated over 12 days)

	Protein-restricted diet with meat	Vegan diet	Recommended intake
Lysine	3,201	1,787	840
Histidine	1,099	1,023	-
Threonine	1,728	1,553	490
Valin	2,176	2,039	980
Leucine	3,102	3,431	770
Isoleucine	1,839	1,970	-
Methionine	1,076	717	-
Phenylalanine	1,753	2,275	210
Tryptophan	445	469	-

Table 2-2. Changes in creatinine (Cr) and urea concentration after dietary changes (mg/dL)

	normal diet	vegan diet	Animal limitation	vegan diet
serum Cr	2.1	2.3	3.5	4.1
Urine Cr	1,151	1,050	997	916
Serum urea	60	45	86	84
Urinary urea	18.4	10.1	10.1	9.9

protein–restricted diet to a whole–vegetarian protein–restricted diet, the serum urea level had decreased from 20.9 mg/dl to 16.1mg /dl (Table 2–2).

In this experiment, there was no problem of hyperkalemia due to the abundant potassium in the vegetables. Hyperkalemia is usually caused by the tissue necrosis that is caused by the leakage of the potassium in the cells, and it is interpreted that only the necessary amount is adequately absorbed by the abundant fiber of the vegetable foods. In addition, the calcium carbonate supplements were associated with the phosphoric acid in the intestines and were discharged into the feces, which was considered to be an important dietary factor.

In addition to the benefits of good nutrition and a variety of the diets, the researchers have listed four reasons why the whole plants are beneficial for the kidney disease. First, the vegetable foods have a high ratio of the unsaturated fats to the saturated fats, and they have beneficial effect on the kidney disease and the lipid metabolism due to the absence of cholesterol. Second, the glomerular filtration rate, the renal plasma flow, the albumin purification, and the immunoglobulin G (IgG) level are lower than those of the animal proteins. Third, the intake of the same amount of protein results in lower acid production regarding the vegetable foods. Fourth, the vegetarian diet can contribute to the lowering of the blood pressure.

2.4. Promoting of dietary fiber on the nitrogen circulations

Three main ingredients of the food we eat are carbohydrates, lipids and proteins. The final products of the carbohydrates and the fats are carbon dioxide and water, but the proteins and the nucleic acids containing nitrogen, which should be released into the body in the form of the nitrogen compounds, such as urea. Ammonia is very toxic, and even if it is 5mg in 100ml of blood, the person will die. Therefore, ammonia is converted in the liver to urea so that it does not harm the body, and it is transported to the kidneys and excreted through the urine. The elements are well–soluble in the water, but they can cause an illness if they are not lost together when they are released.

Physiologically, the elimination of the urea nitrogen in the body occurs through two routes: The urine and the feces. As shown in Figure 2–6, the element is excreted in the urine via the kidneys, and, also, through the large intestine. The element is broken down into ammonia by the intestinal microorganisms, and the human body can reabsorb it for the synthesis of the nonessential amino acids. In turn, protein requirement is reduced. The factor treatment through the large intestine has been reported in many animals, including the mice, the rabbits, and the sheep, and, also, including the humans. It is estimated that approximately from 20% to 30% of the total factor produced in the liver will be hydrolyzed in the large intestine.

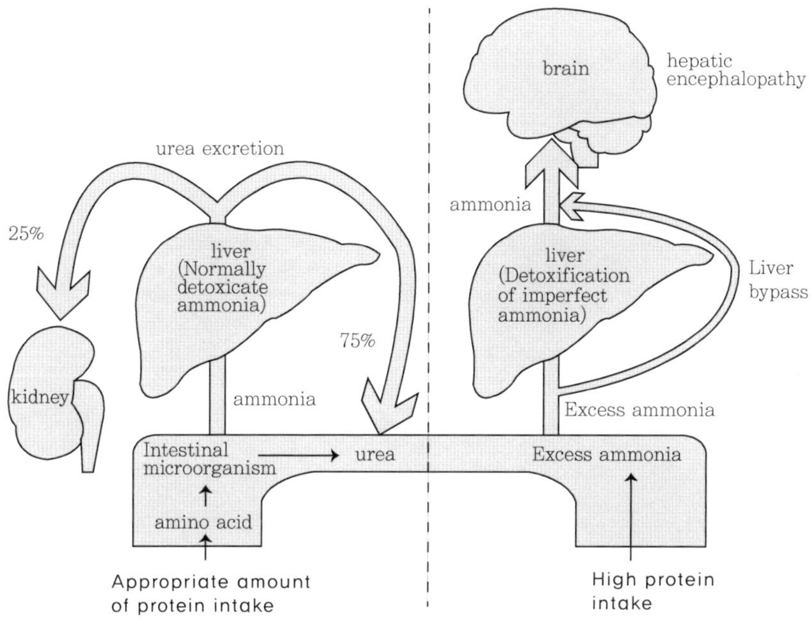

Figure 2-6. Effect of carbohydrate fermentation by intestinal microorganisms on long-term circulation of nitrogen

There are more than 1,000 kinds of microorganisms in the human body at about from 10 billion to 1 trillion per gram. These bacterias are mainly the anaerobes that survive without any oxygen, and they maintain a symbiotic relationship with the human body. They seem to have the sufficient defense against the pathogenic microorganisms that are invading from the outside, and the important nutrients for the bacteria are the dietary fiber that the human body has failed to digest.

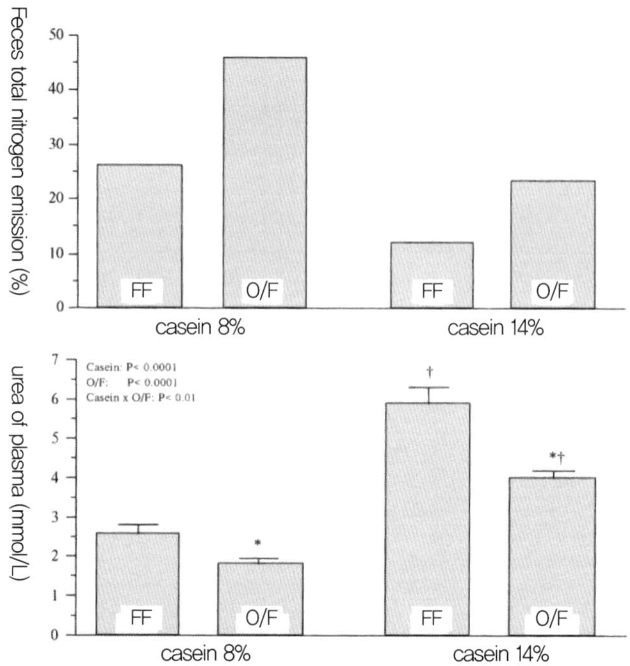

Figure 2-7. Nitrogen efflux and plasma urea concentration in the cecum according to the presence or absence of fiber intake

FF: No fibrin, O/F: Mixed oligo carbohydrate with fibrin

If so, can abundant dietary fiber supply reduce the burden of kidneys? In other words, the dietary fiber will actively multiply the beneficial microorganisms in the intestines, which will use the intestinal elements as the nutrients, and the urea concentration gradients of the intestines and the blood will become larger, resulting in a more elemental transfer from the blood to the intestines (Table 2-6).

Related experiments were reported in 1998. The researchers had fed 8% casein, a milk protein, and they had fed 14% casein to a group of the rats, with the 14% feeding a small amount of urea to the colon. However, when the casein was 8%, when the casein was supplied without the fiber (FF), the amount of the nitrogen discharged from the feces was large (O/F). These results were the same when 14% casein was supplied.

On the other hand, the urea concentration of the plasma was lower than that of the casein supplemented with the dietary fiber. In other words, in the case of the abundant supply of the cellulose, the movement of the elements from the plasma to the large intestine had increased, and the burden on the kidney had been reduced (Fig. 2-7).

Dietary fiber produces short chain fatty acids, such as acetic acid, butyric acid, and propionic acid, through the bacteria in the large intestine as well as the benefits of the removal of the elements, which can be reabsorbed into the body and used as an energy source or a nutrient. Acetic acid, for example, can be used as a source of the amino acids, the heme, the fatty acids, the steroid hormones, the vitamin A, and the citric acid. Patients with a kidney disease need higher calorie intake than protein intake, which is why the dietary fiber has an advantage in kidney.

2.5. Calcium oxalate.

The majority of the kidney stones are the calcium oxalates. The calcium oxalate polymyositis is a complex and diverse phenomenon that is particularly important. The dietary factors, such as oxalic acid, calcium, protein, salt, simple sugars, fat, and fiber, are also important, and the water intake is important as well.

The oxalic acid in the body, which is the material of the uric acid stones, can be divided into the exogenous and the endogenous. Endogenous oxalic acid is directly proportional to the body weight and is synthesized from the two major sources, vitamin C and the glyoxylic acid. Vitamin C is responsible for 40% of the glyoxylic acid and 50% of the endogenous, oxalic acid. If there is enough vitamin B6 in the body, the glyoxylic acid is not converted to the oxalic acid but is converted to the glycine. The exogenous, oxalic acid is found in a variety of the vegetable foods. The spinach, peanut, beetroot, chocolate, parsley, strawberry, wheat, tea, etc. increase the amount of the oxalate in the urine and increase the risk of the urinary stone. The contribution of the dietary oxalic acid to the urine is increased from 20% to 40% [5].

Contrary to the oxalic acid, the higher the intake of the calcium, the lower the risk of the uric acid. This is because it blocks the absorption of the oxalic acid into the body by binding to the oxalic acid in the digestive tract. A study of 45,619 healthy men showed

Table 2-3. Potential kidney burden of various foods(Remer & Manz,1995)

food	Acid load (mEq/100g)	food	Acid load (mEq/100g)
Fruit and fruit juice		Dairy products and eggs	
Apple	-2.2	milk	0.7
raisin	-21.0	yogurt	1.5
Grape juice	-1.0	Cheddar cheese	26.4
Lemon juice	-2.5	Cottage cheese	8.7
Vegetables, grains		Egg (yolk)	23.4
spinach	-14.0	Meat, fish	
broccoli	-1.2	beef	7.8
carrot	-4.9	chicken	8.7
potato	-4.0	Pork	7.9
refine wheat	3.7	liver, sausage	10.6
Brown rice	12.5	salmon	7.1

* *The larger the minus value, the less the burden of mountains. The larger the + value, the greater the burden on height*

that the calcium intake was inversely related to the calcium oxalate osmolality in the natural state.

Protein is also important. An increased intake of 34g of animal protein per day had increased the amount of the calcium in the urine by 23% and the oxalate by 24%, indicating a higher urinary risk. The animal foods rich in sulfur and phosphorus make the body an acidic environment, which releases the calcium from the skeletal system. The released calcium increases the risk of the formation of the new crystals. The calcium oxalate stones were 3.9 times more likely to fracture than the normal objects. On the other hand, a vegetarian diet rich in magnesium, potassium, citric acid, minerals, and phytic acid reduces the uric acid in the urine and alkalizes the body, which inhibits the production of the urinary stones. The high–protein diets above 75 g/day cause hypercalciuria.

2.6. Hyperuricemia, the uric acid stone, the gout, and the vegetarian diet.

Uric acid is synthesized in the purine. Therefore, the foods with the high purine content promote the uric acid production and increase the uric acid concentrationsin the blood and the urine. The reason for the increase of the uric acid concentration in the blood is the excessive uric acid production or the fact that the uric acid is discharged at less than normal–from 80% to 90% of the causations of hyperuricemia due to the emission reduction. However, it is clear that a large amount of the intake would be a problem to the discharge.

Hyperuricemia increases the risks of gout and stone formation. Many foods with the high uric acid are meat, fish, some kinds of

Table 2–4. Increase in gout in western society [6]

year	Subject	gout occurrence (per 1000 people)
1960	Western Europe	3
1978	England	3
1995	England	10

Arthritis & Rheumatism (2004) 50(8):2400–2414

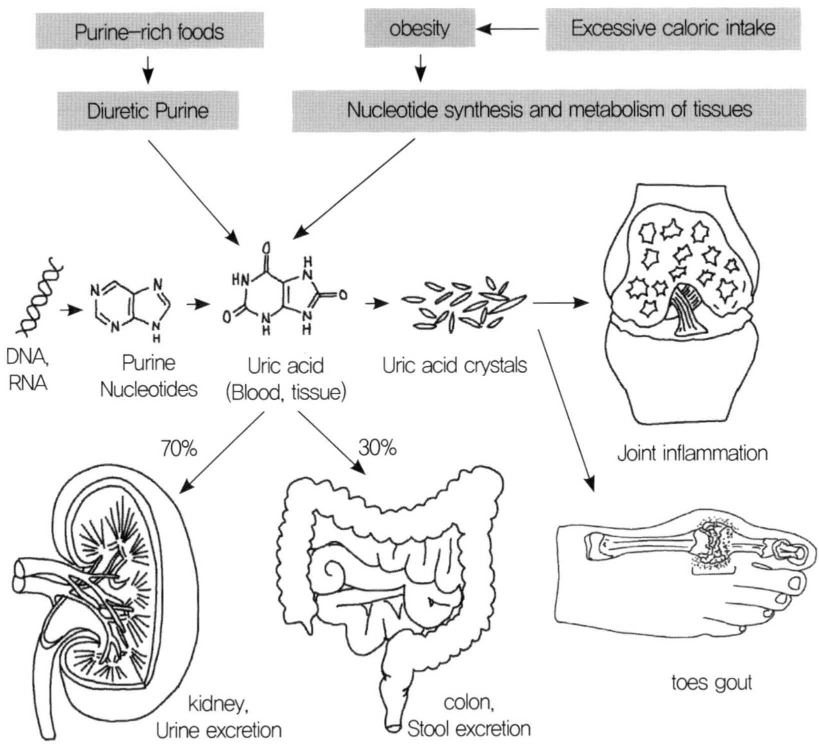

Figure 2–8. Process of uric acid crystal formation and occurrence of gout

Table 2–5. Types of kidney stone

Composition	cause	frequency (%)
Calcium oxalate, phosphoric acid	Metabolism abnormality, naturally	60–80%
Stru Bit	infection	10–15%
Uric acid	Hyperuricemia, hyperuricemia, naturally occurring	5–10%
Cystine	kidney tube damage	1%

BMJ 2004, 328:1420–4

vegetables, all alcoholic beverages and the interiors of the animals. If you eat only the foods that are not strictly purine, you can lower the serum uric acid level by from 15 percent to 20 percent.

Meat – Beef, pork, chicken, turkey, especially the liver.
Fish – Crustaceans, including the molluscs.
Some vegetables – Beans, red beans, asparagus, spinach, and mushrooms.
All alcohols – Especially beer.

The uric acid occurs second after the calcium oxalate stones. Like the calcium oxalate stones, the acidified urine and the less urine are the most important factors in the uric acid stone formation.

Gout causes the crystallization of the uric acid in the joints, causing the irritation, the severe pain, and even disabling the patient to be able to do nothing. Gout is a very common disease that affects at least 1% of the Westerners. But, 40 years ago, the percentage was not that high. Gout has been increasing in the industrialized western societies, and it has now been increasing in the industrialized Asian societies (Table 2–4).

2.7. Vegetarian diet is effective for gout.

Purine, the causative agent of the uric acid, is mainly found in the animal foods and it is, also, found in some plants and alcohol. If so, is there any benefit to the vegetarian diet in preventing hyperuricemia, the uric acid stone formation, and gout? In response to this question, the Siener and Hesse team at a German university answered through an experiment in 2002.

The researchers recruited healthy male volunteers with themean age of 28 years. They were aged from 21 years to 32 years, and, they had been fed a meat–centered, western diet, a normal non–vegetarian diet, and a lacto–ovo vegetarian diet, in turns, for five

Table 2–6. Change of urine composition by diet [7]

	standard	Western diet	Non–Vegetarian	lacto–ovo vegetarian	p
Urine volume (L/24h)	1.29±0.49	1.48±0.38	2.30±.39	2.45±0.76	〈0.001
pH	6.01±0.47	5.95±0.34	6.51±0.22	6.80±0.21	〈0.001
sodium (mmol/d)	159±75	176±40	146±13	102±48	0.045
chlorine (mmol/d)	164±66	169±39	139±17	106±43	0.024
ammonium (mmol/d)	30.8±12.2	38.7±5.1	25.6±6.4	18.7±5.9	〈0.001
Phosphoric acid (mmol/d)	32.6±8.1	35.4±5.5	29.4±3.5	25.2±6.3	0.043
Sulfuric acid (mmol/d)	18.5±9.2	22.5±3.1	18.1±1.9	16.1±3.7	0.004
Creatinine (mmol/d)	16.1±4.4	16.9±2.00	15.3±1.3	13.8±3.2	0.183
Uric acid (mmol/d)	3.59±0.94	3.91±0.67	2.93±0.32	2.58±0.52	〈0.001
RS Uric acid	2.90±2.70	2.71±2.82	0.41±0.41	0.18±0.15	0.009

RS uric acid; relative supersaturation with respect to uric acid ,
Eur J Nutr (2003) 42:332–337

Table 2 -7. The amount and bioavailability of oxalic acid in food

food	Total oxalic acid (mg/100g)	Bioavailability(%)
Soy products	5.6-287	2.2-5.4
spinach	957	0.6-2.4
black tea	4-6	1.9-4.7
chocolate	140	2.6
rhubarb	1,235	4.0

Urol Res (2004) 32:311-316

days each. The Western diet is characterized by the high calorie, the high alcohol consumption, the high protein intake, and the drinking of the water of more than 1.5 liters/day. The normal and vegetarian diets are similar with respect to the calorie intake regarding each nutrient and 2.5L of the beverage is drunk a day.

The relative supersaturation of the uric acid, the pH, the sodium, the chlorine, the ammonium, the phosphoric acid, the sulfuric acid, the creatinine, and the uric acid was measured by measuring the relative supersaturation with respect to the uric acid (Table 2-6).

The mean uric acid production of the meat-centered, western diets was 3.91 mmol/day, which had decreased to 2.93 mmol/day in the normal, balanced non-vegetarian diet, and it had been significantly lowered to 2.58 mmol/day in the vegetarian diet [7]. This is 34% less the meat-based, western diet and 12% less than the normal, non-vegetarian diet.

The amount of salt consumed is, also, an important variable.

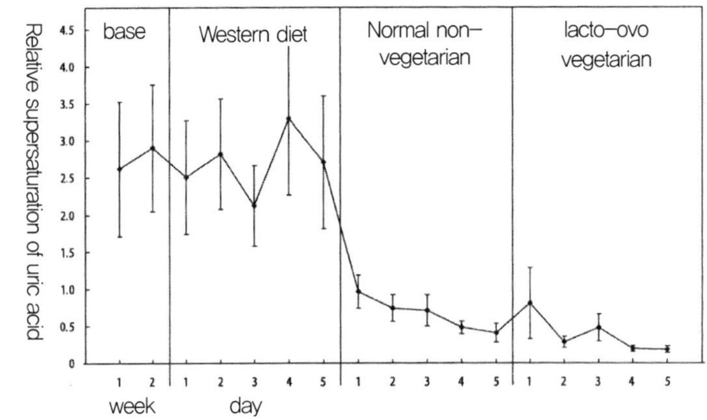

Figure 2-9. Changes in dietary patterns and relative supersaturation of urine uric acid (RS uric acid)

When the intake of the salt (NaCl) had been increased by 2.3 g (100 mmol), the calcium released into the urine was 40 mg. Cock and his colleagues had increased the amount of the dietary salt from 140 mmol to 310 mmol and 34% of the amount of the calcium was released into the urine. The increased urinary calcium increased the risk of the kidney stones.

Increasing the intake of the omega-3 fatty acids can help prevent the kidney stones. The omega-6 fatty acids, which are consumed by the modern humans, increase the arachidonic acid in the phospholipids of the cell membranes, making it easier to absorb the intestinal calcium and, ultimately, resulting in hypercalciuria. The EPA and the DHA, the omega-3, polyunsaturated fatty acids, reduce the arachidonic acid. The normal membrane retention due to the omega-3 normalizes the binding of the kidneys, the digestive tract, and the bone tissues, thereby reducing the production of the calcium oxalate.

The urine volume of more than 2 liters per day significantly lowers the urinary calcium and oxalic acid levels, which prevents the production of the kidney stones.

The pH of the urine, which is, also, a measure of the acid load on the kidneys, had increased from 6.6 in the Western diet to 6.9 in the vegetarian diet, compared to 6.1 in the non-vegetarian diet. The lower the pH, the easier it is to get the stones. The uric acid supersaturation is an important factor in the crystallization of the uric acid. It is high in the Western and meiotic diets, and the risk of the crystallization increases as the pH increases. The change is 2.71 → 0.41 → 0.18, which is 93%, which is 55% less than the normal diet. As the pH of the urine had increased during the vegetarian diet, the urinary ammonia, the sulfuric acid emission, and the phosphoric acid emission had decreased (Figure 2-8).

2.8. Conclusion

For the patients with a kidney disease, the low–protein diet, which reduces the burden on the kidneys by providing the minimum amount of the protein needed by the human body, is more effective than a high–protein diet that exacerbates the kidneys by imposing a strain on the kidneys. The method of supplying the low–fat diets with the animal foods is tasteless, monotonous, high in price, and difficult to purchase by going out to the market. The vegan diet not only solves this problem, but, also, it relieves the burden on the kidneys by reducing the production of the high quality lipids and acids.

In the elderly, the progression of a kidney disease is often linked to diabetes or a heart disease, and it is, therefore, important to regulate the carbohydrates and the lipid supply. The fiber–rich vegetarian diets can improve the blood sugar levels in the diabetic patients, they can reduce the serum cholesterol levels in the cardiovascular patients, and the renal function can be preserved by the complex carbohydrates, rather than the simple carbohydrates. The chronic kidney disease patients often have the high cholesterol, triglyceride, phospholipid, and LDL–cholesterol levels. And the low HDL–cholesterol level in the plasmas have the lipid–lowering effects, so that the lipid supply regulation and the fatty acid balance are, also, important.

Dietary fiber leads to the remarkable results, such as facilitating the urination, reducing the blood lipid, improving the blood sugar control, reducing the risk of colon cancer and increasing the utilization of some cations. It is known that, by increasing the amount of the fermentable carbohydrate and the fiber, the microorganisms in the large intestine are proliferated, and this can increase the nitrogen excretion through the feces. This diet can be particularly attention for the kidney patients with the impaired renal function.

A kidney disease, also, has the problem of the kidney stones. In the industrialized societies where the meat consumption has been increasing. The vegetarian diet is low in purine, which causes the kidney stones, and it is rich in the calcium that blocks the oxalic acid before it is absorbed.

References

1. Chatterjee MR, Quinn LH, Banerjee PP, Poon TC: Rayleigh–Ritz Optimization of the Structure Function for a Kolmogorov Power Density and an Approximate Analytical Solution for the Two-Point Electric Field Correlation Function. Appl Opt 1989, 28:1773–1777.

2. Hansen HP, Tauber-Lassen E, Jensen BR, Parving HH: Effect of Dietary Protein Restriction on Prognosis in Patients with Diabetic Nephropathy. Kidney Int 2002, 62:220–228.

3. Barsotti G, Morelli E, Cupisti A, Meola M, Dani L, Giovannetti S: A Low-Nitrogen Low-Phosphorus Vegan Diet for Patients with Chronic Renal Failure. Nephron 1996, 74:390–394.

4. Parmar MS: Kidney Stones. BMJ 2004, 328:1420–1424.

5. Holmes RP, Assimos DG: The Impact of Dietary Oxalate on Kidney Stone Formation. Urol Res 2004, 32:311–316.

6. Bieber JD, Terkeltaub RA: Gout: On the Brink of Novel Therapeutic Options for an Ancient Disease. Arthritis Rheum 2004, 50:2400–2414.

7. Siener R, Hesse A: The Effect of a Vegetarian and Different Omnivorous Diets on Urinary Risk Factors for Uric Acid Stone Formation. Eur J Nutr 2003, 42:332–337.

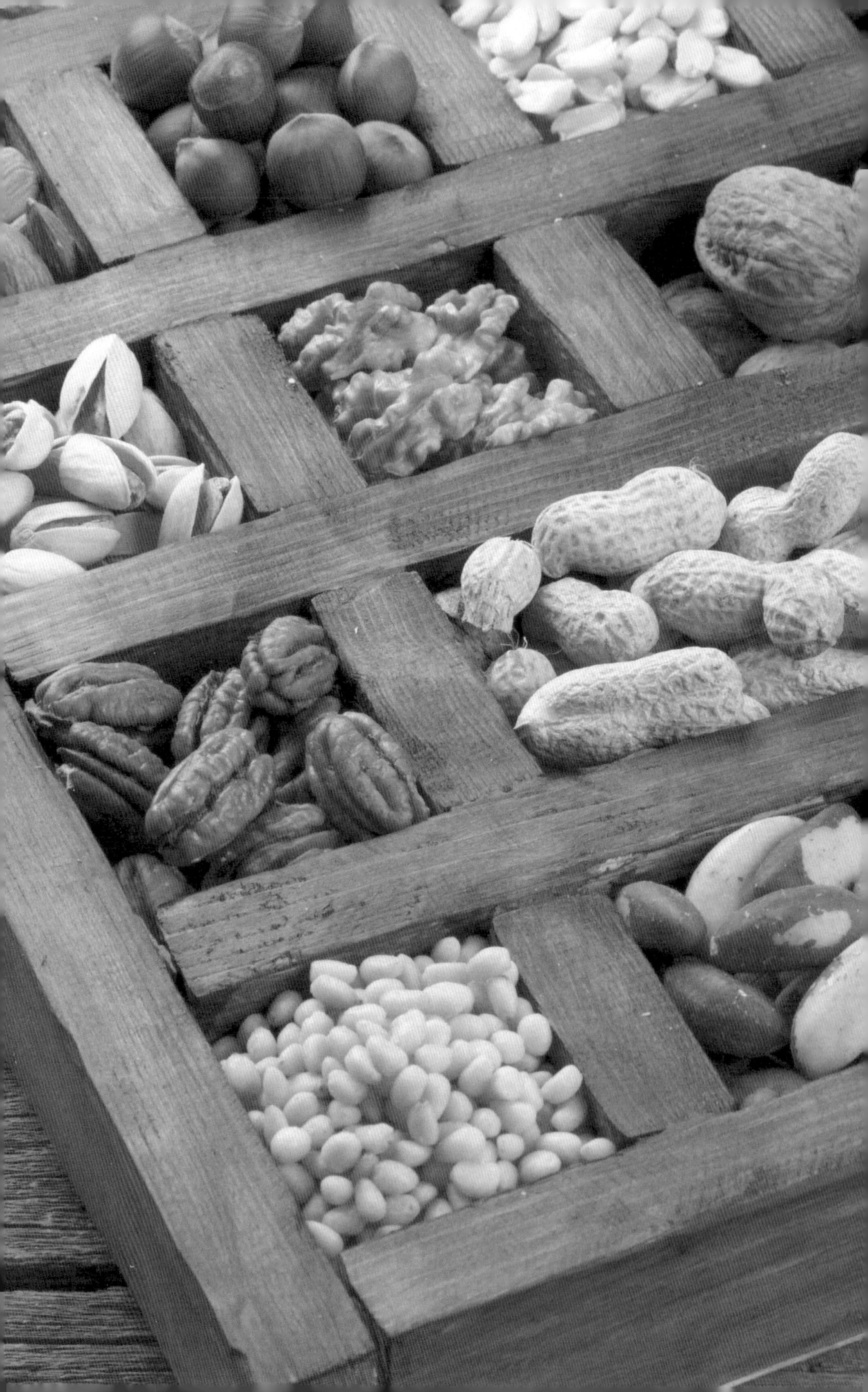

Chapter 3. Cardiovascular System and Vegetarian Diet

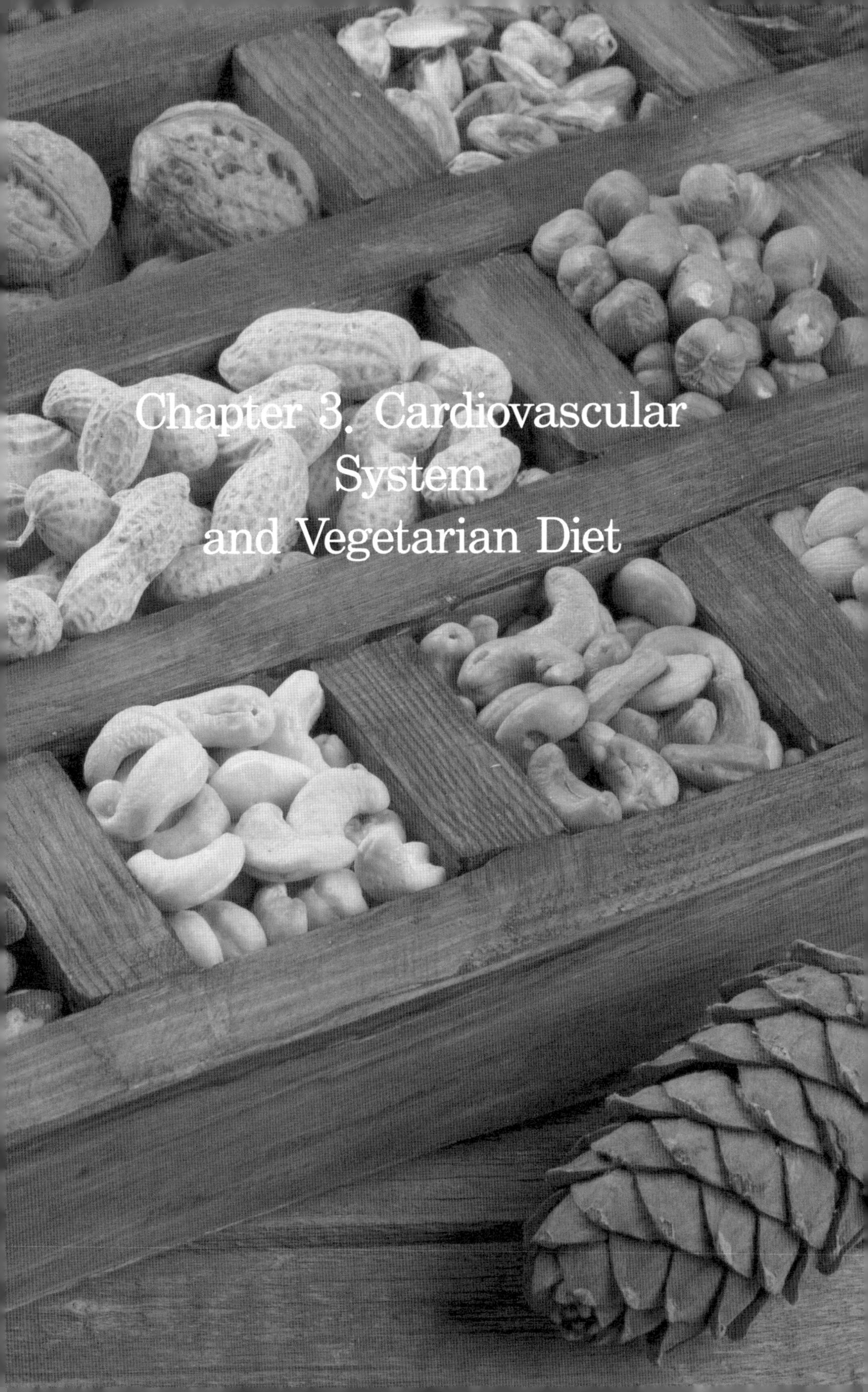

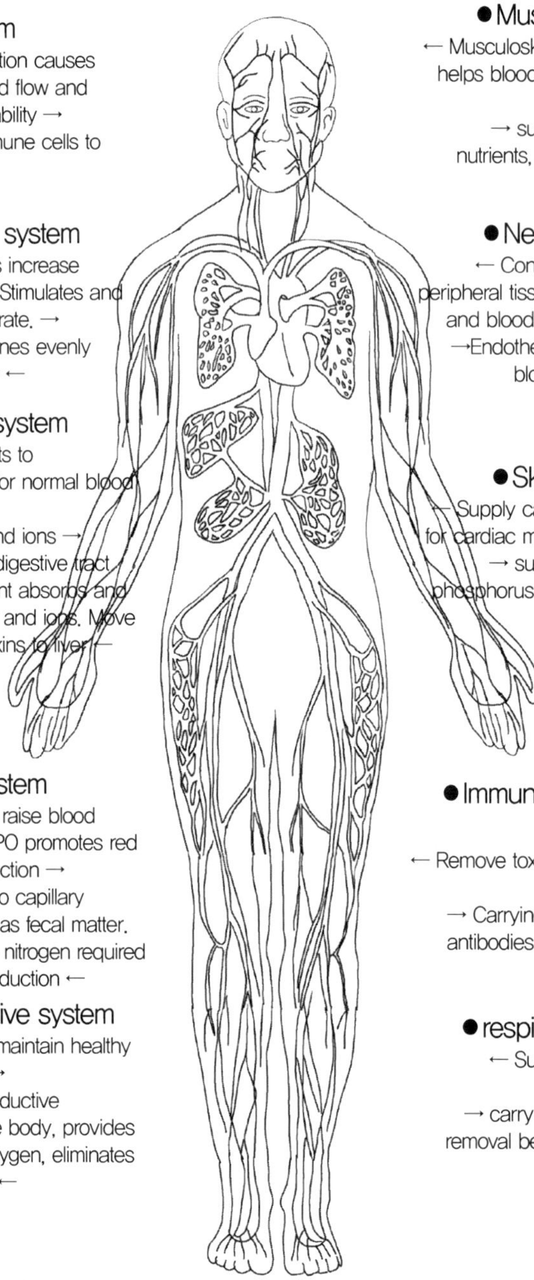

● Skin system

Mast cell stimulation causes changes in blood flow and capillary permeability →
Helps move immune cells to wound area ←

● Endocrine system

Some hormones increase blood pressure, Stimulates and increases heart rate. →
Distribute hormones evenly across the body ←

● Digestive system

Provides nutrients to cardiovascular, for normal blood volume
Absorb water and ions →
It breaks down digestive tract hormone. Nutrient absorbs and transports water and ions. Move nutrients and toxins to liver ←

● Urinary system

Secrete renin to raise blood pressure and EPO promotes red blood cell production →
It carries blood to capillary vessels that act as fecal matter. Re-absorbs the nitrogen required during urine production ←

● Reproductive system

Estrogen helps maintain healthy blood vessels →
Distributes reproductive hormones to the body, provides nutrients and oxygen, eliminates waste and CO_2 ←

● Muscular system

← Musculoskeletal contraction helps blood flow through the blood vessels
→ supply oxygen and nutrients, remove CO_2 and waste products

● Nervous system

← Controls circulation of peripheral tissues by heartbeat and blood pressure control.
→Endothelial cells maintain blood-brain barrier.

● Skeletal system

← Supply calcium necessary for cardiac muscle contraction
→ supply calcium and phosphorus for bone storage

● Immune / lymphatic system

← Remove toxins or pathogens in the blood
→ Carrying and distributing antibodies and aggregating pathogens

● respiratory system

← Supply oxygen and remove CO_2
→ carry oxygen and CO_2 removal between bone and peripheral tissue.

Chapter 3. The Cardiovascular System and the Vegetarian Diet

3.1. The structure and function of the cardiovascular system

The circulatory system consists of three parts: The pump (heart), the solution that transports the substance (blood), and the conduit (blood vessel), also called the "circulatory system". Like the road network in a country, the circulatory system in the body transfers the nutrients and the oxygen to the human body and removes the waste products and the CO_2 generated by the cell metabolism.

The heart weighs only about 300 grams, or one-hundredth of the body weight, but plays an important role in supplying the blood to all the cells in the body, with 60 beats per minute, 86,000 beats a day, and 30 million beats a year. The heart pumps from 5 liters to 6 liters of the blood into the arteries every minute, which means that from 6 tons to 10 tons of the blood are sent to the body a day, and from 150 thousand tons to 250 thousand tons of the blood pass through the heart for the lifetime.

The blood vessels that send blood from the heart to the body are called the "arteries", and the blood vessels that collect the blood that reaches the body and send them back to the heart are called the "veins". The blood vessels near the heart are usually thicker and the blood there moves faster. Because of this, the walls of the arteries have a highly elastic fiber structure to withstand the high pressures of the heart. These fibers stretch to hold the energy in the systole, and the elastic energy in the diastole can push the blood toward each part of the body. Because of the elasticity of the arteries, the flow of the blood is smoother than the flow of the blood in the hard tube.

The diameter of the aorta directly connected with the heart is about 3cm, and the diameter decreases to about 1cm away from the heart. The aorta is divided into the small arteries, which are connected to each organ, and the small arteries branch back to the capillaries and reach the cells of the liver, the kidneys, and the muscles.

The largest aorta in the human body is a resilient artery, with more elastic fibers and with a diameter of more than 1cm. The aortic wall, the pulmonary artery, the subclavian artery and carotid artery, which are directly connected to the heart, are separated.

The middle artery is, also, called the "myocardial artery", and its diameter is the thickest, which is the largest in the human body within from 0.5mm to 1cm. Because it is a blood vessel that distributes the blood to the small arteries that are distributed in the organs of the human body, it is also called the "distribution artery". The small artery regulates the blood flow to the capillaries from 20 μm to 0.5 mm in diameter.

The diameter of the capillary is 7μm ~ 10μm ($10m^{-6}m$), and only one or two red blood cells pass through it. There are a total of from 16 billion to 110 billion capillary blood vessels, and the total length is from 60,000km to 80,000km. The capillary walls are made up of the very thin cell layers, which allow the exchanges of the respiratory gases, the nutrients, and the wastes, such as the oxygen and the carbon dioxide, between the tissues and the capillaries. In the normal cases, the red blood cells and the proteins do not pass through, and the leukocytes can pass through the endothelial cell junctions that constitute the capillaries through the amoeba movement.

This chapter will start with a discussion of the metabolic syndrome to understand why the cardiovascular diseases are soaring in the modern humans and how vegetarianismis beneficial regarding the cardiovascular diseases.

3.2. The importance of the human energy sources and the geology.

In the metabolic syndrome, 'metabolism' mainly means the 'energy metabolism'. Therefore, understanding the supply and utilization of the carbohydrates, the proteins, and the lipids, which are the three major nutrients used as the main energy sources in the human body, is a key factor in understanding the causes of the metabolic syndrome and in understanding its solutions.

Compared to the carbohydrates and the proteins, the lipids have a very high energy efficiency, so the excess energy is stored in the lipid form. It is a normal metabolism that the nutrients remaining after the meal are stored under the lipids under the skin and that the stored lipids are used in the fasting state.

Since the 1950s, the Green Revolution, represented by the nitrogen fertilizer, has led to a 2.6-fold surge in the grain production globally. South Koreans use the grains as the feeds for the livestock, and the modern humans have been overdosed with the chronic, high nutrition. This results in the energy metabolism problems that are different from the previous ones, which are accompanied by diabetes, cardiovascular disease, obesity, kidney disease, blood circulation disorder, and stroke, as well as the competition for the oxidations of the carbohydrates and the lipids.

Can the cause of the metabolic syndrome be identified? The primary cause of the metabolic syndrome is the excessive calorie intake. To understand this claim, we need to look at the nutrients that are used as the calories in our bodies. The common nutrients that the body uses as its main energy sources are the carbohydrates, the proteins, and the lipids. However, there is a large difference in the amount of energy that can be produced per unit mass between these nutrients.

Lipids can produce 9kcal per gram, while the carbohydrates and the proteins produce 4kcal per gram. In addition, the glucose-type carbohydrates, which are the monosaccharides, are converted to the glycogen, a macromolecular polysaccharide, to be stored in the human body. Glycogen must be contained in the liver or the muscle when it contains about 2~3 g of water per gram [1]. On the other hand, the lipids are sufficient if only 10% of the stored fat is present. Therefore, the lipid storage efficiency is increased to 6 times that of the carbohydrates. For example, 5 kg of lipid is sufficient, but, to produce the same calories, it must be at least 30 kg of the carbohydrate.

This had been a great advantage for the early humans who had survived through hunting and gathering. In fact, the high energy storage efficiency of the humans, as well as the lipids, has a very high evolutionary advantage for most animals. So, whatever type of energy you take, the excess calories are stored in the form of the lipids. So, while hibernating, the main energy in the case of the bears is the fat. In the case of the human beings, regarding a man with the body weight of 70 kg, while sitting and working,

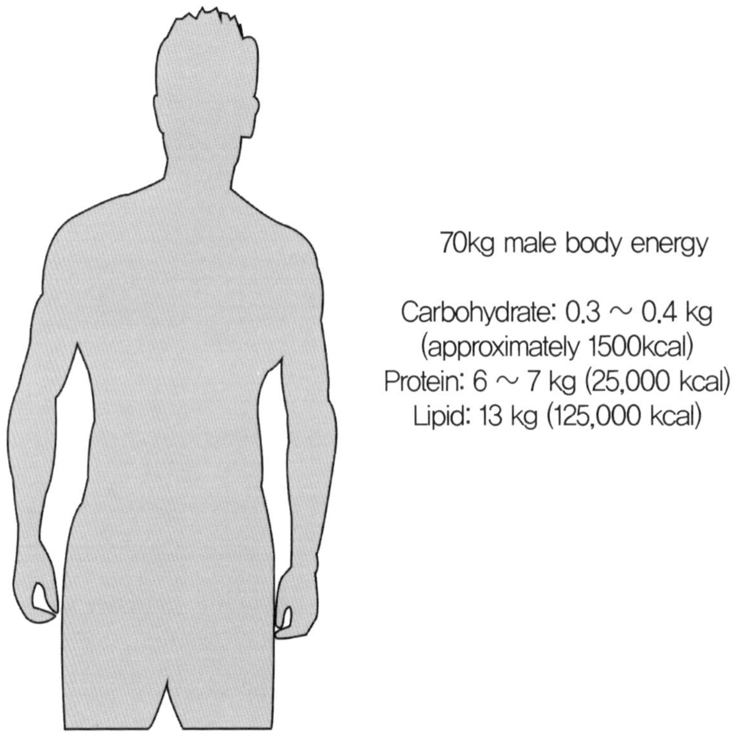

Figure 3-1. Comparison of human energy sources

Table 3-1. Typical personality and energy amount

Compositioin	Mass (kg)	energy (kcal)	Availability (days)
Water and Minerals	49	–	–
protein	6.0	24,000	13.0
Glycogen	0.2	800	0.4
Lpid	15.0	140,000	78
Total	70.0	164,800	91.4

References: Cahill GF. Starvation in man. N Engl J Med 1970;282:668-75

the body carries the carbohydrate of only 300 g (or 400 g), and lipid of 13Kg (125,000 kcal) [1] (Fig. 3-1). In other words, the carbohydrates begin to deplete after from 12 hours to 24 hours, but the lipids can be supplied with the energy to live without any eating for more than two months (70kg, 175cm male). In other words, the lipid has many advantages in terms of the energy efficiency (6 times of carbohydrate), and again, in terms of the evolution or natural environment.

3.3. The energy metabolism is different between the postprandial state and the fasting state.

The postprandial energy state and the energy state while fasting serve as the completely different mechanisms. For example, after meals, the carbohydrates are used as a primary energy source and the insulin is released. On the other hand, in the fasting state, the growth hormone is released, and the energy is supplied by decomposing the lipids stored under the skin. It is known as 'normal metabolism'. The problem, however, is that the excessive energy is consumed to supply the high, caloric, lipid energy from the digestive tract even under the fasting conditions. In order to understand why this is the major cause of the metabolic syndromes, such as diabetes and cardiovascular disease, it is necessary to understand the concept of 'lipoprotein'.

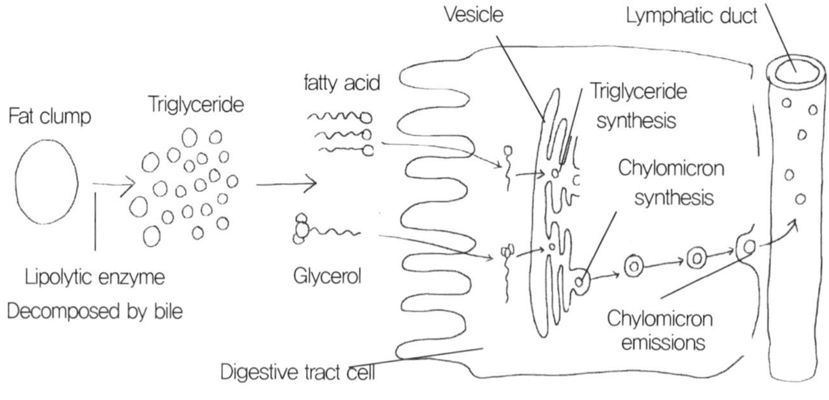

Figure 3-2. Production and migration of triglycerides and free fatty acids, glycerol, and chylomicron

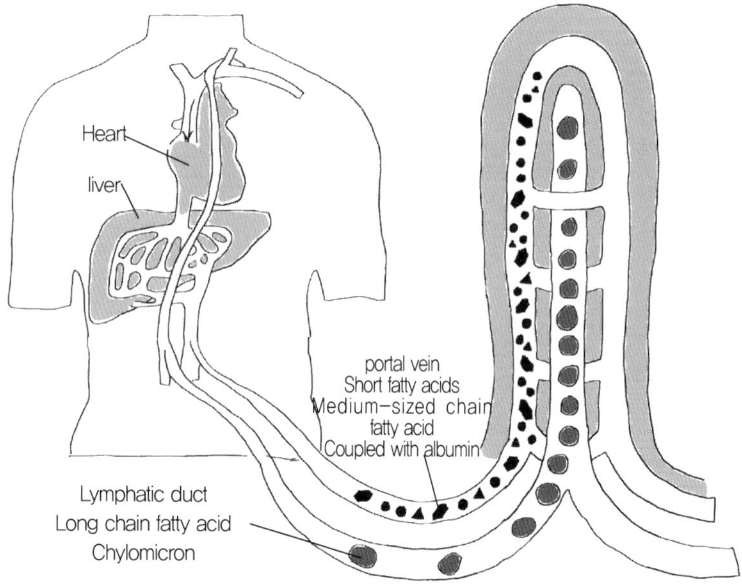

Figure 3-3. The pathway of triglycerides and other nutrients

Short fatty acids and medium chain fatty acids go directly into the portal blood through the intestinal cells and migrate in association with albumin. Long chain fatty acids are formed by chylomicrons, which then migrate to the lymphatic vessels and slowly enter the blood from the chest.

3.4. The importance of the lipid flow and the lipoprotein

The adipose tissue, the viscera, and the liver are the three major organs involved in the production and transport of the lipids in the human body. Between these organs, the lipid transport takes place through the blood, and the lipoproteins play an important role [2].

Water and oil do not mix. Since lipids do not dissolve in the blood, which is the main component of the water, lipids can bind with the water–soluble proteins to move through the blood vessels in order to dissolve. That is, the postprandial triglycerides, which are taken as the food, are degraded by the lipase of the pancreas into the fatty acids and the glycerol and then absorbed by the digestive tract cells. In the gastrointestinal tract, the fatty acids and the glycerol bind again to become the triglycerides, which are surrounded by the water–soluble proteins and which reach the liver through the portal tract in the form of a huge micron. Chylomicron can transfer the triglycerides to the liver, the peripheral and adipose cells, and can make them available as an energy source [3,4].

Unlike the postprandial, in the fasting state, the lipids stored in the adipocytes are degraded into the fatty acids and the glycerol, which are released into the blood, and they arrive in the liver. In the liver, the fatty acids and the glycerol bind again to become the triglycerides and are released from the liver in the form of the Very Low Density Lipoprotein (VLDL), which transports the triglycerides, as an energy source, to the peripheral cells in the blood vessels.(3–

4).

Generally speaking, the triglyceride in the blood is a combination of the chylomicrons, the VLDL, the low-density lipoprotein (LDL), and the triglycerides contained in the high-density lipoprotein (HDL), which can be interpreted as an excessive lipid energy. And the LDL-cholesterol means the cholesterol contained in the lipoproteins which is called the "LDL (low density lipoprotein)".

Figure 3-4 shows a very bulky, chylomicron compared to the VLDL or the LDL. The reason why the chylomicron is noticed in the prevention and healing of the metabolic syndrome is that when the chronic overconsumption of the calories is made, the chylomicron can be continuously supplied from the intestines to the liver in the fasting state without eating. It can disturb the normal metabolic process.

The HDL, the high density lipoprotein, is good. It has the low triglyceride content and the high protein ratio, so that the liver can absorbs the triglyceride and the cholesterol from peripheral tissue mediated by HDL. Therefore, if the amount of caloric intake is low, there is no reason for the HDL to increase. As you will see later, vegetarian diet lowers the LDL, but the HDL does little to change.

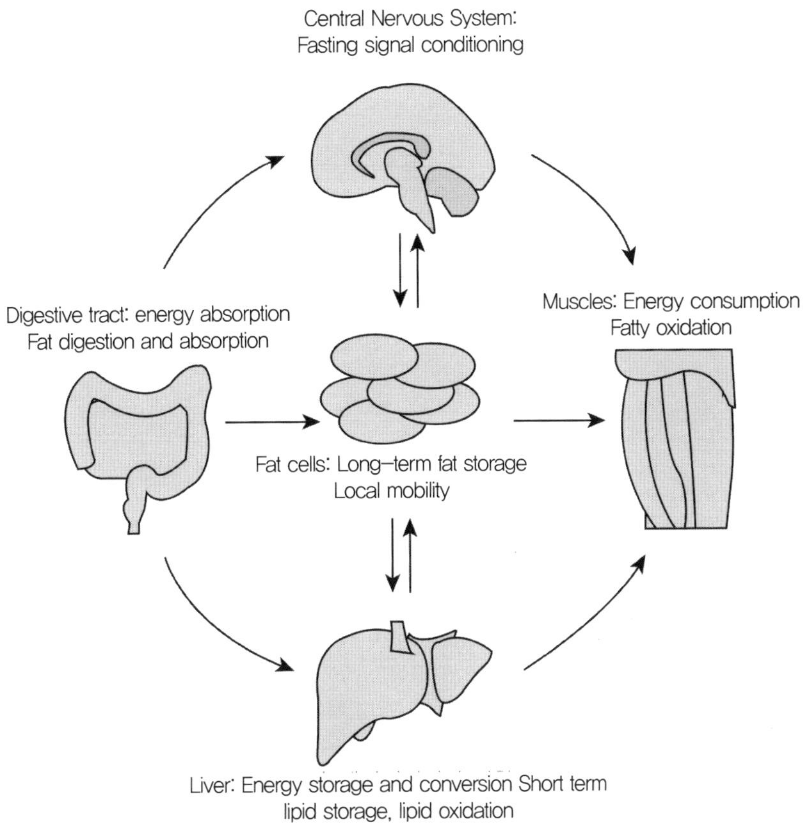

Figure 3–4. Movement of human energy sources

The excess energy is stored in fat and then used for fasting. The triglycerides stored in the fat cells are transferred to the liver in the fasting state, become high–density lipoproteins, circulate throughout the body, and supply fatty acids to the necessary cells. The remaining glycerol becomes a ketone and is supplied to brain cells. Due to the high energy density of lipids, carbohydrates and proteins are also preferred to be stored as fat if they are over–consumed. In particular, insulin is overdosed when consuming white rice or wheat starch lacking fiber, which promotes the synthesis of triglycerides and thus becomes a risk factor for obesity and cardiovascular disease.

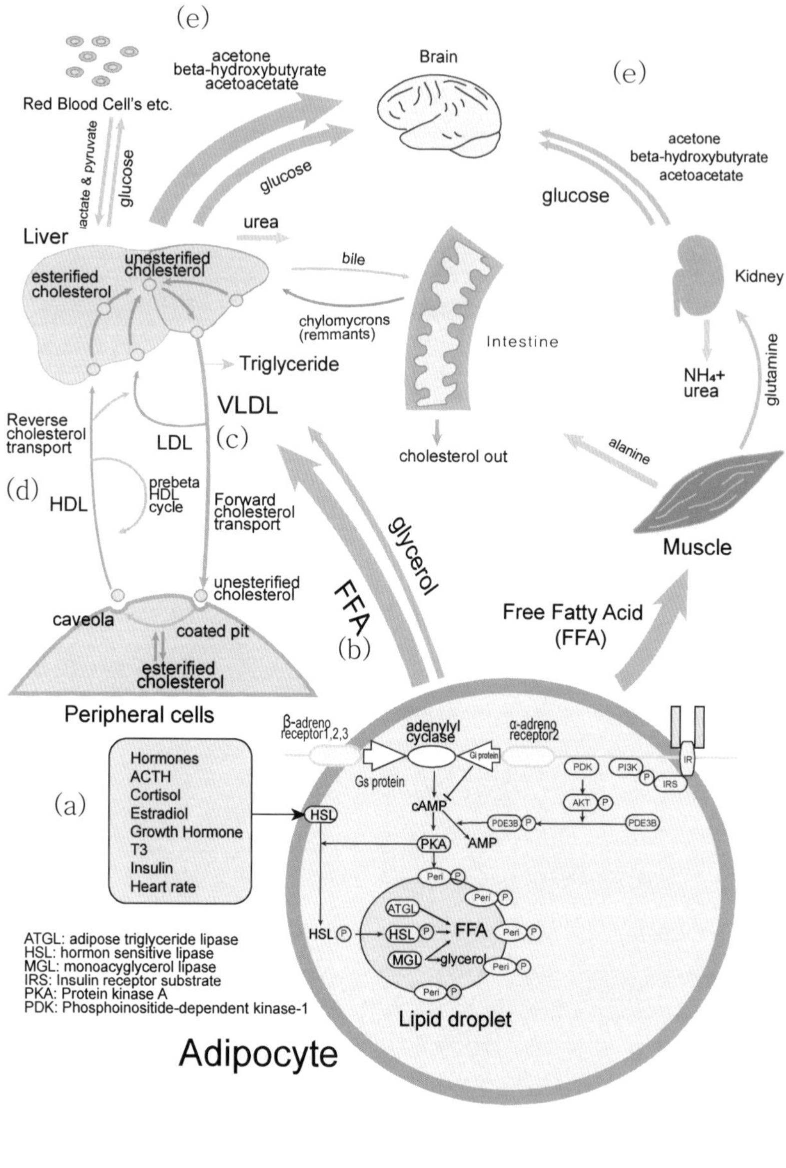

Figure 3–5. Fat migration paths in the fasting state

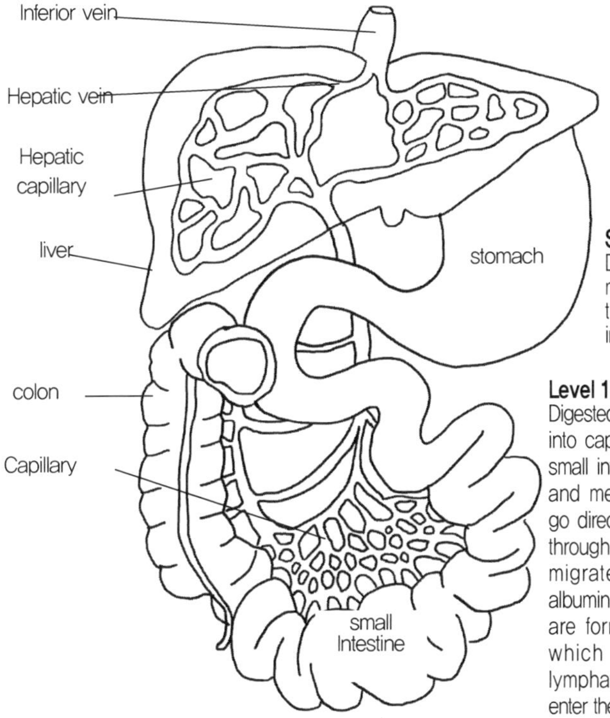

Figure 3–6. Nutrient uptake and migration pathways

◀ Figure 3–5. Commentary

(a) Adrenocorticotrophic hormone (ACTH), cortisol, glucocorticoid, estrodiol, growth hormone, thyroid stimulating hormone (TSH), thyroid hormone , Insulin and the autonomic nervous system affect cellular signals for lipid degradation in adipocytes.

(b) The triglycerides are broken down by the hormones, and the free fatty acids are released into the blood, which is used as an energy source for the cells. Newly synthesized triglycerides in the liver are included as members of very low density lipoproteins and released into the blood.

(c) Triglyceride, which is a component of very low density lipoprotein (VLDL), is converted to low–density lipoprotein (LDL), which is broken down into energy–requiring cells and supplies fatty acids.

(d) LDL moves back to the liver to obtain triglycerides, which are converted into VLDL and released into the blood again.

(e) Glycerol–derived ketones in liver and kidney move to the brain and are used as an energy source.

3.5. Hyperlipidemia and the Randle Cycles: The carbohydrate and the lipid oxidation competition

So, why is excess lipid associated with diabetes? It can be explained by the concept of the oxidation competition of the carbohydrates and the lipids. In other words, our body's energy production is possible by burning the fuel called the "nutrients" in a small generator called the "mitochondria" within the cells. However, the lipids and the carbohydrates compete for the fuel use of the mitochondria (Fig. 3-7, Fig. 3-8). This is called the "Randle cycle" [6].

That is, when an excessive amount of a high-calorie food is consumed, the digestive tract continues to supply the lipid energy not only after the meal but also, in the fasting state. The lipid energy released from intestine collides with the fat energy released from the subcutaneous fat beneath the skin in the fasting state. In the excess fat supply, the cells prefer the fat oxidation rather than the glucose oxidation, leading to the increased blood glucose and insulin level.

Table 3-2. Lipoprotein size and constituents

density (g/mL)	Kinds	diameter(nm)	protein (%)	cholesterol (%)	Phospholipid (%)	Neutral fat and cholesterol ester(%)
〉1.063	HDL	5-15	33	30	29	4
1.019-1.063	LDL	18-28	25	50	21	8
1.006-1.019	IDL	25-50	18	29	22	31
0.95-1.006	VLDL	30-80	10	22	18	50
〈0.95	Chylomicron	100-1000	〈2	8	7	84

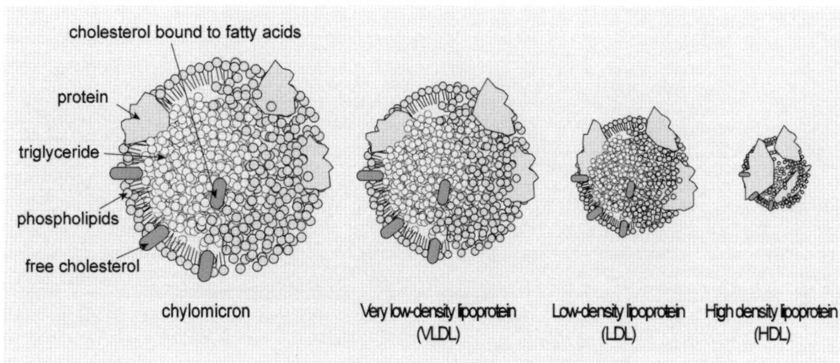

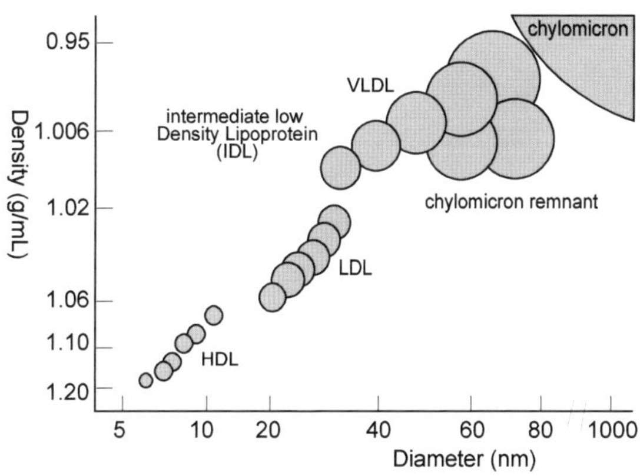

Fauci AS, Kasper DL, Braunwald E, Hauser SL, Longo DL, Jameson JL, Loscalzo JI
Harrison's Principles of Internal Medicine, 17th ed. McGraw-Hill

Figure 3–7. Size and composition of lipoproteins.

Because lipids are nonpolar, they bind with soluble proteins to move in the blood and are called lipoproteins. Chylomicron has a low protein content, a high lipid content, a low density, and a very high volume. On the other hand, high–density lipoproteins have high protein content, low lipid content, high density, and small size.

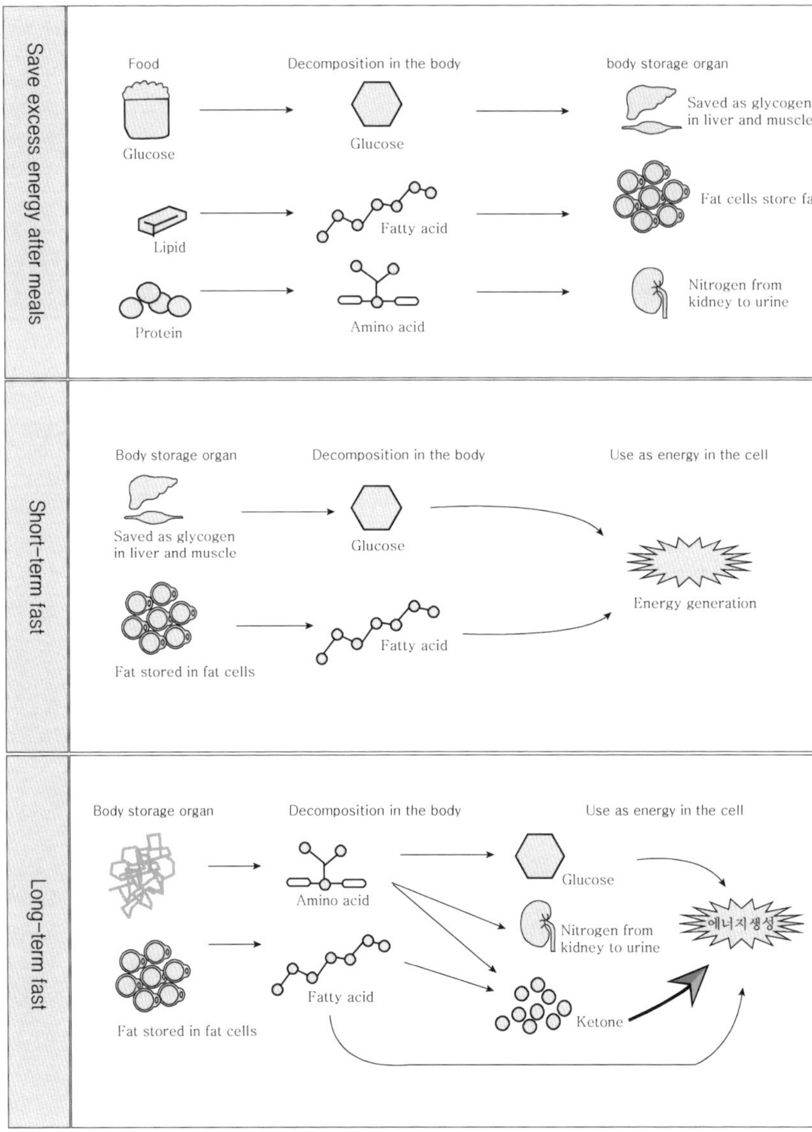

Figure 3-8. Energy metabolism in the postprandial, fasting and fasting state

3.6. The progression of the high caloric intake and the metabolic syndrome.

As the glucose concentration increases, the blood becomes loose and the blood flow slows, which threatens the survival of the peripheral cells, and the body releases more insulin. Insulin is used to tap the cell door and to open the door for glucose. Because glucose does not enter the cell, it makes a lot of insulin that knocks at the door and tries to give a signal, and it becomes hyperinsulinemic. But, our bodies are not machines that can operate infinitely. That is, overproducing the pancreatic cells that are eventually exhausted and broken, they are unable to produce the insulin. So, the diabetics need to take the insulin regularly.

In general, when the neuroendocrine system changes with aging

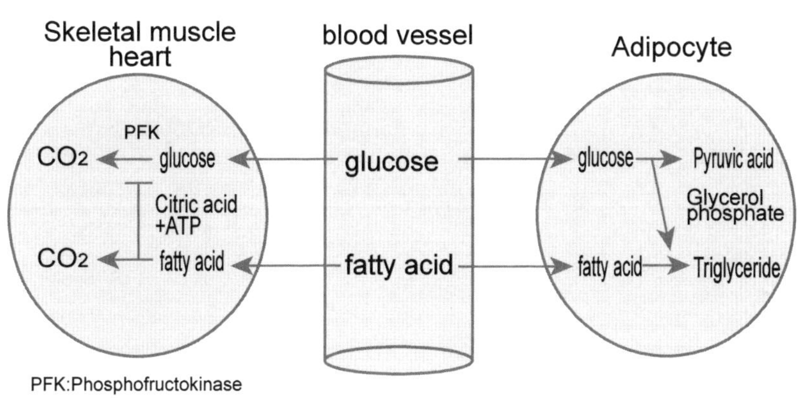

Figure 3-9. Randle cycle diagram in which fatty acid and glucose compete with each other

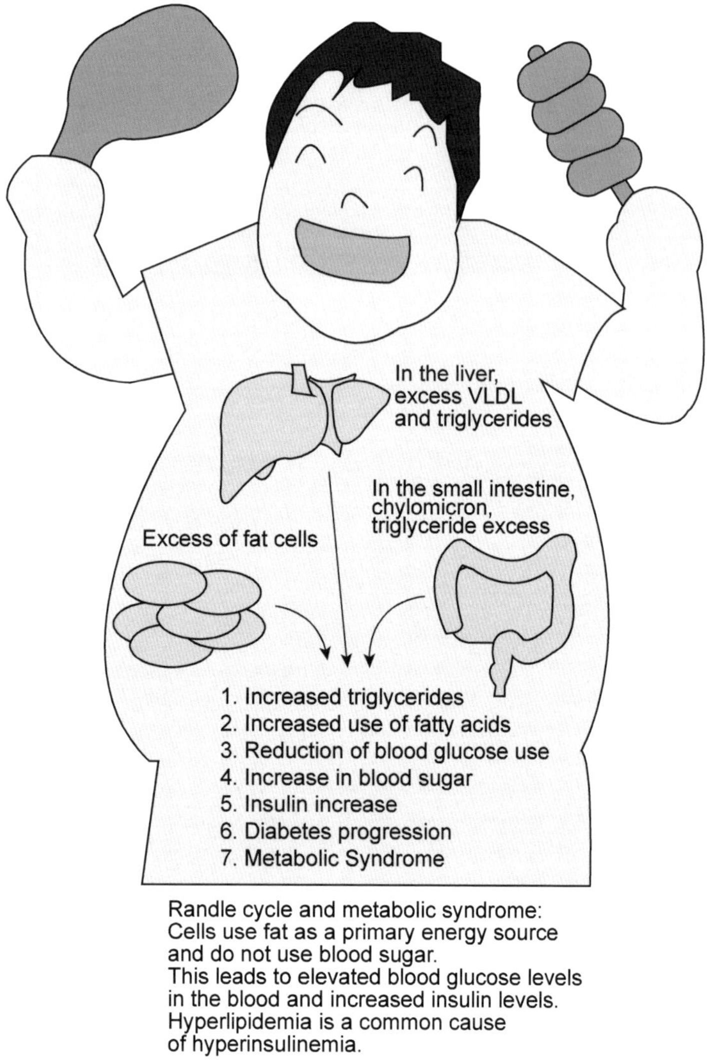

Figure 3–10. Nutrition and Randall Cycle and Metabolic Syndrome

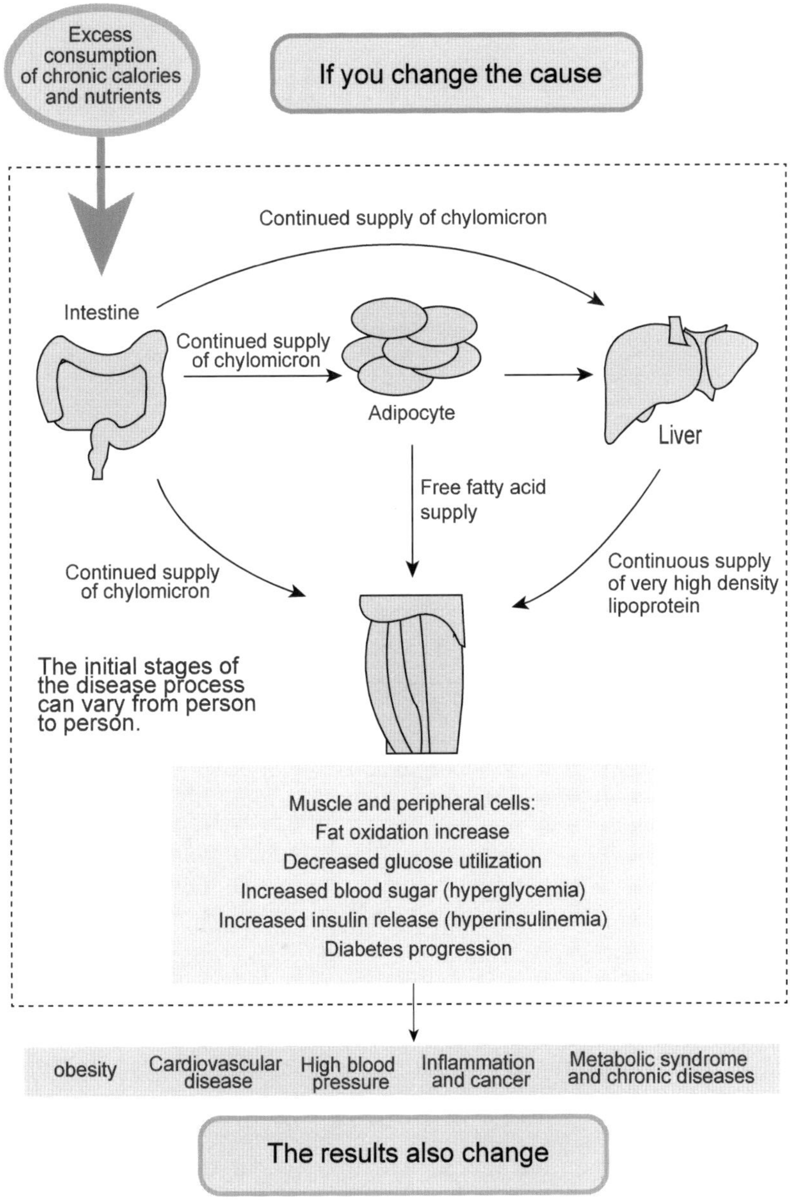

Figure 3-11. Randall Cycle and Process of Metabolic Syndrome

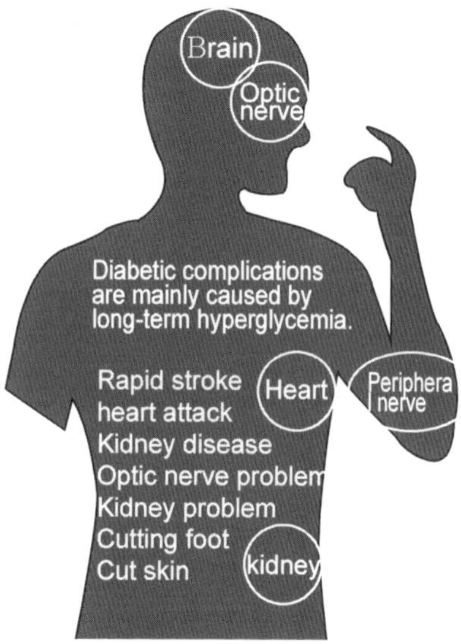

Figure 3–12. Various diabetic complication

and when the excess amount of the energy is continuously supplied, the process is as followed. Increase of the lipids → competition with the carbohydrates and the oxidation competition → the increase in the glucose concentration → the increases in the insulin release → the hyperinsulinemia → the pancreatic damage → the diabetes. This sequence proceeds (Figure 3–13).

This can be interpreted as the general pattern of a very simple metabolic syndrome. Therefore, the fundamental and easy way to resolve the cardiovascular disease, the diabetes and the obesity is not to over–consume the calories. Limiting the calories while having a fullness of the satiety is to reduce or prevent the meat and to eat whole grain.

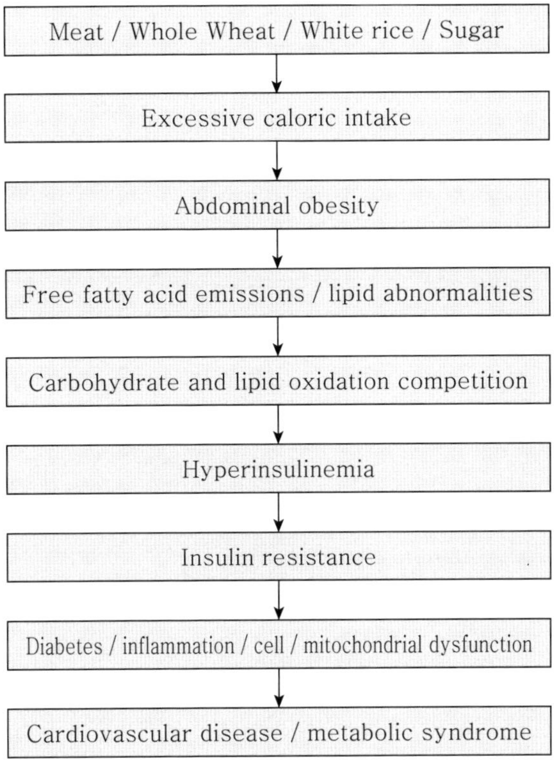

Figure 3-13. Aging, energy overload and the development of metabolic syndrome

Table 3-3. Decrease in size of fat cells due to weight loss

weight	150kg	100kg	75kg
total adipocyte number	75 billion	75 billion	75 billion
Adipocyte size	0.9μg/cell	0.6μg/cell	0.2μg/cell

References: Song, Sook-Ja [Clinical Nutrition, (2001) SamYoung Pub.]

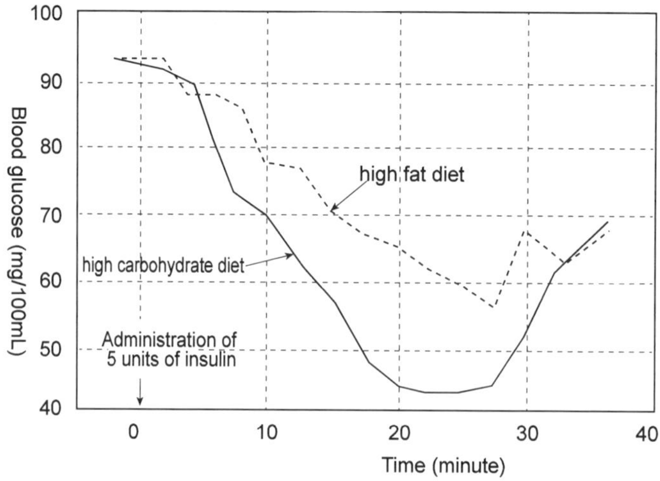

High-fat diet and high-carbohydrate diet insulin-lowering curve (insulin sensitivity test)
In healthy adults, high calorie diet and high carbohydrate diet were fed respectively, and then 5 insulin units were injected. When serum insulin levels were measured, high fat diet was higher than that of high glucose diet.

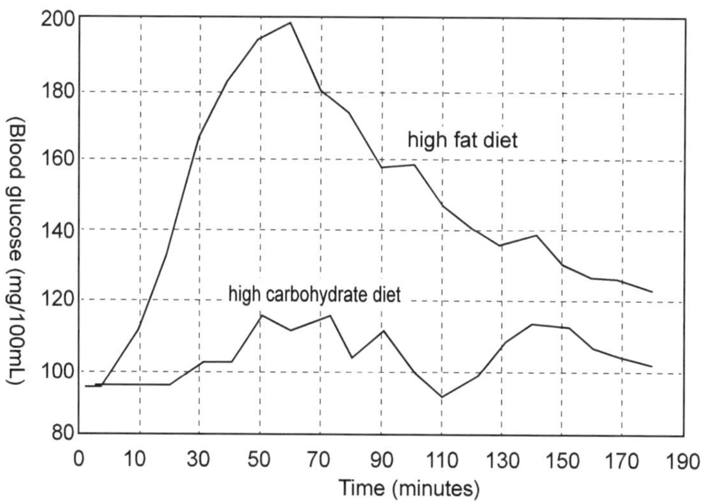

Comparison of glucose intakes during fat and carbohydrate ingestion
When a healthy person consumed the same amount of fat and carbohydrate, 50 g of glucose was fed into the test diet and blood glucose was measured. The fat intake was higher in the case of fat intake and the normal curve was in the case of carbohydrate intake.

Figure 3–14. Aging, energy overload and the development of metabolic syndrome

3.7. The progression of arteriosclerosis

The most common cardiovascular disease among the modern people is arteriosclerosis. So, how does arteriosclerosis occur? Atherosclerosis is a three-stage process (Fig. 3-15). Initially, the fatty streak is the stage in which the fat accumulates in the aortic or middle arterial veins. The second step is the plaque-formation step. When the fat comes into direct contact with the blood, the body activates a self-protective action to coagulate the blood. The arterial wall covers the fat plaque with a fibrous cap to block the deadly effects of the blood clinging to the fat that is stuck. The third step is the formation of the ulcers on the plaques formed, and the platelets, which are the blood-clotting cells, are bound to the exposed fat and the ulcer sites. This results in a complete closure of the arterial wall and the interruption of the blood flow by the thrombus.

If blood flow blocking happens in the coronary arteries, it is called a "coronary artery disease" which include a "myocardial

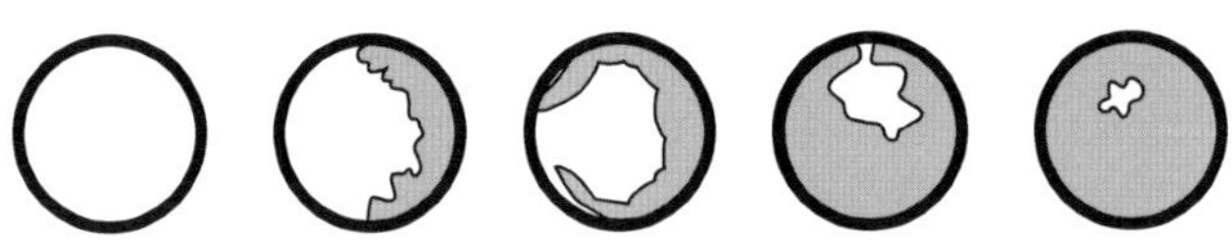

Angina pectoris • myocardial infarction • ischemic myocardial disease • congestive heart failure

Figure 3-15. Progression of atherosclerosis and cardiovascular disease

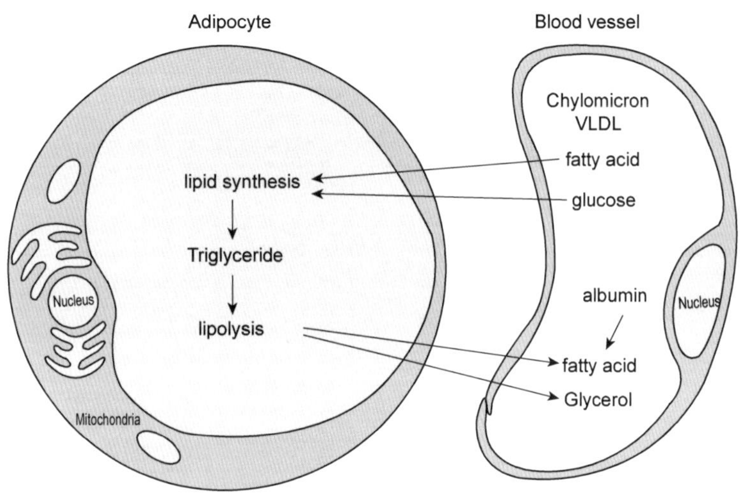

Figure 3–16. Movement of nutrients between fat cells and porch

infarction", and a "heart attack". And when it happens in brain, it is called an "arteriosclerosis in the brain". A serious problem is that the human body does not feel any symptoms until the arteries are blocked by more than half and, sometimes, by up to 70%. The myocardial infarction, the ischemic, myocardial disease, and the symptoms of the congestive heart failure occur in succession when the artery is occluded by more than 60%, and, eventually,when the vessel is completely blocked, resulting in death.

Angina is caused by a lack of the blood supply to the heart muscle, resulting in pain, pressure, and tightness in the middle or left side of the chest. Ischemic heart disease is a cardiac dysfunction caused by a lack of the blood supply to the heart muscle. The repeated aggravation and improvement without a complete closure is referred to as 'angina pectoris', and, if the cardiac muscle dies because of the blocked blood supply, it is called an "acute myocardial infarction".

Congestive heart failure is a heart failure that does not provide enough blood to the human body, which, in turn, reduces the supply of the nutrients and the oxygen to the body, and the metabolism of the body cells accumulates the wastes. This is because the brain is unable to function because due to the seizure and the kidneys pour the urine into the body. The lungs become difficult to breathe, and the bronchitis and the asthma will occur. There are many causes of these cardiovascular diseases, but the important factor is that they are the forms of atherosclerosis.

Atherosclerosis occurs not only in the heart muscle but, also, in all the arteries of the human body. If arteriosclerosis occurs in the brain, it is called stroke. If it occures in kidney's artery, it is called a kidney disorder. And, if it occurs in the reproductive system, the person becomes impotent. In addition, when a hardening occurs in the peripheral arteries supplying the blood from the arms and the legs, the oxygen and the nutrients are not supplied to the peripheral cells, the waste products are not removed, and even a cutting is sometimes carried out.

3.8. Atherosclerosis and cholesterol

The cause of atherosclerosis, which causes a damage due to a blood circulation disorder throughout the body, is the fat that accumulates on the walls of the arterial blood vessels as described above. Its main ingredient is cholesterol.

In fact, cholesterol is a major component of the cell membranes, the brain cells, and the various hormones in the human body, so the body synthesizes from 900mg to 1,200mg per day, which is more than the required amount of cholesterol. Therefore, there is no reason to be fed with food. Rather, when cholesterol is introduced through the food, the human body cannot deal with the excess cholesterol. After it is saturated within the human cells, it accumulates in the blood vessel walls and proceeds to arteriosclerosis as described above.

Figure 3-17 shows the results of a 1990 study of 35,000 people aged from 35 to 57 in the United States. As the blood cholesterol had increased from 150 mg/dl, the number of the coronary artery deaths had increased [10].

A comparative study of 19 countries in the world shows the same results. The average cholesterol level in Japan was less than 200 mg/dl, with 100 deaths per 100,000 people, while it was over 230 mg/dl in the UK, Ireland, and Denmark.The number of the coronary artery disease deaths was more than 300 per 100,000 [11]. Based on these results, the adequate cholesterol level to prevent

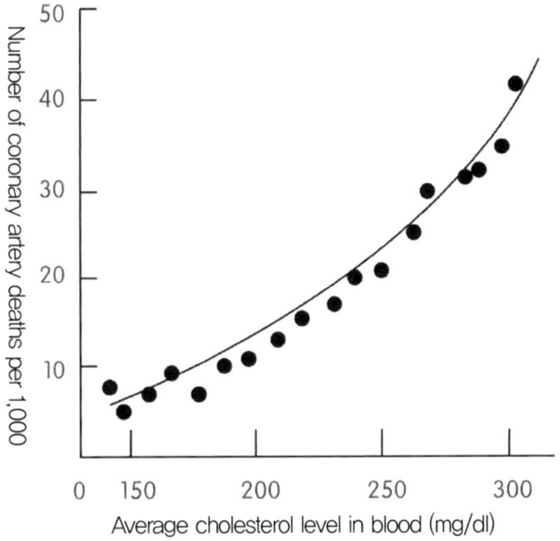

Figure 3-17. Proportion of blood cholesterol and coronary death rate

a heart disease may be less than 150 mg/dl. In his book, "Wellness Lifestyle," Dr. Nile recommends the goal of cholesterol to be "to become 100 + years old" [12]

3.9. Colin Campbell's Study in China

The Chinese Study [13] of Colin Campbell is a good description of the relationship between the diet and the illness. In the early 1970s, the Chinese Prime Minister Ji, Eun-rae had been in a dangerous state with cancer. Campbellinvestigates the death rates for 12 cancers in 800,000 people in 2,400 regions across China to gather the information. The large-scale research project, which had surveyed 650,000 people, showed a cancer incidence that was up to 100 times different depending on the region. Campbell learned about this during a conversation with the Chinese scholar Chen. In the case of the United States, such information could be excluded because Campbell could not see such a difference. He eventually convinces the US government and gets the support.

Campbell got the vast amount of the data regarding 48 diseases and 367 factors through the blood and the survey from 65,500 adults in 65 regions of China. He had gathered the urine and had collected the information about the food that their family had eaten for three days (Table 3-4). The results were as follows:

First, Americans get, on the average, from 15 percent to 16 percent of their total calories from protein. More than 80% of the protein intake is 70 g from animal. On the other hand, the percentage of the protein in the Chinese rural areas is only 9% ~ 10%, and the animal protein is 10% and 7.1g. As a result, the cholesterol level had to be different: the American average was

Table 3-4. Comparison of Chinese and American Food Intake

nutrient	China	USA
Calorie (kcal/day)	2,641	1,989
Total fat (calorie ratio)	14.5	34~38
Dietary fiber (g / day)	33	12
Total protein (g / day)	64	91
Animal protein (caloric ratio)	0.8	10~11
Iron (mg / day)	34	18

215 mg/dl, while the Chinese average was almost 100 mg/dl ~ 127 mg/dl. For 85% of the Chinese, it was 150 mg/dl.
What is interesting in hisstudy is that, when the blood cholesterol falls from 170 mg/dl to 90 mg/dl, the incidence of most cancers, including the liver cancer, the rectal cancer, and the colorectal cancer, drops. Campbell adds, in his article, that he is referring to Caldwell as a doctor.

"I did not see an example of death from a heart disease among those who were 150 mg/dl."

3.10. Vegetarianism and the myocardial infarction.

Cholesterol is inserted between the cells and the cell membranes to tighten the cell membranes and is an essential component of the five steroid hormones. Because of this, the human body synthesizes more than the necessary amount of the cholesterol within the cell, and there is no reason to receive any cholesterol as food. However, the animal foods that are often on the table contain cholesterol, which causes cholesterol to build up slowly and steadily in the blood vessel walls. Although the amount of the daily accumulation is small, arteriosclerosis cannot be avoided if this process is carried out for several years or decades. On the other hand, the vegetable foods do not have any cholesterol, but they are rich in fiber, and they play a role in removing the excess cholesterol (Table 3-5).

Cholesterol is the main barrier to the coronary artery vessels, and cholesterol is always included in the animal foods. On the other hand, the vegetable foods have no cholesterol. The inference that the vegetarian diet is beneficial to the coronary artery disease is natural.

In 1992, a related experiment was conducted at a hospital in India. The researchers diagnosed the patients with acute myocardial infarction in the hospital. And then they divided into two groups within two or three days, One group being fed the previous meat diet and the other group being fed with reduced meat, egg, butter and hydrogenated oil. At this time, the fat intakes of the two groups had been equal to from 24% to 26% of the total calorie intake. The intakes of the fruits and the vegetables had been three times higher in the vegetarian diet group than in the normal diet group, and the intakes of the fiber, vitamin C, vitamin E, carotene, and potassium had been high in the vegetarian group while the intakes of the saturated fat and the cholesterol had been low.

The carbohydrate intake had been changed from the simple carbohydrates, such as white wheat, to the complex carbohydrates of the whole wheat. After 12 weeks, the vegetarian diet became lower in body mass, the LDL cholesterol, blood pressure and blood glucose compared to the normal diet group, while the HDL cholesterol, which is beneficial to the human body, had been increased.

Low-density lipoprotein (LDL) is a light cholesterol carrier that transports cholesterol to blood vessels and causes the coronary artery disease. On the other hand, the high-density lipoprotein

Table 3-5. Food and Cholesterol (mg/100g)

Food	Cholesterol level	Food	Cholesterol level
Pickled salmon roe	510	Cheese	80
egg	470	chicken	80
Cattle liver	240	pig	60
herring	230	mayonnaise	60
eel	240	Vegetables, Grains, Fruits	0

Herring fish and eggs have higher cholesterol levels than chickens and pigs.

(HDL) removes the surflus cholesterol accumulated in the blood vessels and moves it to the liver, thus allowing the body to use the cholesterol to produce more bile. Thus, a decrease in the LDL and an increase in the HDL are a very good indication that the myocardial infarction is being treated. These results had led to a 36% reduction in the incidence of the coronary artery disease, a 42% reduction in the coronary artery deaths and a 38% decrease in the myocardial infarction in the vegetarian diet group compared with the normal diet group.

3.11. The Mediterranean diet and myocardial infarction

The total lipid intake of the Mediterranean diet is 38%, which is not significantly different from that of the west. Instead of decreasing the saturated fat, it is replaced with the vegetable oils, such as the olive oil and the sunflower oil. However, a study of the effects of the Mediterranean diet on the coronary artery mortality following a myocardial infarction are similar to those of the Indian vegetarian diet. In 1994, the Rhein–Echinard Heart Research Institute provided a Mediterranean diet of which the oil was replaced with the vegetable oil rich in the polyunsaturated fats, such as the omega–3 fatty acid, instead of the animal fat to the severe myocardial infarction patients.

In this diet, the beans and the plants, the whole wheat bread, the fruits and the vegetables had been increased while the meat,

Table 3-6. Mediterranean diet and food, nutrition, blood changes

	increase	decrease	Not changed
Dietary change	Fruits, vegetables, beans, Whole wheat, vegetable oil, fiber	Meat, butter, cream, cholesterol	Total fat (31-33%) Cheese, fish
Blood change	Vitamin C, Vitamin E Oleic acid, Linolenic acid (omega-3) EPA, DHA	Linoleic acid (Omega-6)	cholesterol, LDL, HDL, Trans fatty acids, Platelet aggregation

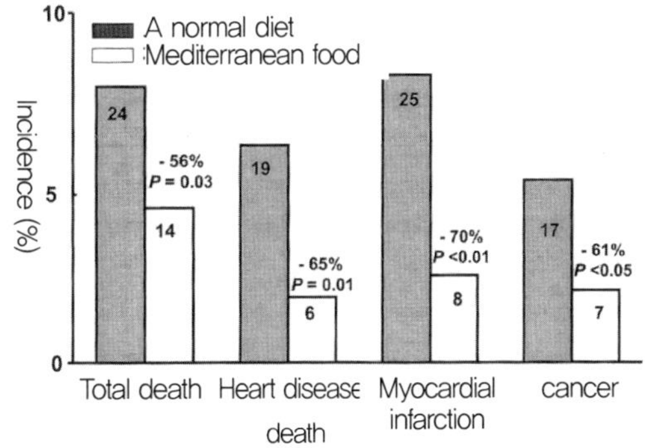

Figure 3-18. Improvement of cardiovascular disease in Mediterranean diet

butter and cream had been decreased. The total fat intake had remained at 31% (Table 3–6). As a result of these diets, the levels of the oleic acid, the alpha–linolenic acid, the EPA (eicosapentaenoic acid), and the antioxidant vitamins had been elevated in the serum components of the patients, and the total plasma lipid levels had remained unchanged (Table 3–6, Fig. 3–18).

After 27 months, the dietary group with the Mediterranean diet had decreased by 65% compared with the other dietary group, and by 61% in terms of the incidence of cancer [15].

3.12. The nuts and the Ischemic heart disease.

The results of various epidemiological studies show that the lipid composition is an important element of the vegetarian diet that is beneficial for the prevention and treatment of the cardiovascular diseases. In particular, the legumes and the nuts, important for the vegetarian diet, contain the plentiful amounts of the polyunsaturated fats, including the omega-3 fatty acid. They are beneficial for the cardiovascular health, and which reduce the platelet aggregation. Vitamin C, vitamin E, beta-carotene and the phytochemicals are, also, rich in antioxidants. These ingredients lower the LDL, the cholesterol that is harmful to the human body,

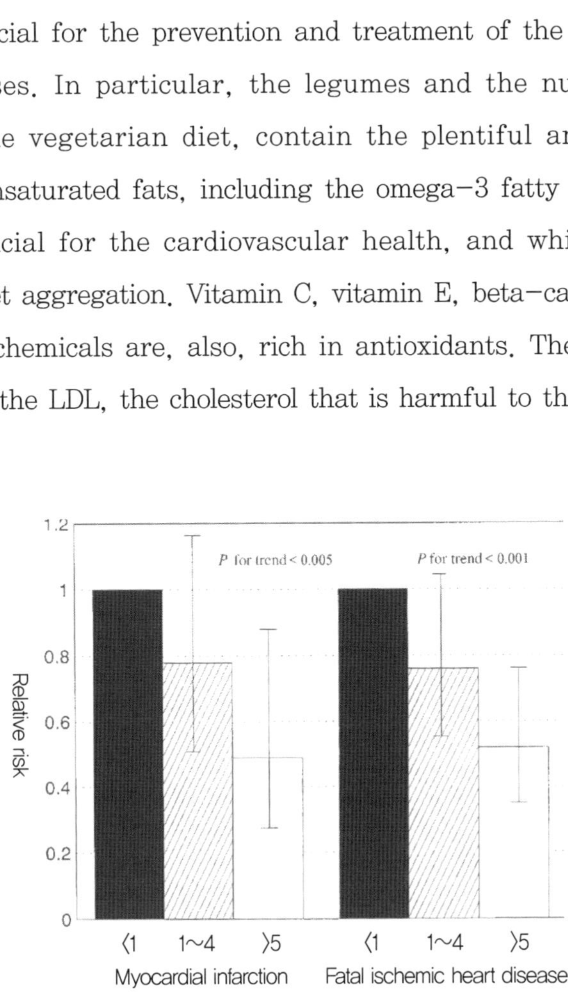

Figure 3-19. The higher the frequency of nuts intake, the lower the relative risk of heart disease (the number of meals per week)

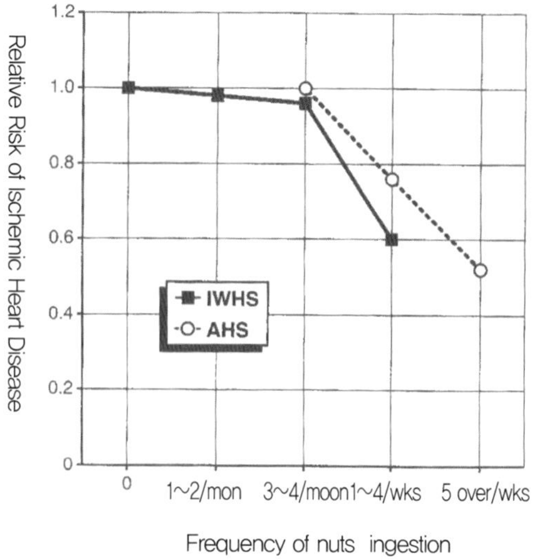

Figure 3-20. Improvement of cardiovascular disease in Mediterranean diet

and prevent the ischemia of the blood vessels. The folate-rich food lowers the homocysteine levels that are harmful to the ischemic heart disease.

In 1992, a large epidemiological study of 34,198 Californians showed an inverse relationship between the nuts intake and the myocardial infarction, the ischemic heart disease mortality. As shown in Figure 3-20, the group who ate the nuts from 1 meal to 4 meals a week showed the reduced myocardial infarction rate by 22%, compared to the group who ate the nuts less than once a week, and 51% compared to the group that ate the nuts five times a week.

3.13. Fiber prevents the occurrence of the cardiovascular diseases

Fiber is a component that cannot be digested by the human body and is not absorbed but is excreted in the feces. In the old nutrition, it was not used for energy, and it could not find a special function. However, fiber, now, has a beneficial effect in lowering the serum cholesterol and the LDL cholesterol. Two effects of fiber are known. One is to block the long-term circulation of the cholesterol, and the other is the action of the bacteria in the intestines.

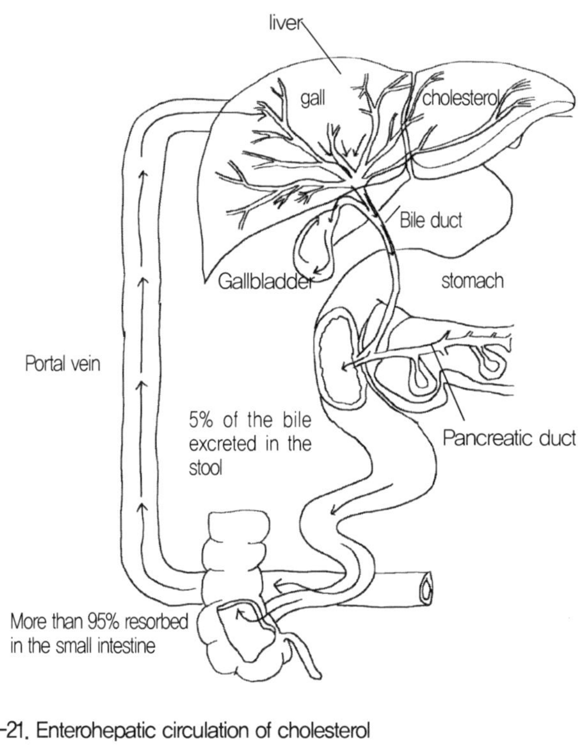

Figure 3-21. Enterohepatic circulation of cholesterol

First, the body synthesizes the bile in the liver to absorb the lipid, stores it in the gallbladder, and secretes the bile from the gallbladder when needed. The main ingredient of the bile is the cholesterol. Fiber is adsorbed by this cholesterol and leaves the feces. However, when less fiber is consumed, the secreted cholesterol is reabsorbed in the ileum, which is the last part of the small intestine, resulting in a higher cholesterol level in the body (Fig. 3–21).

Second, the bacteria that ferment the cellulose produce the acetic acid, the propianic acid, and the butyric acid, which inhibit the cholesterol synthesis. Are these fibers actually effective against heart disease?

In 1986, 43,757 healthy men aged from 40 years to 75 years had been studied for the relationship between dietary fiber and the risk of the coronary heart disease. 131 dietary items were followed up for 6 years to investigate 734 cases of myocardial infarction. In 1996, the researchers published the results of the analysis. According to the degree of the fiber consumption, the group with the highest

Table 3–7. Water soluble fiber intake and serum LDL–cholesterol

Ingested water–soluble fibrous material	Changes in serum LDL–cholesterol
Placebo (0g)	0.8% increase
5g	5.6% decrease
10g	6.8% decrease
15g	14.9% decrease

Table 3-8. Daily intake of soluble fiber for lipid-lowering effect

Food	Intake(g)
Baked beans	100g~150g
oat	57~140g
pectin	6~40g
gum	8~36g

J Am Diet Assoc 94:425,1994

intake of fiber (average 28.9g) was compared to the lowest group (12.4g). The relative risk was 0.59. It was concluded that fiber is a very powerful factor in preventing myocardial infarction.

In another 1992 study, cholesterol was lowered with the increasing fiber intake. In Table 3-7, the serum cholesterol had been lowered by 15% when 15 g of fiber had been added per day. The results of these four-week experiments showed that the serum cholesterol level had increased by 0.8% when a placebo was administered, but it had decreased by 5.6% in the 5g daily fiber intake, by 6.8% in the 10g intake, and had decreased by 14.9% in in the 15g LDL-cholesterol intake [18].

The recommended amount of fiber is usually from 25g to 30g for adults including 6g to 10g in the case of water soluble fiber. The cellulose, the lignin, the pectin, thegum, the seaweed polysaccharides, and some hemicelluloses are abundant in the legumes, the nuts, the grains, the fruits and the vegetables have high cholesterol clearing effects. Of course, these fibers will be more effective when consumed through food (Table 3-8) [19].

3.14. Saturated fats and the cardiovascular diseases

Cholesterol is a major factor in the development of a cardiovascular disease, but there is a stronger factor–the saturated fat. The representative research on this is Dr. Kiz's study in the 1960s. According to his formula, the body's total serum cholesterol level is influenced not only by the cholesterol, itself, but, also, by the content of the saturated and polyunsaturated fats.

Usually, the saturated fats are solid at the temperatures we live in every day, and the unsaturated fats are in the liquid form. Often, the lipid of the meat is called the "fat", and the lipid of the plant is called the "oil", but their compositions are the same. They show the difference between a solid and a liquid due to their slight difference

Table 3-9. Types and ratios of fatty acids in food

Food	Fat in 100g of food (g)	fatty acid (%)		
		Saturated fatty acid	Unsaturated fatty acid	P/S ratio
almond	54	8	92	2.21
peanut	51	18	82	1.49
Walnut	64	11	89	6.90
Corn oil	80	18	82	?
beef	5~25	50	50	0.09
Pork	5~15	39	61	0.17
milk	3.5	62	38	0.11
butter	81	62	38	0.11

P / S ratio: ratio of polyunsaturated fat (P) to saturated fat (S) in food in structure. The problem is that, if our diet contains a lot of saturated fat, the body will produce a lot of cholesterol, whereas the intake of the polyunsaturated fat will reduce the amount of the cholesterol.

Dr. Kiz, the author of the studies on the relationship between saturated fat and cholesterol, says that the cholesterol synergistic effect of the saturated fat is twice the effect of reducing the polyunsaturated fats. Thus, if the P/S value of the saturated fat (S) to the unsaturated fat (P) in the food is higher than 2.0, the blood cholesterol level is lowered, while, if it is lower than 2.0, the blood cholesterol level is increased.

In Table 3-9, the fat composition table of the various foods reveals that the plants, especially the nuts, are mostly unsaturated and that the animal foods have very little unsaturated fat. Naturally, the P/S value of the meat is low, and it causes a greater burden of the cholesterol, as well as the cholesterol from the saturated fat.

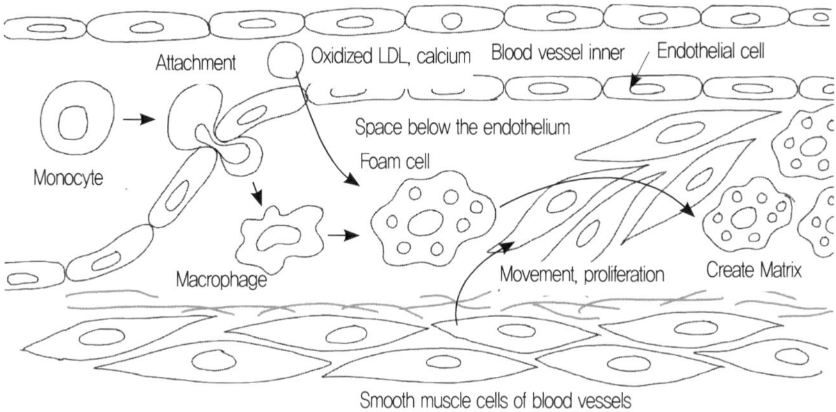

Figure 3–22. Vascular occlusion of oxidized fats

When heat is applied to meat or oil at high temperature, it easily bonds with oxygen in the air. The rancid fat excites the macrophages, etc., into the blood vessels, causing them to go under the blood vessels, where the macrophages are flocculated into foam cells, depositing calcium and the like, creating plaques, blocking the blood vessels, and eventually being exposed to various cardiovascular diseases. The various inflammations of the human body are associated with rancid lipids.

3.15. The percentages of the local vegetarians and the non-vegetarians.

In 2001, we examined the amounts of the saturated fat, the cholesterol and the unsaturated fat in the blood of the vegetarians and the non-vegetarians in Australia. As shown in Table 3-10, the total blood cholesterol and LDL-cholesterol levels were significantly lower in the vegetarians compared to the non-vegetarians. The saturated fat levels of the vegetarians were lower than those of the non-vegetarians, while the saturated fat content in the blood of the predators was 49.6 mg/100ml, while that for the vegan diet was 39.9 mg/100ml [20].

As a result, the vegetarian diet will have a lowering effect on the total cholesterol due to the reduced saturated fat, and it will, also, help prevent and treat heart disease.

Table 3-10. Fatty acid composition in blood according to dietary type

fatty acid	Carnivorous prefer (18)	Meat Meal (60)	lacto-ovo vegetarian (43)	vegan (18)
Average age	34.2	38.3	34.9	33.0
Total cholesterol (mmol/l)	4.59	4.50	3.60	3.52
LDL (mmol/l)	2.94	2.93	2.11	2.14
HDL (mmol/l)	1.08	1.09	1.03	0.96
Saturated fatty acid (mg/100ml)	49.6	49.3	43.0	39.9
Monounsaturated fatty acid(mg/100ml)	15.3	15.2	13.3	12.5
Polyunsaturated fatty acid (mg/100ml)	49.9	51.3	46.4	44.7
Total fatty acids	115	116	103	97

Clinical Science (2001) 100, 25-32

3.16. . The function of iron

One of the major shortcomings of the vegetarian diet in classical nutrition is the lack of the iron absorption. The iron of vegetarian diet is less prone to the iron deficiency because it is less absorbable than the animal heme iron. However, modern nutritional science suggests that the excessive iron dampness due to the heme iron in animal foods can be a major cause of cancer, diabetes, and cardiovascular disease etc. This is because the iron can catalyze the chain reaction of reactive oxygen. The mechanism of the occurrence of the various diseases, including the metabolic syndrome due to an iron overload, is introduced. Next, we will compare the blood iron contents of the vegetarians and the non–vegetarians, and then we will examine their relevance to the metabolic syndrome.

Could there be life on Earth without iron? Iron generates a magnetic field in the center of the earth to defend the earth from the ionized particles poured out of the sun and the space by creating an earth magnetic field. Interestingly, the organisms, especially the higher animals, have iron, which catalyzes the numerous chemical reactions to help maintain life. This function involves a transition metal that helps the iron to chemically react well.

Iron provides the electrons well to the other atoms, such as oxygen, nitrogen, and sulfur. As a result, iron is often present in a cationic state, in which two electrons or three electrons are lost. Iron plays a role in the oxygen transfer and the

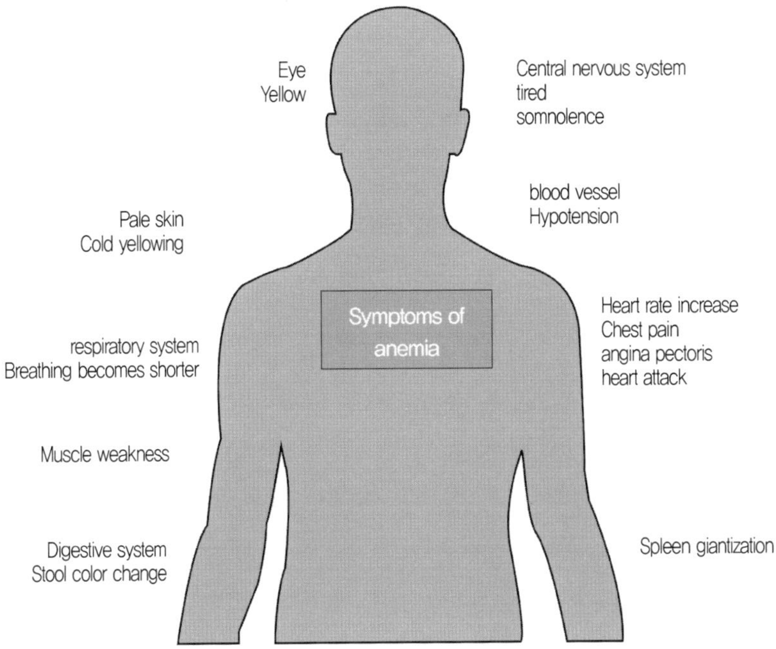

Figure 3-23. Symptoms of anemia

Table 3-11. Foods rich in iron

food	Low	medium	plenty
grain	Oatmeal, rice, whole wheat	corn flour, wheat flour	
fruit	Apple, avocado, banana, grape, peach, plum	mango, pineapple	guava, lemon, orange, tomato
vegetable	Eggplant	carrots, potato	broccoli, cabbage, cauliflower Pumpkin, cabbage,
beverage	Tea, coffee	red wine	white wine
nuts	Almonds, coconut, walnuts		
Beans			Seolitee, Baektae, Mungo
Seedling			Sesame seeds, pumpkin seeds

oxidative metabolism, such as peroxidase and hydrogen peroxide decomposition enzyme, and, also, acts as a component of the various proteins. However, the largest amount of the iron in the body functions as the oxygen-carrying hemoglobin, accounting for 64% of the iron in men and 73% of the iron in women (Table 3-12). Therefore, when the iron is scarce, the oxygen transport is reduced, resulting in a decrease in the metabolic activity and the psychological helplessness.

Iron rich foods include broccoli, pumpkin, cabbage, tomatoes and lemons, as well as carrots, potatoes and corn (Table 3-11).

3.17. The circulation and intake of iron in the human body

Normally, an adult body contains from 3 g to 4 g of iron. Most of the iron in the body is present in the bone marrow and the reticular endothelial system (Figure 3-24). The reticuloendothelial system is known as the mononuclear phagocytic system. In 1924, the German pathologist Aschoff observed that the cells in the endothelium underwent a strong predation (eating bacteria, viruses, and dead cells). Since phagocytosis is mainly caused by the macrophages in the endothelial cells, Carr was suggested to be the mononuclear cells or the macrophages in 1973. Mononuclear cells float in the blood, and some become differentiated into the macrophages, such as the lymph nodes, the bone marrows, the liver, the spleen, the brain, the pancreas, and the male and female reproductive organs. Many human organs contain the macrophages and can range from 10% to 15% of the total cells.

The splenic cells of the spleen destroy the old red blood cells and recycle the hemoglobin. That is, hemosiderin is made to synthesize the hemoglobin in order to make the new, red blood cells. For adults, the liver and the bone marrows contain the iron from 100 mg to 300 mg, respectively. The bone marrow consumes 24 milligrams of iron per day to produce between 200 billion red blood cells and 300 billion red blood cells. Then, the aged red blood cells are taken back by the macrophages, and the iron is recovered again. And the macrophage delivers the iron to the transport

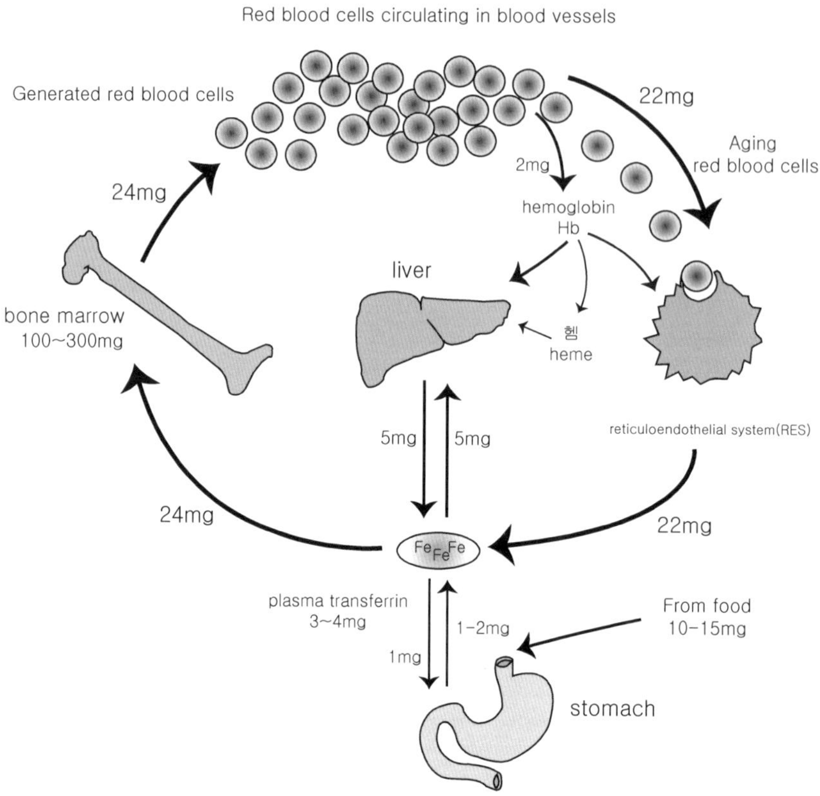

Figure 3-24. Recirculating pathway of erythrocyte iron by macrophage system (per day)

The human body produces and kills more than 1,000 times the number of cells that make up the body for a lifetime. Assuming a lifespan of 100 years, it will produce and die 10 times more of the body's cells each year. If the dead cells are not cleaned quickly, inflammation is triggered. Inflammation is a major cause of a variety of diseases, including cancer, diabetes and cardiovascular disease. Thus, for the health of the human body, as much as the generation of cells is an important process, the dead cells are cleaned smoothly. Major cells that clean dead cells swallow dead cells with macrophages and use them as nutrients. When the fat and nutrients are in excess, the sweeping action of the hungry macrophages slows or stops. In the fasting state, sleep helps macrophages efficiently eat dead cells from the body. An intermittent fasting of about once a month helps to clean the cells regularly and helps the health. For cancer, most cancer cells die because of fasting for two weeks.

Table 3-12. Iron function and storage of human body

	male adult, mg (%)	female adult, mg (%)
	function	
hemoglobin	2300 (64)	1700 (73)
Myoglobin	320 (9)	180 (8)
Heme enzyme	80 (2)	60 (3)
non-heme enzyme	100 (3)	80 (3)
	storage	
ferritin	540 (15)	200 (9)
hemosiderin	230 (6)	100 (4)
transferrin	5 (<1)	4 (<1)
total sum	3575 (100)	2314 (100)

protein called the "plasma transferrin", thereby giving to the bone marrow 22 mg of iron daily (Fig. 3-24).

Human body has total of 3~4g iron. 0.03% of total iron, 1mg is lost through the red blood cells that go out of the blood vessels like the mucous cells, the bile, and the menstrual. Therefore, 1 mg of iron should be absorbed through the diet to maintain a constant concentration of the iron in the body. If you ingest 10mg~15mg of iron through food, 1mg~2mg of it will be absorbed into your body

3.18. Blood iron, dental diabetes.

Iron can easily oxidize (lose electrons) and reduce (get electrons) reversibly as a transition metal. This may play an important role in the pathology of cancer, diabetes, and the cardiovascular diseases, and, therefore, the studies on the toxicity due to the excessive intake of iron have recently been made. Oxygen in the body usually changes into the two molecules of water by combining with four electrons and four hydrogen cations. However, the high reactivity of iron produces a wide variety of the strong, reactive oxygen. The partially reduced, free radicals can impair the structure and function of organisms, including the genes and the proteins, by creating the toxic hydrogen peroxide, the superoxide anion, and the hydroxyl radicals [21– 23]. The gene disruption can be associated with the development of cancer, diabetes, and the various diseases, and the damaged cells can enter into a vicious cycle that, again, produces the reactive radicals.

These reactive oxidant materials produce the additional and more reactive peroxide radicals through the successive reactions, in which the iron acts as a catalyst for these reactions. This is called a "metal catalyst, harbor–vise reaction" [21].

$$Fe^{3+} + O_2 \rightarrow Fe^{2+} + O_2$$

$$Fe^{2+} + H_2O_2 \rightarrow Fe^{3+} + 2OH + OH^-$$

$$O_2^- + H_2O_2 \rightarrow O_2 + \cdot OH + OH^-$$

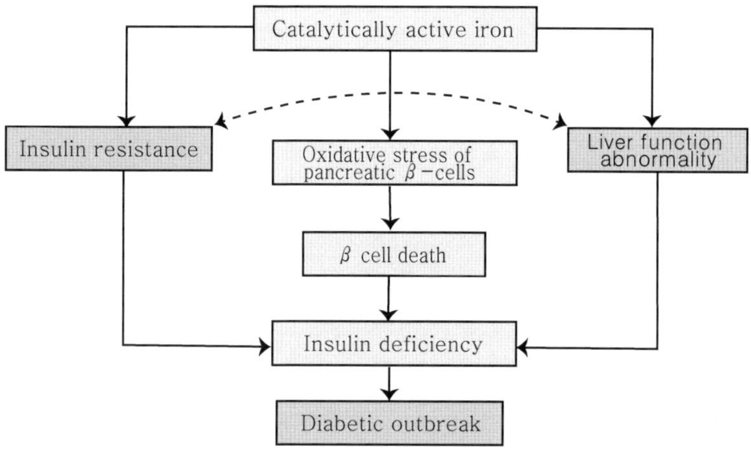

Diabetes Care, (2007)30:1926

Figure 3-25. Excessive iron-onset mechanism of diabetes

Because of this high reactivity of iron, the organisms moderately control the iron, including the concentration control and the storage proteins. In addition, it has a variety of the reducing enzymes to defend itself against the toxic radicals.

There is debate that iron may be involved in the development of diabetes started from several clinical observations. First, a lot of the type 2 diabetes was found in the people with the excessive iron. Second, chelation therapy or phlebotomy can lower the iron content in the body to improve the diabetic symptoms. Third, the frequent donations or the reduced iron storage improves the insulin secretion

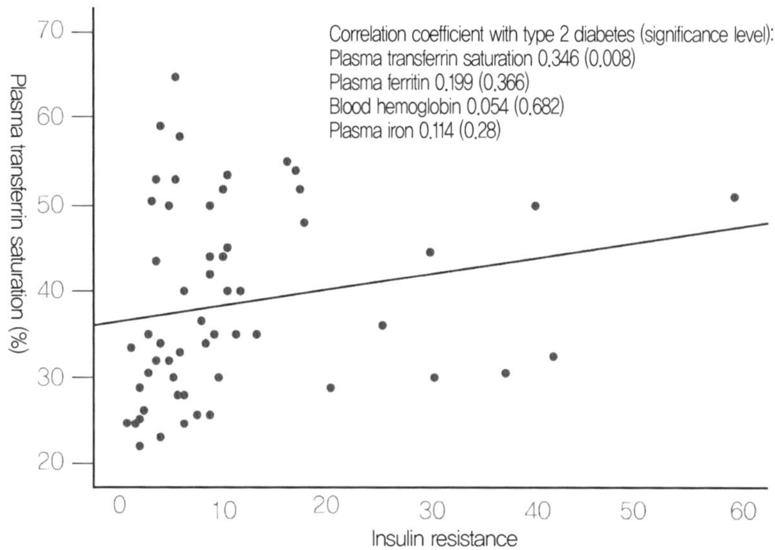

Figure 3–26. Correlation between plasma transferrin saturation and insulin resistance

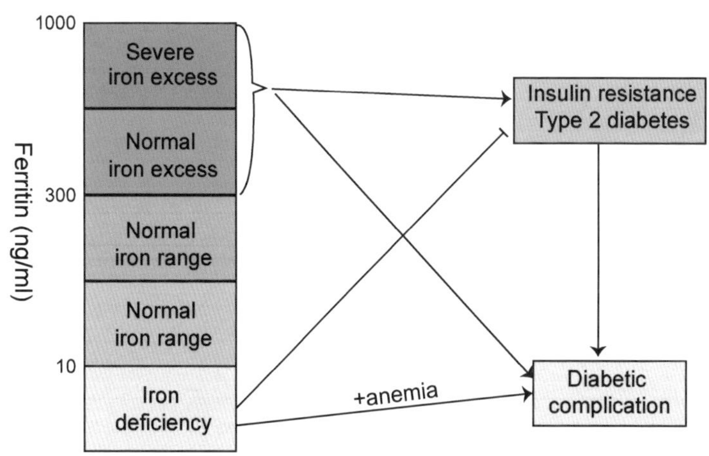

Figure 3–27. Diabetic complications of iron overload and diabetes insulin resistance

and the insulin sensitivity [24, 25].

There are three reasons for the increased possibility of diabetes due to the iron overload: First, the animal studies have shown that iron overload reduces the insulin release by damaging the beta cells of the pancreas [26]. As you know, the beta cells are the insulin-secreting cells, which are very vulnerable to the oxidative damage by the radicals.

Second, the pancreas more easily accumulates the bivalent cations than the other body organs, therefore, more exposed to the risk of the radicals [27]. Excessive iron may not only damage the pancreas, but may, also, increase the insulin resistance by impairing the function of the liver or the abdominal, mast cells [28, 29]. The most representative example of this is genetic hemochromatosis. People with this hereditary disease accumulate the iron in the various tissues of the body, including those in diabetes, the liver diseases and arthritis. Sixty percent of the patients with the type 1 genetic hemochromatosis have diabetes [30].

3.19. Hemolysis, meat, and diabetes

In 1985, the first study to report the association between meat consumption and type 2 diabetes was carried out [31]. As shown in Table 3-13, when ingesting meat twice a week, the prevalence of diabetes mellitus was 2.7 times for males and 2.3 times for females. In the diagnosis of the death due to diabetes, the proportion of the diabetes increases as the amount of the meat consumed increases

Table 3-13. Increased meat intake and diabetes

	Relative risk		
	Meat intake	male	female
Prevalence of self-administered diabetes (1960)	〈1 day/week (vegetarian)	1.0	1.0
	1+ day/week (non-vegetarian)	1.7 (1.2–2.4)	1.4 (1.1–1.8)
	〈1 day/week	1.0	1.0
	1–2 day/week	1.4	1.1
	3–5 day/week	1.5	1.2
	6+ day/week	2.7	2.3
death due to diabetes	〈1 day/week (vegetarian)	1.0	1.0
	1+ day/week (non-vegetarian)	1.9 (1.2–3.1)	1.1 (0.8–1.6)
	1 day/week	1.0	1.0
	1–2 day/week	1.6 (0.9–2.7)	1.3 (0.9–2.0)
	3–5 day/week	1.6 (0.8–3.0)	1.2 (0.7–1.8)
	6+ day/week	3.6(1.9–7.1)	0.6 (0.3–1.2)

In parentheses, 95% confidence interval

3.20. Ferritin and transferrin

Ferritin is a protein that stores iron in most cells and is present in the cells of birds, bacteria, plants, and animals. Ferritin is a major iron storage molecule as a buffer that can be used when the cell is deficient in iron or in excess of iron. Iron is very reactive in size and must be safely stored well in order not to damage the individual, and this role becomes a ferritin protein in the cell. Ferritin has the same structure as an empty sphere with an outer radius of from 12 nm(nano meter, 10^{-9}m)) to 13 nm and an inner radius of from 7 nm to 8 nm, which can store about 4,500 iron particles (Fig. 3-28). Iron is usually stored in a solution in a trivalent cation state. If the

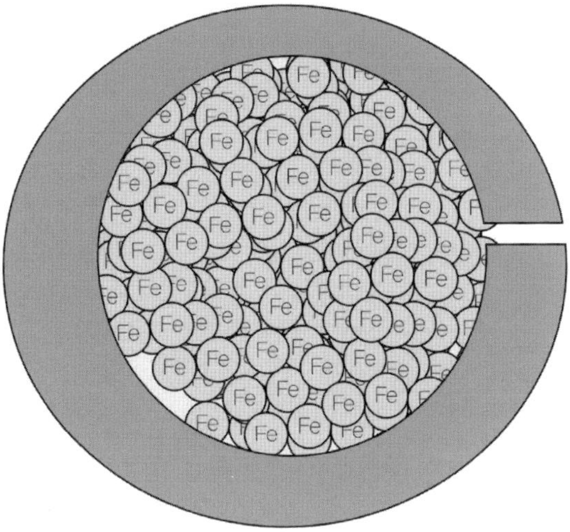

Figure 3-28. Section of ferritin

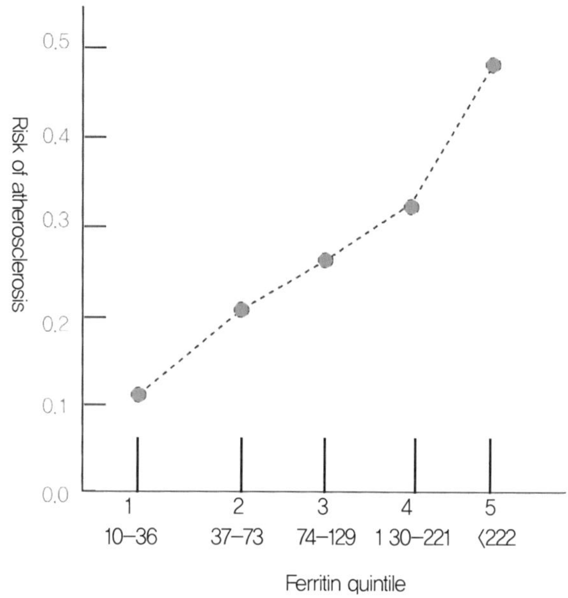

Figure 3–29. The risk of atheroscleros is with the ferritin quintile

iron is needed, the divalents are reduced to the cations and then released.

Ferritin is usually in the cell but is released into the blood in small quantities as needed to transport the iron. Thus, the ferritin in the blood can be used for the indirect diagnosis of the iron deficiency or the iron excess. Figure 3–29 shows that, when the ferritin content is divided into the quintiles, the risk is more than four times higher than that of the first group with the lowest risk of atherosclerosis. When a vegetarian diet, especially a vegan diet, is used, the ferritin content falls within a stable range, which is higher than the anemic baseline.

3.21. The cardiovascular diseases and the iron excess

Similar to diabetes, studies of the cardiovascular diseases and the iron overload began to be reported in the 1980s. In the patients with genetic hemochromatosis (hemochromatosis), the cardiovascular diseases had frequently progressed, and the iron chelation had lowered the blood iron levels, leading to the improvements of the cardiovascular diseases [33, 34]. As shown in Figure 3-30, when divided into 8 groups according to the ferritin levels, with the 4th group as 1, the risk of the carotid plaques was increased to 1.6 in the group that had consumed the most

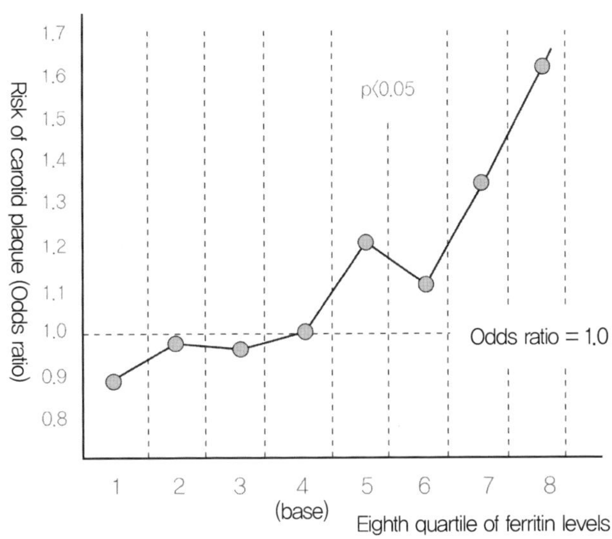

Figure 3-30. Increased plasma ferritin levels and increased risk of carotid plaques

3.22. Vegetarianismis more effective regarding the cardiovascular diseases than the low–fat meats.

The long–lasting, type 2 diabetes often causes the serious complications, such as the cardiovascular diseases, the kidney diseases, the optic nerve damages, the cranial nerve damages, and even the life–threatening complications. A variety of the epidemiological studies and the clinical prescriptions indicate that proper diet is important for the improvement of the type 2 diabetes.

Many studies suggest that the vegetarian diet can help with the proper blood glucose control. Andrew et al. [35] had investigated whether the low–fat, vegetarian diets could be effective regarding the type 2 diabetes. The researchers recruited the volunteers through the Georgetown University Medical Center and the local community and randomly divided them into two groups. In a six–week dietary experiment, one group of seven people had been provided the vegan diets, while the other group of six people had been provided the traditional, low–fat diets, and two of which fell out of the experiment and, eventually, became four.

10%~15% of the total calories in the diets was provided as protein and less than 10% was fat. And the carbohydrates ingested the fiber–rich, whole grains. The low–fat diet group was recommended to eat fish and poultry rather than red meat, and all nutrients except vitamin B12 were met by the recommended amounts. After 12 weeks, the fasting plasma glucose in the vegan group had decreased by 28% from 10.7 mmol/L to 7.75 mmol/L (195 mg/

Table 3-14. Increased plasma ferritin levels and increased risk of carotid plaques

	vegan group		Low-fat dietary group	
	Before experiment	After 12 weeks	Before experiment	After 12 weeks
weight (kg)	96.7 (13.3)	89.5 (14.4)	97.0 (22.9)	93.2 (22.2)
Fasting blood sugar (mmol/L)	10.74±2.85	7.75±2.07	9.86±1.63	8.64±0.20
Glycosylated hemoglobin (%)	8.3±1.7	6.9±1.1	8.0±1.1	7.0±0.6
cholesterol (mmol/L)	5.26±1.09	4.63±1.32	5.56±0.61	4.93±0.46
High density lipoprotein (mmol/L)	1.15±0.32	0.95±0.28	1.12±0.17	1.10±0.17
Triglyceride (mmol/L)	2.12±0.78	1.87±0.63	2.29±1.92	1.85±1.14
Systolic blood pressure (mmHg)	136.6±10.0	126.2±14.9	149.5±21.6	130.6±11.9
Diastolic blood pressure (mmHg)	84.0±4.5	78.2±9.7	86.0±15.8	75.4±11.6
Microalbumin (mg/24hrs)	434.8±565.5	155.2±182.6	82.9±114.6	169.2±298.0

dL to 141 mg/dL) (Table 3–14). On the other hand, there was a significant difference ($P < 0.05$) from the whole vegetarian diet by 12%, from 9.86 mmol/L to 8.64 mmol/L (179 mg/dL to 157 mg/dL), in the low–fat diet group. Also, the weight of the vegan diet group had decreased by 7.2kg, and the low fat diet group had showed a decrease by about twice as much as that of the group of 3.8kg. This weight loss is even more remarkable because it was an experiment that does not limit the calorie intake in the dietary intake.

3.23. The iron levels of the vegetarians and the non–vegetarians

If you look only at the amount of iron intake, the vegetarian diet has more than animal based diet. And, the non–heme iron of the vegetarian diet has a very wide absorption spectrum, which varies ten times from 2.0% to 22.5% depending on the condition of the human body.

However, the absorption rate of animal heme iron is only about twice at from 26% to 47%. This difference has a significant effect on the human body. If the amount of the non–heme iron ingested as a meal is increased from 1.5 mg to 6.0 mg four times, the rate of the absorption by the human body decreases from 18% to 6%, by one–third. The total amount of the iron actually absorbed is 1.5 mg × 0.18 = 0.27 mg and 6.0 mg × 0.06 = 0.36 mg, and a certain range of amount enters the human body without any significant difference.

Whereas 1.5 mg or 6.0 mg of the animal heme iron is absorbed into the human body by 20% of the iron ingested, the amount of the iron is very different from 0.3 mg to 1.2 mg. Therefore, the absorption of the hemp iron is 4 times different. The excessively–taken iron in the heme iron is used in the body and remains in the cells and the tissues to accumulate, which causes the oxidation and causes the various diseases. The list includes type 2 diabetes, cancer, cardiovascular disease, etc. In fact, according to a study comparing the vegetarian and non–vegetarian ferritin, the vegetarian's ferritin levels were lower than those of the non-vegetarians, but were in the stable range. Ball and Barrett had examined the amount of the iron ingested and its internal status in 50 vegetarian women and 24 non-vegetarian women who were aged from 18 years old to 45 years old in Australia.

The average daily intake of iron was 10.7 mg for the vegetarian females and slightly higher than 9.9 mg for the non-vegetarian females, but the mean serum ferritin level was lower for the vegetarians. Serum ferritin level of vegetarian diet group is higher than the anemic level (Fig. 3-27). It can be understood that a vegetarian diet absorbs the iron at a level that prevents the risk of the deficiency while preventing the risk of the excess toxicity.

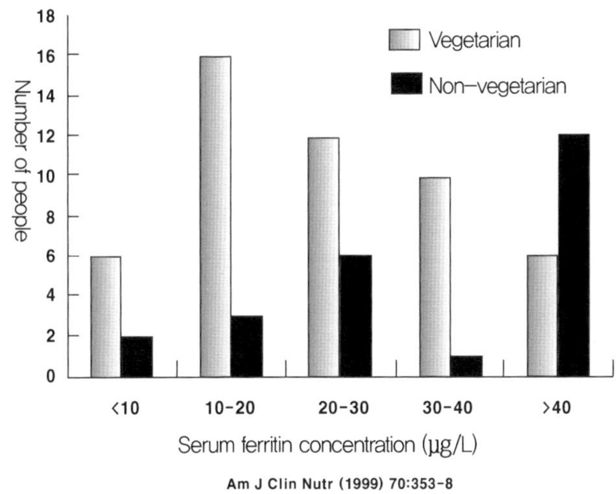

Figure 3-31. Serum ferritin levels of vegetarians and non-vegetarians

Table 3-15. Iron content of food

food	Iron content (mg)
1 cup peeled beans	5.0
1 peeled potato	2.8
One bean burrito	2.5
1 cup tomato sauce spaghetti	2.3
10 apricot dried ones	1.7
1 cup of oatmeal	1.6
cup of spinach	1.5
2 teaspoons of cocoa powder	1.5
Whole wheat bread 1 piece	1.2
1/4 cup of peanuts	0.8
Broccoli half cup	0.7
Blueberry half cup	0.5
Pea 1/4 cup	1.3

3.24. The metabolic syndrome and the excess energy dissipation

The major cause of the metabolic syndrome is that the amount of the calories consumed is excessive and accumulates in the body. Thus, the over–stored energy is the key to the treatment of the metabolic syndrome. It is possible through vegetarian diet, but a faster method is through fasting. If the lipid produces 9 calories per gram and consumes 1800 calories per day, the amount of the lipid that decreases through a single fast is about 200 grams. So, if you take a 10–days fast, you will lose 2 kg of the body weight. You may feel like there is not a big effect. However, fasting does not only have the effect of removing the excess calories from the lipid stored in the lipid cells. Rather, it breaks down the garbage that is accumulated inside the cells and makes the cells of the body healthy. This process is called "autophagy" and is the subject of the 2016 Nobel Prize in Medical Physiology.

Fasting, which blocks the nutrients supplied from the outside of the cells, stimulates the cells to supply the energy from the cells in order to breathe. In this process, the garbage inside the heart cell and the blood vessel cells is decomposed and recycled into the nutrients of the cells. And the heart cell and blood vessel cells become healthy. In addition to the cardiovascular, the beta cells of the pancreas that make up the insulin also make the pancreatic cells become healthy by breaking down the garbage in the cells.

Fasting has the effect of improving the metabolic syndrome by removing the fats in the abdomen. Before discussing the cytological process of Autophagy, we will first look at a few cases of diabetes and the cardiovascular diseases that are cured by fasting.

3.25. Fast food and the vegetarian diet for the diabetic patients

The following cases are presented through the favors of the authors as the parts of the contents of deceased Professor Song SookJa's "Natural healing diet" (Oblige, 2011). .

The following is a question–and–answer session with a 64–year–old male, diabetic patient with the weight of 80 kg.

Patient: I'm a 64–year–old woman, and my blood sugar is checked every day, which is, sometimes, over 200. This is even when I'm taking the insulin. Today, I ate a lot of Chinese food outside and got the blood sugar of 230.

Professor Song : Do you have any other complications?

Patient: I received a dialysis prescription for my kidney failure. I can hardly see through one of my eyes.

How long have you been losing weight?

Professor Song : Diabetes is a disease caused by eating a lot of wrong foods. It's no use trying to prescribe insulin without losing weight.

Patient: Is there any way?

Professor Song : Food is medicine. Because I am ill and because I have the wrong food, I need to eat well so that I can get better. Diabetes gets worse if you do not drink as much as you can at the current weight. Then, heart disease, cerebral infarction, kidney failure, blindness, paralysis, foot rot disease, etc., cannot be listed as many of the symptoms are alive, but I will not be able to die even if I cannot die. I am a nutritionist and I think that fasting in diabetes is a bit dangerous, but, if you can do it, you need to fast and lose weight. Fasting relieves the kidneys, so you do not have to dialysis it right now. Also, because the body fat is consumed, the blocked blood vessels are pierced and the blood circulation is good, and the blood vessels leading to the eyes are also punctured, and the symptoms that cannot be seen can be solved. Although the person who dances is not a doctor, because he is an expert in that area, you can solve the serious problems that you are experiencing when you lose the weight through dance. First of all, we will lose the weight at the dancing club and come back and let you know about the dietary life.

Twenty days later, the consultation started again.

Patient: I was so successful.My weight was so good because I lost 15kg to arrive at 65kg. I lost a lot of the blood sugar, and it fell to 150 or less immediately after breakfast. What should we do in the future?

Professor Song : Good. First of all, if you do not lose weight, you will not be able to start your natural healing. The causes of diabetes are overeating and binge eating, and overeating is caused by eating the refined foods, such as white rice, white flour, sugar, and the oil without the fiber. If you eat the moderately uncooked, natural food, you will feel full and satisfied, and you will not try to eat more. And the fiber is the insulin that the sky gave. Since the white rice and the white flour have no fiber, the diabetics should think of them as the poisons. On the other hand, the brown rice and the whole wheat are rich in fiber.

With this kind of a mind, in the future, you should eat the meals that give you the feeling of fullness and that do not make you obese. To do so, remove all the meat, the fish, the eggs, and the processed tablets. When eating, first, eat a plate of the raw vegetables, ingest the fat and the protein, and the soybeans,the sesame seeds, the brown rice, and the grains should never be eaten with white boiled rice. And you have to chew slowly. After an hour of eating, if you have the normal blood sugar level of 130mg/dl or more, then you should eat less boiled rice. You can have the habit of matching the numbers.

Patient: What should I do if I have too little energy or am undernourished?

Professor Song : Do not worry. Even if you eat less, the brown rice grains, the soybeans, the sesame, and the raw vegetables are never lacking in nutrition. The focus of the calories we have set in the hospitals is to influence the postprandial blood glucose levels. If the postprandial blood glucose level is high and if you have to avoid the urine, it is more important than eating the calories you need and then eating only enough to avoid the urine.

If you eat more, you are not cheerful. In diabetes, when the insulin action is not working properly, the extra saccharide is poured into the urine. That's it. It is possible to control the diabetes without any physical exertion because the extra saccharide is used just enough. Consider the postprandial blood glucose and, if it is higher than normal, reduce the amount of the food through the unconditional fiber meal.

3.26. The fasting and vegetarian healing of women in their 60s who have undergone a cardiac surgery

Patient: One of them was operated on because three of the cardiovascular vessels were blocked. The other two are listed below. I read the professor's writing accidentally in the press, and he said that the diet and the natural remedies can solve without a surgery.

How long have you lost the weight?

Patient: It is 70kg in weight and 160cm in height.

Professor Song : If you lose 55kg, you do not need any surgery. Because I have a lot of weight, I have a lot of fat in my body, so the fat mass and the red blood cells are getting tangled in the blood, so I have a lot of blood circulation. The blood vessels that supply the blood to the heart of your patient, the coronary arteries, are blocked by the blood, and the blood is not able to pass. Then, the blood vessels cannot carry oxygen and the nutrients, so the heart becomes hardened, therefore, causing the infarction and the angina that do not work well. So, in the hospital, remove the blood-clotting blood that blocks the blood vessels or put a balloon in the narrowed blood vessels to widen the blood vessels to pass the blood.

Patient: Is it possible to have such an effect without any surgery?

Professor Song : It is possible to remove the blocking of the blood without any surgery. But, the nutrients pass through the throat. They are the fat and the protein that emit the energy of our bodies and the heat from our bodies. So, you can use the nutrient mass as a nutrient.

Patient: What should I do?

Professor Song : If you exercise fast enough for a couple of days while eating the fast food, you will run out of energy, and you will be consuming the energy from your body. When a person needs 2,000kcal of energy per day, he or she should consume enough calories in the fat and the body tissues of the body, and, when they only eat the fruits, they use the fruits for the energy, and the supplements are consumed in the body fat as well. When combined with exercise, you will be able to consume the large amounts of the body fat and the blood as the energies.

Patient: It is easy and simple to listen to. How do you practice it?

Professor Song : First of all, please have two spoonfuls of the perilla powder and fruit this evening. The fruits are easy to digest and the vitamin C helps strengthen the blood vessels. There are many vitamins and the omega-3 fatty acids in the perilla. It, also, cleanses the blood vessels and strengthens them.

Patient: What is the fruit, and how much is it to eat?

Professor Song : I do not care about any fruits, but I prefer the seasonal fruits. Even if you eat as much as you want, you can eat only a few calories. Chew your perilla well or grind it. And sunbathe in the woods. If you walk with a longbreath, the oxygen is supplied enough to accumulate the body fat and heat, so that the blood vessels that block are, also, consumed as the energies. Sunshine, also, turns the cholesterol into the vitamin D, which helps clean the blood vessels. You, also, need to drink a lot of water.

Patient: When should I eat boiled rice?

Professor Song : You will have to eat the fruits a little longer because you weigh 70kg. You should abstain until you reach 50kg. Try to eat the fruits, and the perilla powder. If you think it is hard to tolerate, chew the boiled brown rice with half the air.

Patient: Do not eat vegetables?

Professor Song : If you eat the vegetables as a side dish, you have to eat salt, but this is harmful to the cardiovascular disease. Cardiovascular disease can be a cause of sudden death if you have the symptom of constipation, so please follow my diet so that you can get enough fiber. At dinner, add the boiled beans, the cucumber, and the onions in a seaweed in the poached water. Add a bowl of the perilla powder and the tomatoes with a grilled sauce.

Patient: You should have a side dish when you eat the boiled rice. Is it not possible without a side dish?

Professor Song : It is no good to eat salty food until the health is restored. I chew the boiled rice separately, and I chew the vegetables and the fruits separately. It's like eating a Western dish instead of a Korean dish. I eat the fruits first, eat the green pepper, and then eat the boiled brown rice. Or the whole grain-baked bread is, also, good. The boiled brown rice is, also, good. They will satisfy your taste.

Patient: I'll do what your professor says.

After 10 days, the consultation was done again.

Patient: Thank you, professor. I lost 6kg of weight. I went to the hospital today and found one of the two blocked blood vessels. One of the remaining blood vessels is not open, so I have to undergo a surgery immediately.

Professor Song : Did you get the date of the surgery?

Patient: I forgot it. The surgical procedure is terrible. What should I do?

Professor Song : If one of the two has been opened, you can have one of the others opened. Do what you have done so far. I'm still 64 kilograms in weight, so, if I lose 10 kilos, I will definitely have one opened.

Patient: Do I have to eat the boiled, brown rice that I do not want to eat again? Is there any way of breaking the blood vessels while eating meat?

Professor Song : If you do not eat meat and only use a purely vegetarian diet, it will help you a lot. But, if you want to eat it, you should eat only 50g (three or less chopsticks) of the lean meat. If you cannot control this, the high protein intake will result in the production of the body fat and the blood. No matter how much fat there is, there is not much fat, but the animal fat is very harmful to the cardiovascular disease. Anyway, even if you have a surgery, you should be careful to drink water for a few days.Would it not be easier to abstain from fasting and eating fruit?

Patient: But, should I not eat boiled rice?

Professor Song : There are only the saccharides and the lipids in the white rice and no nutrients. When the saccharides and the fats exert their power and heat in the body, they cannot produce the power and the heat without the vitamins and the minerals. They are synthesized into the body fat, and they produce the blood sugar and the cholesterol in the blood. In addition, the relative lack of the vitamins and the minerals affects the physiology of the human body, destroys the homeostasis, weakens the immune system, makes the blood vessels poor, and exacerbates the cardiovascular diseases, such as arteriosclerosis and cerebral hemorrhage.

Patient: All right. I had not known why I had so much terrible and terrifying angina so far. I heard it from you, and, now, I see it. I do not think it's a good idea to have expensive medicine and surgery. I am confident that the vegetarian diet will restore my health, and I do not think I will ever eat meat.

3.27. Three ways of the deaths of the cells

The body of an adult consists of about 50 shells to 60 shells of the cells. But, the first is just a single cell. The sperm and the egg combine to make one fertilized egg, one becomes two, two become four, and they continue to divide into the cellsthat are dedicated to the function of each tissue in the body. The lifespan of one cell is usually from 10 months to 12 months, depending on its location. The intestinal cells last from three days to one week, and the brain cells and the cardiac cells last almost a lifetime. Here, we are wondering. How does the cell continue to divide and keep the size of our body constant? In other words, in order to maintain a certain state and size of our body, not only the cell divisions, but, also, the cell deaths, and the post-death treatments are important.

There are three methods of the cell deaths in our body, two of which are called the "Programmed Cell Death" (PCD). Type 1 is called "apoptosis" (apoptosis), and type 2 is called "autophagy-type cell death". The third cell death is called "necrosis" and is characterized by an inflammatory response. Since 1980, the cell death process has been studied by many scientists, and the cell-signaling mechanisms have been vigorously studied regarding the cells. In the 2000s, more attention had been paid to the studies on the atrophy-type cell death and the cell necrosis. 'Autophagy' is a compound word of auto + phargy. 'Auto' has the meaning of 'self' and 'phargy' has the meaning of 'to eat'. When the nutrients are not

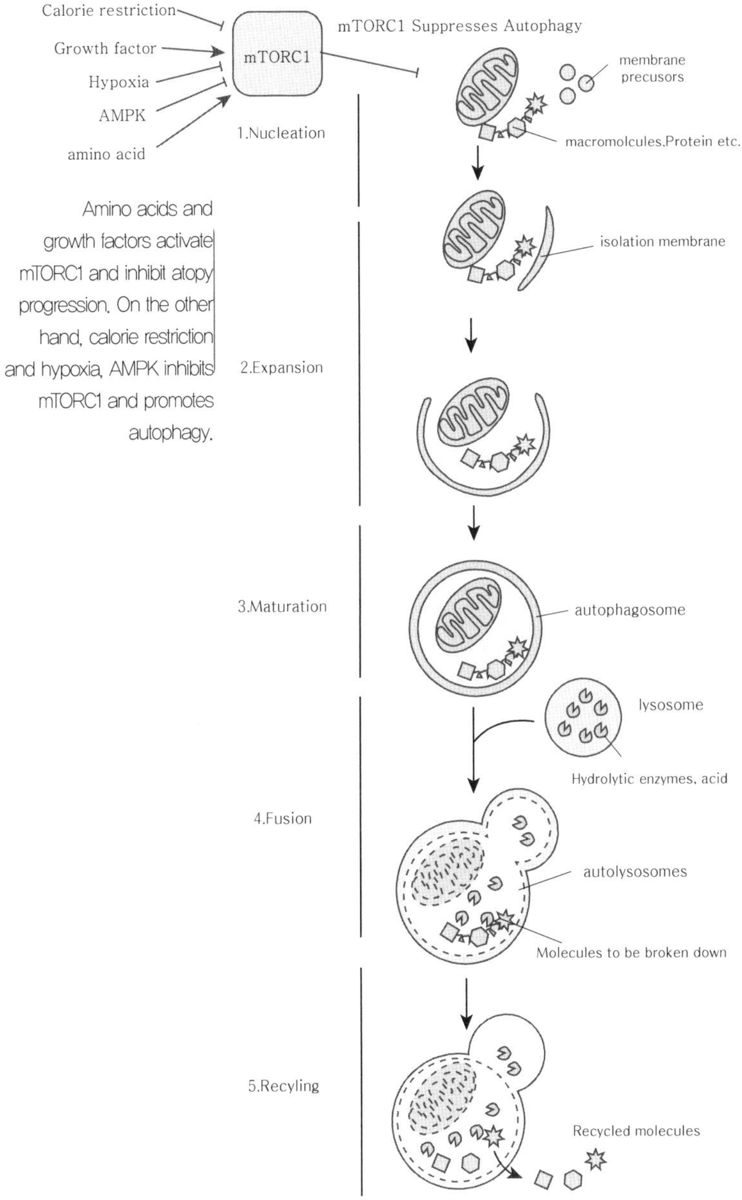

Figure 3–32. Regulatory factors and process of atopy. (Arrow Table → Promotes, Bar Table ⊣ Suppresses)

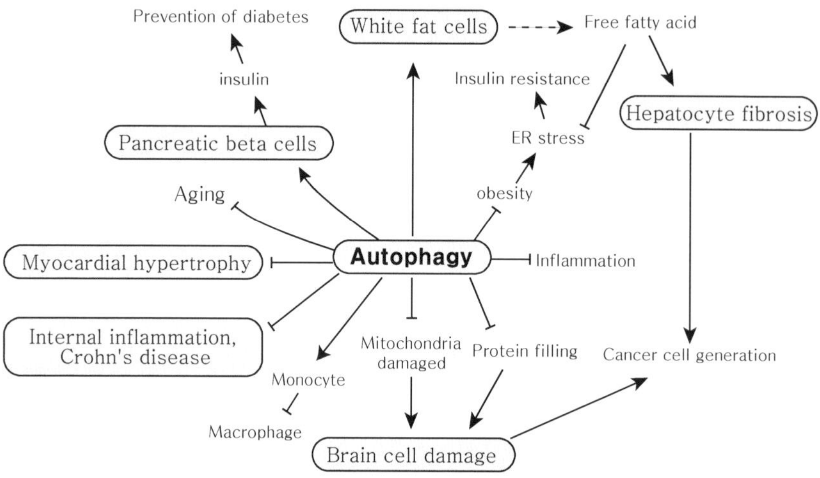

Figure 3-33. Prevention of Metabolic Syndrome in autophagy

supplied from outside the cell, the cells begin to look for the energy sources in the cell to survive on their own. In this situation, the first degradation is a spoiled protein or a broken cellular organelle that is useless or damaged inside the cell. This includes the chunks of the clumps of the protein, such as the amyloid beta in the brain cells, which are considered to be the main causes of dementia, and the mitochondria damage and release the free radicals.

3.28. . The regulatory factors and the progression of Autophagy.

'Autophagy' is a word devised by Dr. Dub, who received the Nobel Prize in Physiology in 1974 for discovering the lysosomes [1]. In 2016, Professor Osumi received the Nobel Prize in Physiology on the theme of Autophagy. Autophagy is a process of decomposing and recycling the components inside the cytoplasm, which is a key process for maintaining the cell homeostasis. Atrophy is promoted when the starvation, the increased reactive oxygen species, or the endoplasmic reticulum are stressed out of the cells [2]. In other words, Autophagy is a process of decomposing and recycling the waste inside the cells to survive in starvation, but it is also a process of maintaining the health of the cells by removing the garbage in the cell. It is important to remove the garbage from the cell, such as the damaged protein or the damaged mitochondria, which can damage the cell nucleus by releasing the free radicals in an uncontrolled state which can lead to the diseases, such as cancer, diabetes, and cardiovascular disease.

The autophagy process can be divided into five stages: The nucleation, the expansion, the maturation, the fusion, and the recycling (Fig. 3-28). Nucleation is the formation of a precursor of the film. The second is the process of encapsulating the damaged proteins or the macromolecules as they expand. The third process, the maturation, is the process of making the autophagosome completely surrounded by the membrane, and, in the fourth, the atopagosomes are fused with the lysosomes to become the autolysomes. Finally, the lysosomes contain the acid and the proteolytic enzymes, which break down the proteins into the basic amino acid units, making them go into a state where they can be recycled [3].

Autophagy is rapidly activated and progressed when the supply of the nutrients and the growth factors from the outside of the cell become insufficient. When the nutrient supply is limited, the ATP, a common energy unit of all organisms, is reduced, which activates the intracellular material called the "AMPK" [4]. The restriction of the amino acids also promotes the autophagy by deactivating the mTORC1, an intracellular substance. On the other hand, when the amino acids are abundant, the particularly branched amino acids, such as the leucine, activate the mTORC1, which in turn inhibits the autophagy [5].

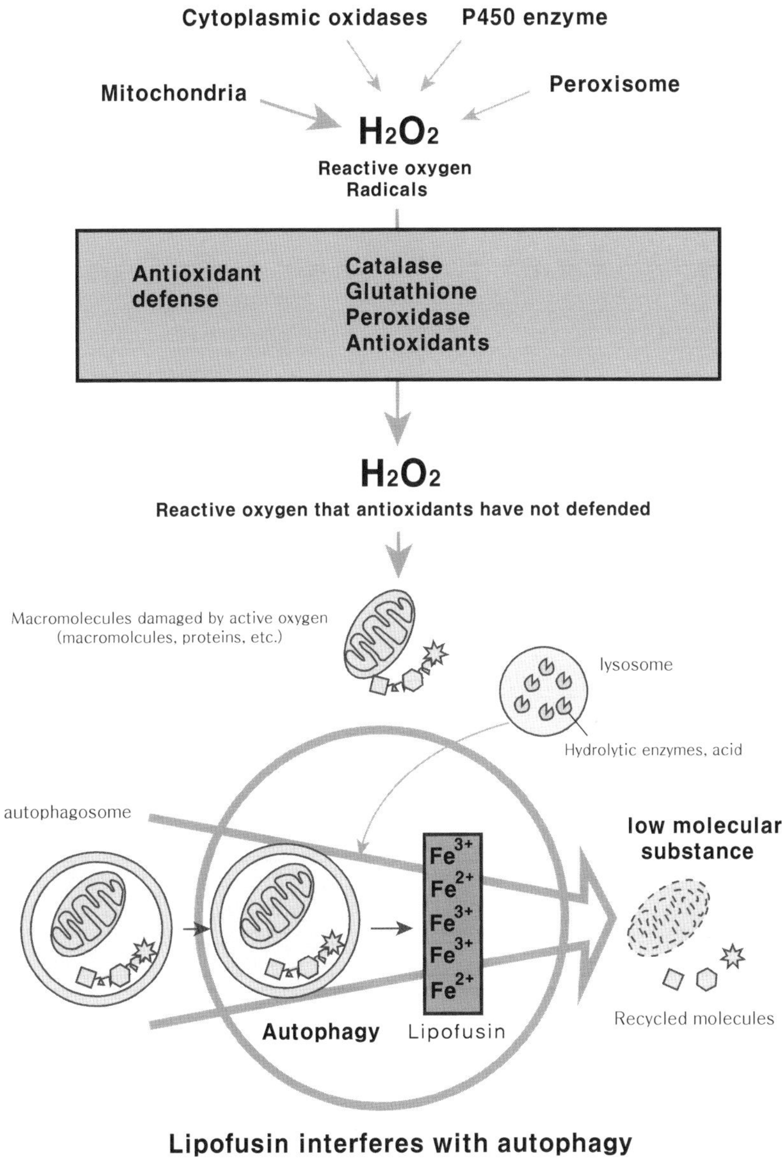

Figure 3-34. Autophagy suppression effect of lipofuscin

3.29. The prevention of the metabolic syndrome in Autophagy

Autophagy, which starves the cells and cleans them, has been reported to be effective for the cardiovascular disease and diabetes. Limiting the supply of the glucose to the cardiomyocytes leads to the progression of the atrophy, which begins to degrade the damaged proteins and the damaged intracellular organs. In this process, the cardiac cell deaths are reduced and the resistance to the myocardial ischemia and the tolerance are improved [6] (Figure 3–29). When fasting, the glucose is depleted, the triglycerides stored in the fat cells are broken down into the free, fatty acids. and the glycerol is used as an energy source. The increased levels of the free, fatty acids inhibit the mTORC1, which, in turn, promotes the autophagy process [7]. However, a high–fat diet will increase the blood triglycerides and the cholesterol level, which will, rather, damage the autophagy. This is because the prolonged exposure to the fat suppresses the fusion of the autophagosome and the lyso–

Table 3–16. Comparison of the Quantity of Ketone Diet and General Diet [37]

ingredient	A normal diet	*Ketone diet*
carbohydrate (C)	62	*3*
Fat (F)	6	*72*
protein (P)	27	*15*
calorie (kcal/g)	4.4	*7.2*
F / (P + C)	0.07	*4*

* F / (P + C) ratio: fat / (carbohydrate + protein)

som [4].

The type-2 diabetes is characterized by dyslipidemia, insulin resistance, and damage to the pancreatic beta cells. These symptoms consistently result from the over-feeding of the nutrients [8]. The Autophagy maintains the insulin production by stably maintaining the size, structure and function of the beta cells. If the glucose and the fat are continuously supplied and the beta cells are overloaded to synthesize the insulin, the oxidative stress increases in the beta cells, causing the protein to become entangled and causing the beta cells to be in danger. At this time, limiting the nutrients will reduce the risks of injury and the deaths of the beta cells by activating the autophagy mechanism [9].

Diabetic patients often have a larger left ventricular size and a thicker ventricular wall [10]. A massive and rigid heart wall cannot release the blood properly, which causes a heart disease. Studies have shown that the diabetic, myocardial disease occurs when the autophagy-associated genes are damaged [11]. Therefore, it is possible to hypothesize that the activation of the Autophagy will protect the functions of the heart [4].

Diabetes, hyperlipidemia, and insulin resistance impair the function of the endothelial cells and smooth the muscle cells [12]. When the LDL lipoprotein particles invade and oxidize these cells, the inflammatory cells come in to thicken the blood vessel walls and to block the blood vessels with an inflammation. The mononuclear cells enter the blood vessels, differentiate into the macrophages, and become the bubble cells again. The foam cells die in the blood vessels and combine with the calcium flowing in the blood vessels to form the plaques, which is a common process for atherosclerosis [13]. Studies have shown that autophagy is further promoted in the conditions such as the inflammatory cytokines, the hypoxia, theoxidized LDL, and the metabolic stress [14]. In addition, a damage to the Atg5's, one of the autophagy genes in the macrophages, has rapidly increased the risk of the vascular, plaque formation [14]. Thus, limiting the nutrients to the macrophages through fasting makes it possible to assume that the macrophages activate the atrophy and inhibit the vascular, plaque formation. This results in an improvement of the heart and the blood vessels [61].

3.30. The iron overproduction and the autophagy inhibition of the lipofuscin.

Immediate elimination is important when the several cellular organelles, such as the mitochondria, in a single cell are destroyed because, when they malfunction, they can make the active oxygen destroy the surrounding cellular material and, ultimately, mutate it into the cancer cells. Therefore, it is natural that the cells of the human body will have a large burden when such an autophagy-holding mechanism does not work. Scientists report that, as the aging process progresses, the rate of the autophagy formation rapidly slows down. One of the major causes is the accumulation of the lipofuscin in the cell, such as an unbreakable plastic lump (Fig. 3-30). Lipo-leucine inhibits the progression of the atrophy, which is a cell-scavenging activity, which leads to a further increase of the reactive oxygen species in the cell, which, in turn, leads to the oxidation of the intracellular substances, which eventually leads to the death or the malfunctioning of the cell [15].

When this phenomenon occurs in the brain cells, Alzheimer's Disease and Parkinson's Disease can progress to dementia, and this process can occur in all cells of human body, such as the myocardial cells, the hepatocytes, and the beta cells of the pancreas. One of the major components of lipofuscin is iron (Fe), and, from this point of view, the excessive intake of iron is very dangerous. To prevent anemia, it should not be inadequate, but it is not necessary to accumulate too much of it in the human body.

3.31. The metabolic changes in the fasting process.

Fasting was performed in the 1950s and in the 1960s as the treatment of obesity. According to these studies, the food supply through the food ends after about 5 hours after the ingestion of the food. From this point onwards, the human body begins to supply the glucose by opening up the reservoir called the "glycogen in the liver", which is linked to thousands of the glucose. That is, the glucose supply through the glycogen starts after the end of the glucose supply through the food, peaks at the end of two hours, and the glucose supply through the glycogen is exhausted after 30 hours of the food intake.

Five hours after the meal, which is the end of the supply of the glucose through the food intake, the lipids of the muscle proteins and the fat cells in the body are degraded, and they are converted to glucose. In less than two days, you will begin to lose the glucose supply. Your body will use the β(beta)–hydroxy butyrate as the main energy source.

According to these studies, the brain cannot use glucose as a fuel in a long–term fasting. The reason is that you cannot go on with your muscles as your protein breaks down and feeds you with glucose. Because of this, in the long–term fasting, the use of the glucose in the brain decreases sharply and, instead, the ketone bodies, such as the β(beta)–hydroxybutyric acid, are used as the main energy sources.

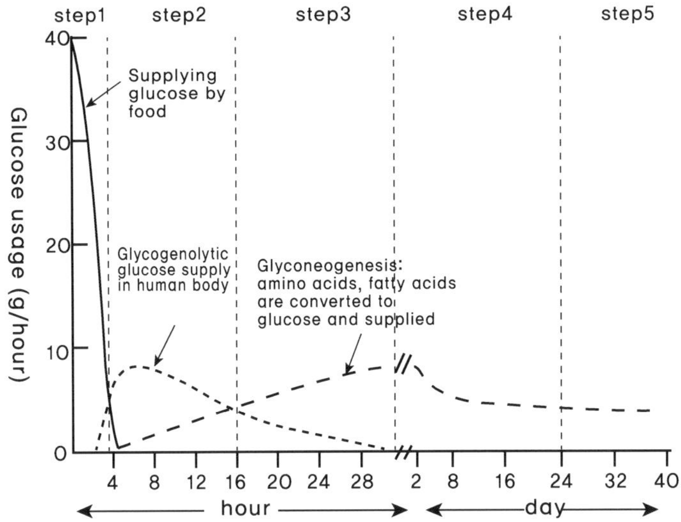

	step1	step2	step3	step4	step5
Source of blood sugar	Food	Glycogen glyconeogenesis in liver	Glyconeogenesis in liver Glycogen	Glyconeogenesis in liver Glycogen	Glyconeogenesis in liver Glycogen
Tissue in the body using glucose	All tissue	All organizations except the liver Muscle, fat tissue use rate is decreased	All organizations except the liver Muscle, fat tissue use rate is decreased	Brain, red blood cells, kidney water quality, use of glucose in some of the muscles	Use in the brain at a reduced rate, Red blood cells, kidney medular
main energy source of the brain	Glucose	Glucose	Glucose	Glucose, ketone	ketone, glucose

Figure 3-34. Patterns of Glucose Production and Utilization in Fasting Process [36]

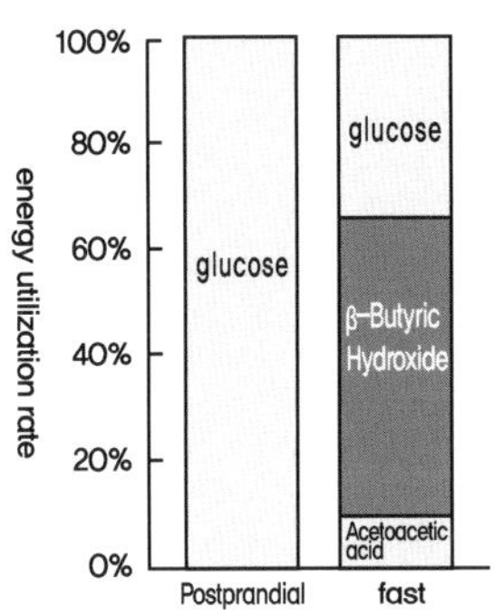

Figure 3-35. Patterns of change in utilization of glucose and ketone during fasting [36]

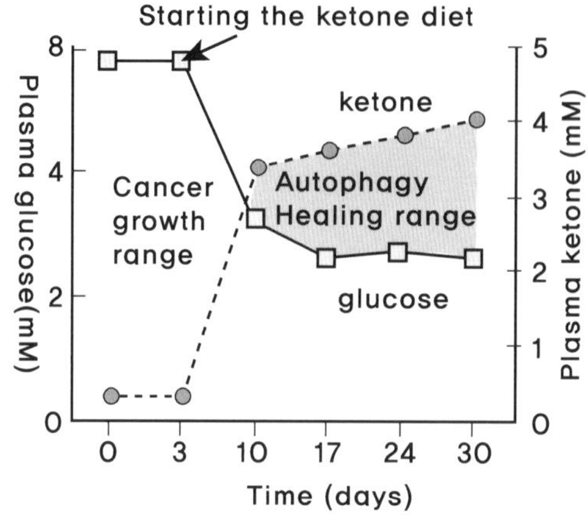

Figure 3-36. Blood levels of ketones and glucose in cancer healing begins [37]
Multiplying glucose mM by 18 results in mg / dL. Ketone mM is mg / dl multiplied by 10.41[38].

3.32. Conclusion

The main causes of the cardiovascular disease in the human body are the blood vessel accumulation and the vascular occlusion of the cholesterol. Because of this, the blood is not properly supplied and the blood vessels are ruptured, resulting in the disorders, such as those of the heart, the brain, the kidney, the peripheral organs, etc.. An easy way to reduce the cholesterol intake is to go on a vegetarian diet.

The vegetarian diet is not only free of cholesterol, but, also, it has the very low content of the saturated, fatty acids that act to produce the cholesterol in the body. In addition, the fibrous material excretes the cholesterol excreted in the bile to excrete through the function. Especially, the beans and the nuts contain the omega-3 fatty acids and the polyunsaturated fats in abundance to reduce the platelet aggregation that can occur during arteriosclerosis.

The antioxidants, vitamin C, vitamin E, the beta carotene, and the phytochemical lower the LDL cholesterol and prevent the oxidation of the cholesterol to prevent the ischemia of the blood vessels. The folic acid lowers the homocysteine levels to prevent a heart disease. It can be seen that the simple choice of the veggies offers a variety of the benefits to the cardiovascular system.

References

1. Cahill GF, Jr.: Starvation in man. N Engl J Med 1970, 282:668–675.

2. Lagrost L, Gambert P, Athias A, Lallemant C: Metabolic role of human apoprotein A-IV. Adv Exp Med Biol 1991, 285:109–115.

3. Buttet M, Traynard V, Tran TT, Besnard P, Poirier H, Niot I: From fatty-acid sensing to chylomicron synthesis: Role of intestinal lipid-binding proteins. Biochimie 2013.

4. Black DD: Development and physiological regulation of intestinal lipid absorption. I. Development of intestinal lipid absorption: cellular events in chylomicron assembly and secretion. Am J Physiol Gastrointest Liver Physiol 2007, 293:G519–524.

5. Arner P: Differences in lipolysis between human subcutaneous and omental adipose tissues. Ann Med 1995, 27:435–438.

6. Boden G, Jadali F, White J, Liang Y, Mozzoli M, Chen X, Coleman E, Smith C: Effects of fat on insulin-stimulated carbohydrate metabolism in normal men. J Clin Invest 1991, 88:960–966.

7. Randle PJ, Garland PB, Hales CN, Newsholme EA: The glucose fatty-acid cycle. Its role in insulin sensitivity and the metabolic disturbances of diabetes mellitus. Lancet 1963, 1:785–789.

8. Boden G, Chen X: Effects of fat on glucose uptake and utilization in patients with non-insulin-dependent diabetes. J Clin Invest 1995, 96:1261–1268.

9. Chrousos GP: Stressors, stress, and neuroendocrine integration of the adaptive response. The 1997 Hans Selye Memorial Lecture. Ann N Y Acad Sci 1998, 851:311–335.

10. Stamler J, Wentworth D, Neaton JD: Is Relationship Between Serum Cholesterol and Risk of Premature Death from Coronary Heart Disease Continuous and Graded? Findings in 356,222 Primary Screenees of the Multiple Risk Factor Intervention Trial (MRFIT). Jama 1986, 256:2823–2828.

11. Simons LA: Interrelations of Lipids and Lipoproteins with Coronary Artery Disease Mortality in 19 Countries. The American Journal of Cardiology 1986, 57:G5–G10.

12. 네들리 니: 웰빙 생활습관. 서울: 시조사; 2005.

13. Campbell TC, II TMC: The China Study. BenBella Books; 2006.

14. 캠벨 콜, 캠벨 토: 무엇을 먹을 것인가. 열린과학; 2012.

15. de Lorgeril M, Renaud S, Mamelle N, Salen P, Martin JL, Monjaud I, Guidollet J, Touboul P,

Delaye J: Mediterranean Alpha-linolenic Acid-rich Diet in Secondary Prevention of Coronary Heart Disease. Lancet 1994, 343:1454-1459.

16. Fraser GE, Sabate J, Beeson WL, Strahan TM: A Possible Protective Effect of Nut Consumption on Risk of Coronary Heart Disease. The Adventist Health Study. Arch Intern Med 1992, 152:1416-1424.

17. Kushi LH, Folsom AR, Prineas RJ, Mink PJ, Wu Y, Bostick RM: Dietary Antioxidant Vitamins and Death from Coronary Heart Disease in Postmenopausal Women. N Engl J Med 1996, 334:1156-1162.

18. Haskell WL, Spiller GA, Jensen CD, Ellis BK, Gates JE: Role of Water-Soluble Dietary Fiber in the Management of Elevated Plasma Cholesterol in Healthy Subjects. Am J Cardiol 1992, 69:433-439.

19. Glore SR, Van Treeck D, Knehans AW, Guild M: Soluble Fiber and Serum Lipids: a Literature Review. J Am Diet Assoc 1994, 94:425-436.

20. Li D: Relationship Between the Concentrations of Plasma Phospholipid Stearic Acid and Plasma Lipoprotein Lipids in Healthy Men. Clin Sci (Lond) 2001, 100:25-32.

21. Halliwell B, Gutteridge JM: Role of free radicals and catalytic metal ions in human disease: an overview. Methods Enzymol 1990, 186:1-85.

22. Moldovan L, Moldovan NI: Oxygen free radicals and redox biology of organelles. Histochem Cell Biol 2004, 122:395-412.

23. Fridovich I: The biology of oxygen radicals. Science 1978, 201:875-880.

24. Jiang R, Ma J, Ascherio A, Stampfer MJ, Willett WC, Hu FB: Dietary iron intake and blood donations in relation to risk of type 2 diabetes in men: a prospective cohort study. Am J Clin Nutr 2004, 79:70-75.

25. Fernandez-Real JM, Lopez-Bermejo A, Ricart W: Iron stores, blood donation, and insulin sensitivity and secretion. Clin Chem 2005, 51:1201-1205.

26. Cooksey RC, Jouihan HA, Ajioka RS, Hazel MW, Jones DL, Kushner JP, McClain DA: Oxidative stress, beta-cell apoptosis, and decreased insulin secretory capacity in mouse models of hemochromatosis. Endocrinology 2004, 145:5305-5312.

27. Andrews NC: The iron transporter DMT1. Int J Biochem Cell Biol 1999, 31:991-994.

28. Dandona P, Hussain MA, Varghese Z, Politis D, Flynn DM, Hoffbrand AV: Insulin resistance and iron overload. Ann Clin Biochem 1983, 20 Pt 2:77-79.

29. Dongiovanni P, Ruscica M, Rametta R, Recalcati S, Steffani L, Gatti S, Girelli D, Cairo G,

Magni P, Fargion S, Valenti L: Dietary iron overload induces visceral adipose tissue insulin resistance. Am J Pathol 2013, 182:2254–2263.

30. Witte DL, Crosby WH, Edwards CQ, Fairbanks VF, Mitros FA: Practice guideline development task force of the College of American Pathologists. Hereditary hemochromatosis. Clin Chim Acta 1996, 245:139–200.

31. Snowdon DA, Phillips RL: Does a vegetarian diet reduce the occurrence of diabetes? Am J Public Health 1985, 75:507–512.

32. Schafer AI, Cheron RG, Dluhy R, Cooper B, Gleason RE, Soeldner JS, Bunn HF: Clinical consequences of acquired transfusional iron overload in adults. N Engl J Med 1981, 304:319–324.

33. Borgna–Pignatti C, Cappellini MD, De Stefano P, Del Vecchio GC, Forni GL, Gamberini MR, Ghilardi R, Piga A, Romeo MA, Zhao H, Cnaan A: Cardiac morbidity and mortality in deferoxamine– or deferiprone–treated patients with thalassemia major. Blood 2006, 107:3733–3737.

34. Fabio G, Minonzio F, Delbini P, Bianchi A, Cappellini MD: Reversal of cardiac complications by deferiprone and deferoxamine combination therapy in a patient affected by a severe type of juvenile hemochromatosis (JH). Blood 2007, 109:362–364.

35. Nicholson AS, Sklar M, Barnard ND, Gore S, Sullivan R, Browning S: Toward improved management of NIDDM: A randomized, controlled, pilot intervention using a lowfat, vegetarian diet. Prev Med 1999, 29:87–91.

36. Cahill Jr, G.F., Fuel metabolism in starvation. Annu. Rev. Nutr., 2006. 26: p. 1–22

37. Seyfried, T.N., 암은 대사질환이다(암을 보는 새로운 시각)(양장본 HardCover). 2015: 한솔.

38. Meidenbauer, J.J., P. Mukherjee, and T.N. Seyfried, The glucose ketone index calculator: a simple tool to monitor therapeutic efficacy for metabolic management of brain cancer. Nutrition & Metabolism, 2015. 12: p. 12.

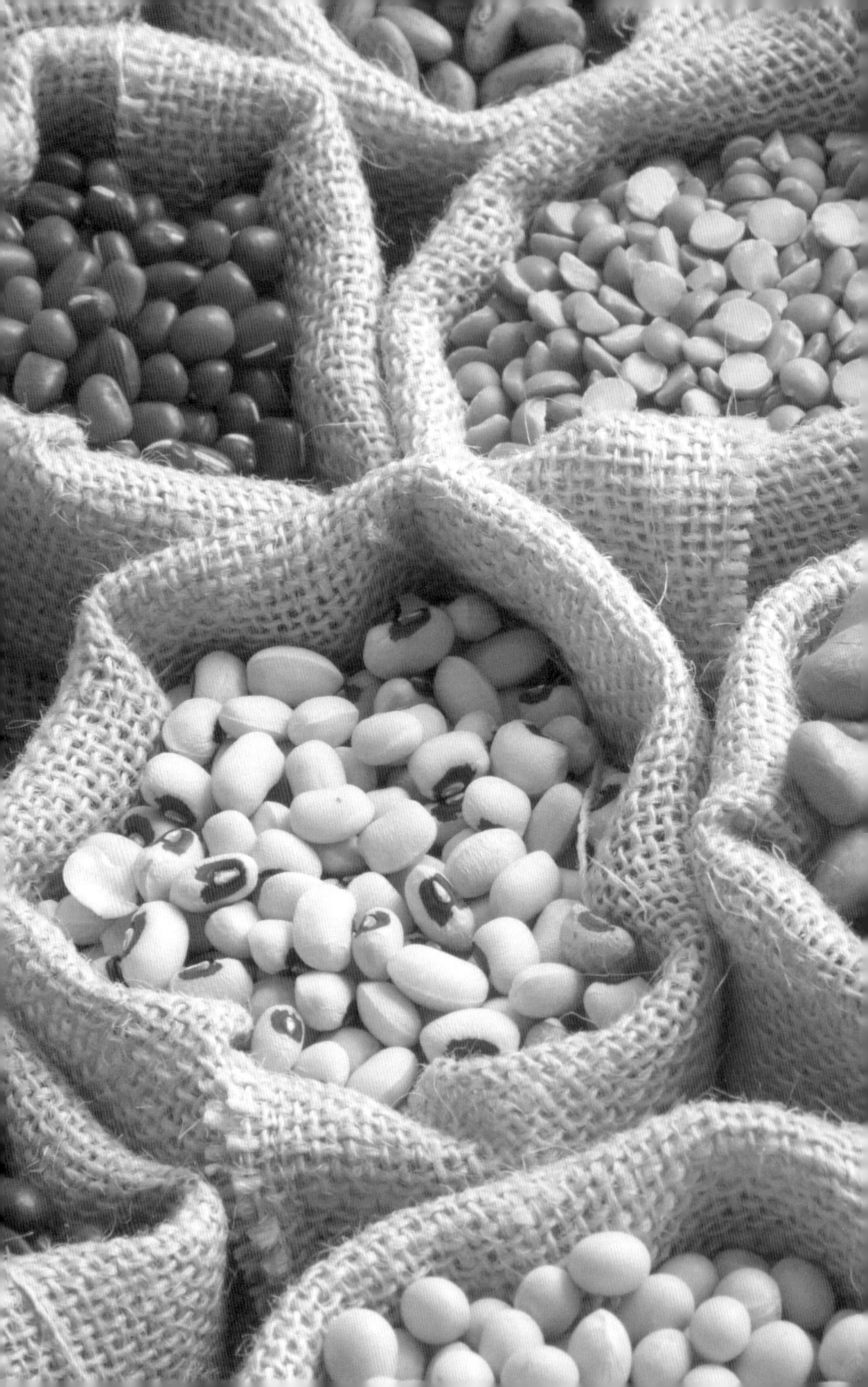

Chapter 4. Digestive System and Vegetarian Diet

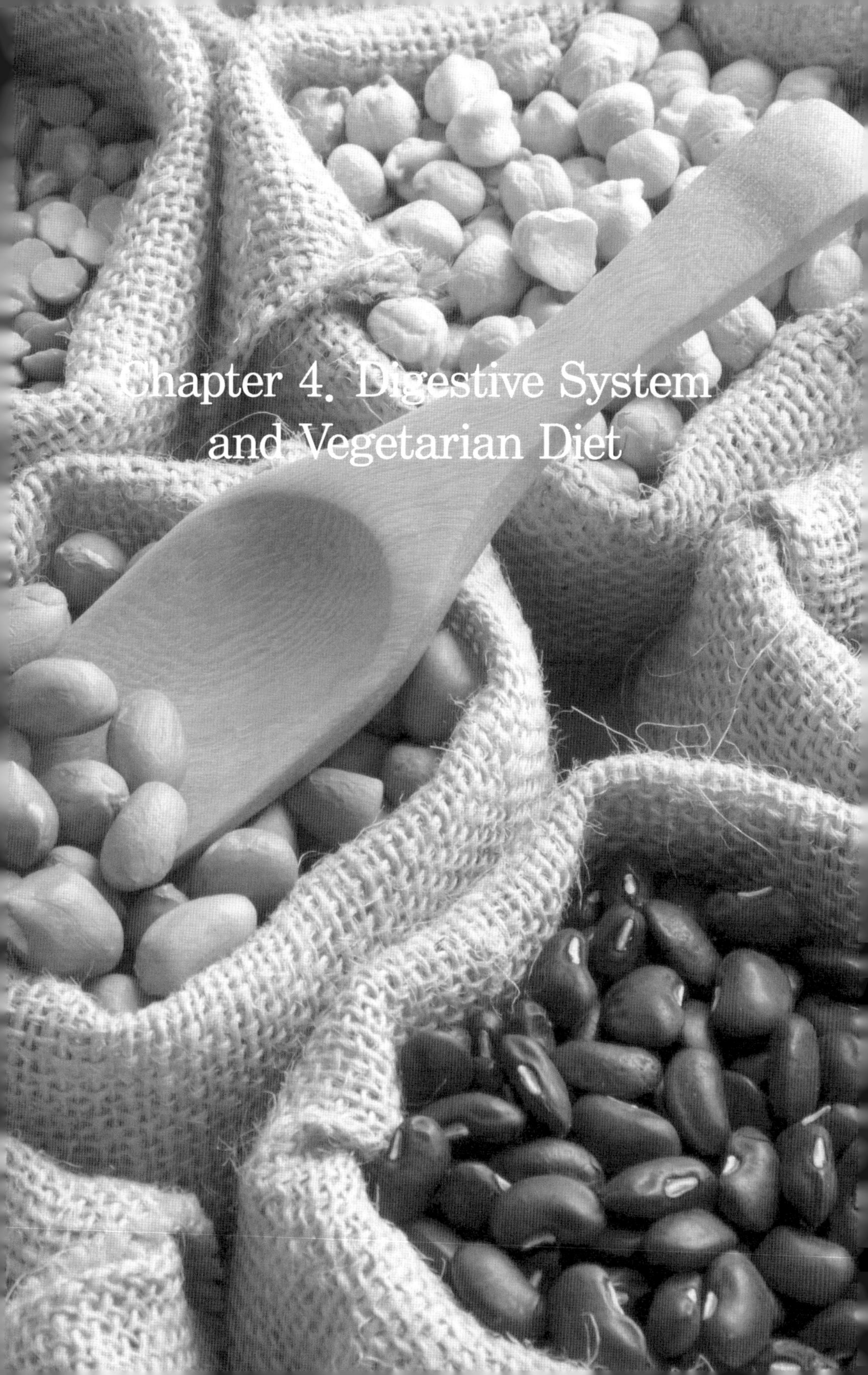

● **Skin system**

Vitamin D_3 required for calcium and phosphate absorption →
Allow lipids to be stored in skin fat cells ←

● **Endocrine system**

Growth Hormone, Thyroid Hormone Control Bone Growth →
Endocrine system (brain, chest, pelvis) protection ←

● **Cardiovascular system**

Hormone secretion of the digestive tract. Carries nutrients, water and ions from the nutrient absorption site →
Absorb liquid to maintain normal blood volume. The liver carries the heme ←

● **Urinary system**

It releases toxic substances absorbed by epithelial cells of digestive tract. Remove impurities from the liver →
The pressure of the digestive organs against the diaphragm limits the suction and supports the discharge. ←

● **Reproductive system**

Provide nutrients needed for the production of germ cells ←

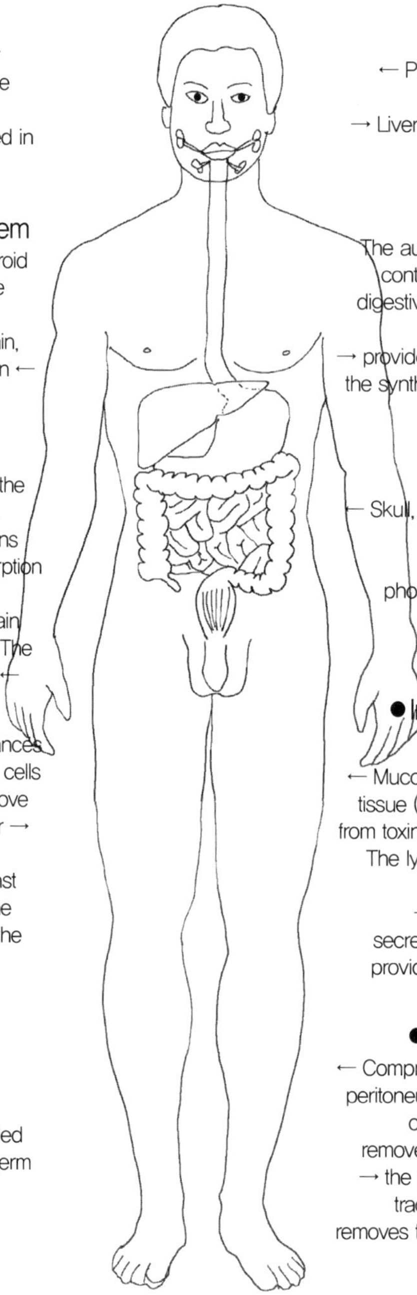

● **Muscular system**

← Protect digestive tract from abdominal cavity
→ Liver regulates blood glucose and fatty acids

● **Nervous system**

The autonomic nervous system controls the movement of the digestive tract and the secretion of digestive enzymes.
→ provide materials necessary for the synthesis of neurotransmitters

● **Skeletal system**

← Skull, ribs, spine pelvis protect the digestive organs.
→ Absorb calcium and phosphate required for bone matrix

● **Immune / lymphatic system**

← Mucosa–associated lymphoid tissue (MALT) protects the body from toxins absorbed by the tube. The lymphatic system absorbs lipids.
→ The acid and enzyme secretion of the digestive tract provides a pathogen defense.

● **respiratory system**

← Compression of the pleura and peritoneum through compression of the respiratory muscles removes the respiratory system
→ the pressure of the digestive tract against the diaphragm removes the suction and supports the discharge

Chapter 4. The digestive system and the vegetarian diet.

4.1 . The structure and the function of the digestive system

The energy required for the normal activities of the more than 50 trillion cells in the human body is produced by the metabolism of the cells. Cells need two things to produce the energy: One is oxygen and the other is the organic matter, such as the carbohydrates, the fats, and the proteins. The respiratory system supplies oxygen to all cells of the body through the cardiovascular system, and the digestive system supplies the organic matter through the cardiovascular system and the lymphatic system. In this case, the organic materials supplied are, also, used as fuel, but they are, also, used as the components of the human body.

The digestive system consists of the digestive tract and the ancillary organs. The digestive tract consists of the mouth → the pharynx → the esophagus → the stomach → the small intestine → the large intestine. The accessory organs consist of the digestive tract, such as the teeth, the tongue, the salivary gland, the liver, and the pancreas. In other words, the digestive tract is the place where the digestion occurs, and the digestive tract digestion tube helps the digestive tract secrete. Like the alveoli of the respiratory system, the surface of the digestive tract is cilia, like the small carpet hair, which greatly increases the surface area and increases the absorption of the nutrients. The digestion is accomplished by a combination of the following steps.

Ingestion : The food enters the digestive tract through the mouth.

Mechanical processing : the physical cutting and mixing through the digestive tract.

Digestion : In the digestion through the epithelial cells, the food is chopped off by the chemical degradation of the enzymes.

Secretion : Water, acids, enzymes, buffers, salts, and the like are secreted by the organ that makes the digestive juices.

Absorption : The organic substances, the electrolytes, the vitamins, the water, etc. migrate into the body via the digestive tract epithelial cells.

Excretion : Extra water is removed from the body. The waste from the digestive tract and the digestive fluid producing organ is discharged into the intestinal tract. The life span of most gut epithelium cells is short, from a few days in the esophagus to six days in the large intestine. By the epithelial stem cells, the digestive tract cells are constantly renewed and fragmented to compensate for the loss of the continued surface cells.

4.2. The importance of the intake

The first step for a healthy vegetarian diet is to eat the whole grains. When eating a variety of the grains, such as brown rice, whole wheat, and barley, you can eat a healthy vegetarian diet by including it with the embryo and the fiber. The answer to why the weight gain is important is to understand the evolution of the human beings and the changes in the fibrous isotope production during the course of the civilization.

Through the process of the hunting and the gathering on the dietary fiberous islands, the agriculture after 10,000 years ago, the industrial revolution, and the irrigation, the inventories of the human flesh began to decrease rapidly. And the homeostasis that had been maintained in the adaptation of the human body to the natural environment for a long time was broken. As a result, the modern people are paying for a lot of diseases. Therefore, the first step to healing the unwanted diseases is to return to the natural diet, and the important item is to consume the whole grains. First, I will look at the definition of 'fiber'then look at the changes in the fiber intake, and examine the effects of the fiber.

The name 'fiber' refers to the rough extraction of the plants with the acid and the alkali, followed by what is called the "crude fiber". In 1920, Lawrence developed the concept of 'the unavailable carbohydrates', and, in 1953, Hipsley included the cellulose, the hemicellulose and the lignin as the dietary fibers. In 1972, Trowell

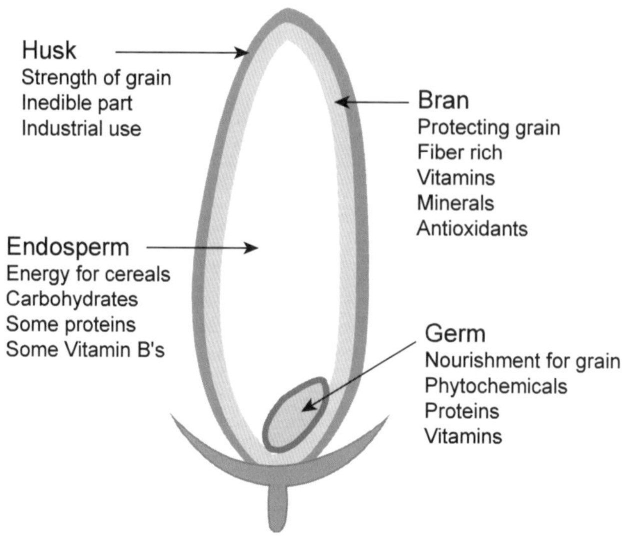

Figure 4–1. Structure of whole grains (brown rice). White rice contains only seafood.

Table 4–1. Comparison of nutrients between brown rice and white rice

nutrient	Brown rice	refine rice	nutrient	Brown rice	refine rice
protein	7.2g	6.5g	nicotinic acid	5.1mg	1.5mg
Lipid	2.5g	0.4g	Pantothenic acid	1.2mg	0.4mg
carbohydrate	76.8g	77.5g	Biotin	4μg	2μg
Ash	1.2g	0.5g	folic acid	15μg	8μg
Dietary fiber	1.3g	0.4g	vitaminB6	1.0mg	0.5mg
calcium	41mg	24mg	Inositol	120mg	10mg
phosphorus	284mg	147mg	Choline	110mg	60mg
iron	2.1mg	0.4mg	Benzoic acid	32mg	14mg
magnesium	120mg	50mg	vitaminK	10mg	1mg
vitaminB1	0.54mg	0.12mg	vitaminE	1.0mg	0.2mg
vitaminB2	0.06mg	0.03mg	Phytic acid	240mg	41mg

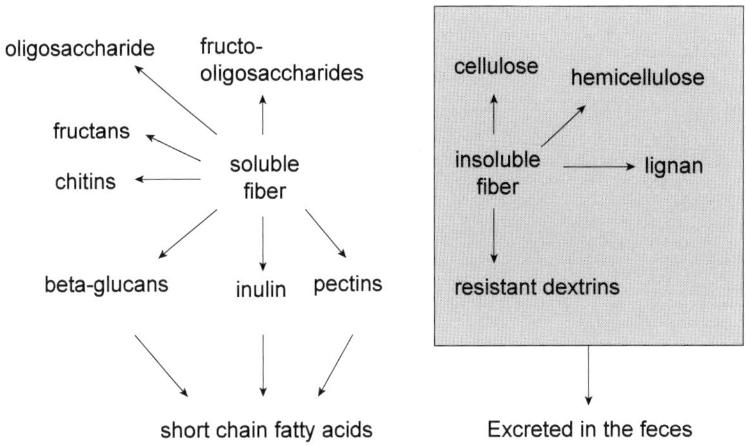

Figure 4–2. Types of fiber

defined 'dietary fiber' as 'a plant material that is not hydrolyzed by the human, digestive enzymes", thereby, including the physiological concept.

The soluble fiber includes the pectin, the guar gum, the alginic acid, the carrageenan, and the polydextrose, and the insoluble dietary fiber includes the lignin, the cellulose, the hemicellulose, and the chitin. In most foods, the soluble fiber accounts for one–third and the insoluble fiber accounts for two–thirds.

4.3. Changes in the dietary fiber intake.

According to the Klicks study, humans had consumed a wide range of the natural foods, including the vegetables, the seeds, the nuts, the roots, the flowers, the pollen, and the small amounts of the animal food, which had accounted for over 24% of the diet (Fig. 4-3).

As the human cultivation began 10,000 years ago, the nutrients consumed by the mankind have changed to a range of the monotonous foods restricted to a few grains [1]. At this time, however, the harvested grains were not purified as they are now, and almost all of the fiber was contained, so about 12% of the whole food had been consumed. As the Industrial Revolution took place, a stone quarry was devised, a rough dietary fiber was removed from the grain, and the grains had been supplied, and the proportion of the dietary fiber had been reduced by about 6% of the total food.

The decisive removal of the dietary fiber is almost complete since the introduction of the high-performance, roller mills made of iron 100 years ago. With the high-performance grinder with the structure of a roller, the grains were changed into the simple carbohydrates which were almost purely white, and only about from 0.15% to 0.24% of the fibrils was contained [1]. It is, also, associated with a growing number of the chronic diseases, such as the cardiovascular disease, diabetes, and cancer.

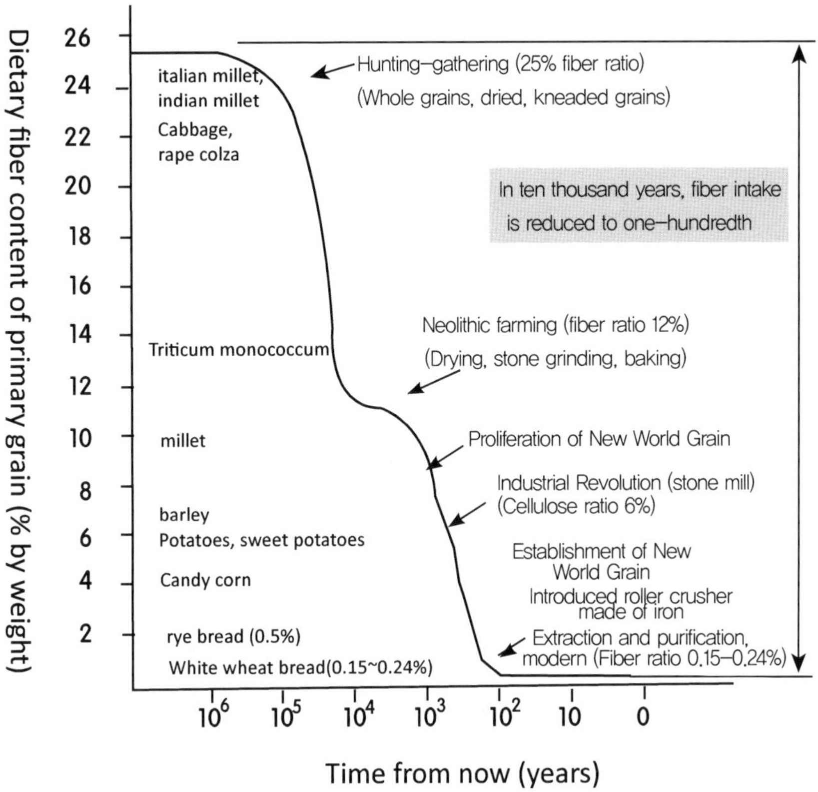

Figure 4–3. Changes in dietary fiber intake of mankind

4.4. Discovery of dietary fiber

Until 1965, the dietary fiber was almost of no interest in relation to the human nutrition. At that time, there was a lack of food, and one of the essential nutrients, such as the vitamins and the minerals, was discovered, and the study of the deficiency had been active. That is, the dietary fiber, which is not decomposed by the human enzyme and which is not absorbed into the body, had been treated as having been unnecessarily discarded.

The indulgence of the fiber has gained the widespread attention from the general public and the researchers since the report of Bucket, Trowell, and Walker in Africa. During his stay in Uganda in the 1960s, Bucket found that the Africans had eaten a more staggering number of the fibers than the Westerners. In addition, the stools had been easily discharged without any discomfort. He described them in the epidemiological report as follows:

"It is common in the United States and the United Kingdom to see the people who have been eating the vegetable foods like their ancestors in Africa.Regarding these people, I had rarely seen many diseases,such as coronary heart disease, diabetes, varicose veins, obesity, diverticulitis, appendicitis, gallstones, cavities, hernias, and diaphragmatic hernias,. The Westernized diets are small in volume and dense in calories, so the food that the Westerners eat cannot easily enable our digestive tracts to remain healthy. [2]"

They found that the African, indigenous people are healthy, while the civilized Western populations have a variety of cancers, the differences in the diseases regarding the dietary fiber intake, etc. In 1975, they published a book entitled, "Refined Carbohydrate Foods and Diseases" [3]. Since the publication, the many advantages of fiber have been reported by many researchers (Fig. 4-5). In other words, the beneficial effects and the mechanisms of the functions of the fiber in the gastrointestinal physiology, the chemistry, the classification and the analysis of the dietary fiber, the kinds of the dietary fiber, the cardiovascular diseases regarding the dietary fiber, the colon cancer, and the metabolic syndrome were revealed.

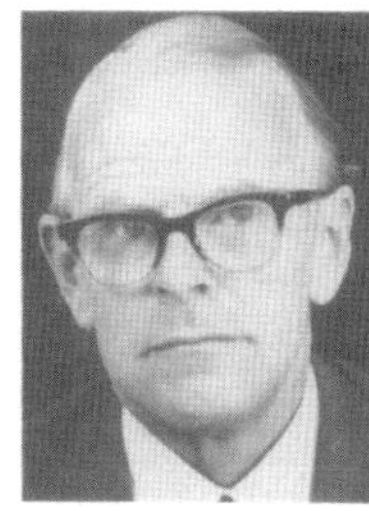

Figure 4-4. Burkitt

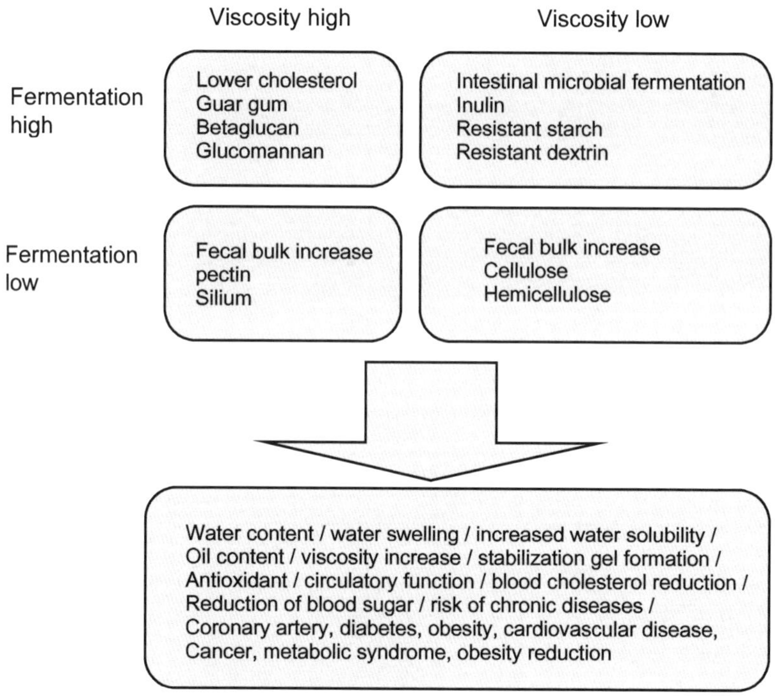

Figure 4–5. Types of fiber and beneficial functions

4.5. The volume and the rate of movement of feces

There is no doubt that the dietary fiber in the healthy people increases the volume of the stools and increases the number of the bowel movements, while making the stiffness of the stools thin. In addition, the increased intake of the dietary fiber by the ingestion of brown rice or whole wheat reduces the length of the intestinal transit time and increases the weight of the stool (Figure 4-6(a)). Regarding the benefits of the fiber intake, especially, in the patients with constipation, the effect is very large. In addition, the greater the amount of the feces, the fewer the incidence of the colorectal cancer (Fig. 4-6(b)). This is likely to be related to the proliferation of the toxic microorganisms and the release of the toxic substances as the stools stay in the large intestine(Fig. 4-7).

The importance of the water intake.

When the two liquids are separated by a selectively permeable membrane, the water moves to a higher concentration. The cell membrane of the digestive tract serves as a sort of a selective membrane, and all the water moving across the digestive tract is moved by the osmotic gradient. The movement of the water due to the osmotic pressure is very rapid, and, therefore, the liquid in the cells surrounding the digestive tract and the liquid inside the digestive tract have the same concentration. In other words, energy is not needed in the processes of the absorption and excretion of water in the human cells, but it is needed only regarding the difference in the concentration.

The human, epithelial cells continuously absorb the nutrients and the ions in the digestive tract, and, as the digestion and the absorption proceed, the solute concentration in the digestive tract gradually decreases. And as the solute concentration decreases, the water moves from the digestive tract to the surrounding tissues, and the osmotic balance is maintained, which is why most of the water is absorbed in the large intestine. Every day, 2000 ml of water enters the digestive tract in the forms of food and drink, and 7000 ml is secreted from the stomach, the digestive tract, and the pancreas and through the bile secretion. However, only 150 ml is discharged in the feces.

Sometimes, even though the fiber-rich foods are eaten, the amount of the feces is not increased, or even the symptoms get

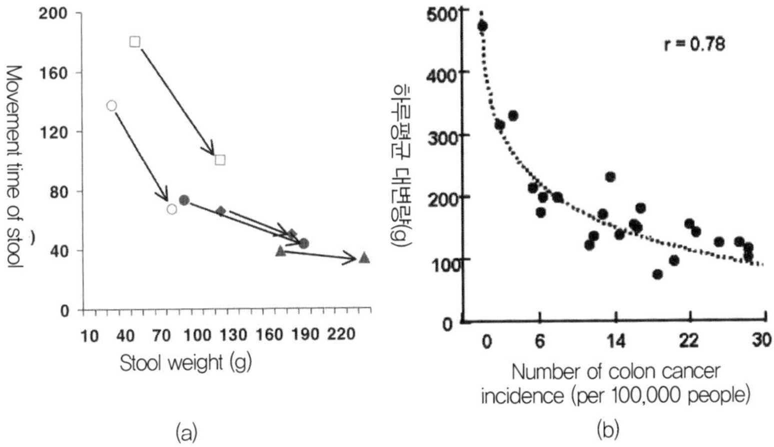

Figure 4-6. Stool weight rate Colorectal cancer incidence

(a) As the weight of the stool increases, the moving speed increases. (b) In the figure, the correlation coefficient r is 0.79. The squared value of r is 0.624, which means that 62.4% of the causes of colorectal cancer can be explained by the amount of feces.

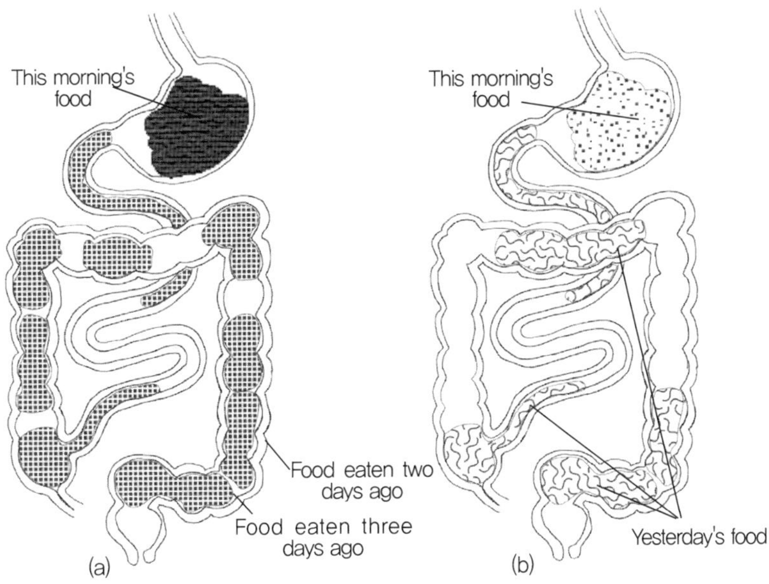

Figure 4-7. Difference between food lacking fiber (a) and abundant food (b)

worse. Even if the content of the water in the feces changes slightly, the stiffness of the stool changes significantly. This is because the body loses the moisture through the large intestine. According to reports, when the healthy volunteers reduced the daily intake of water from 2500ml to 500ml, the number of the bowel movements per week had decreased by 4.9 ± 0.3 from 6.9 ± 0.9. The weight of the stool had, also, decreased from 1.29 ± 0.20 to 0.94 ± 0.17kg for one week.

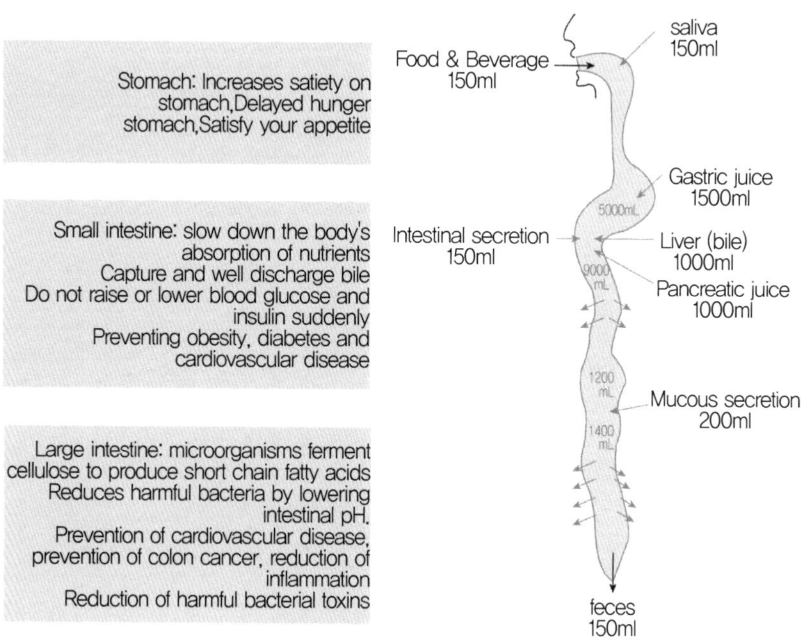

Figure 4–8. Secretion and absorption of water in the digestive tract

4.6. The effect of the cellulose on the glucose metabolism

Each fiber has a different ability to regulate the rate of the absorption of sugar and the hormone responses. Jenkins and colleagues used the concept of "glycemic index" to compare the ability of the various, carbohydrate–containing foods to control the blood sugar. Studies have shown that the diets containing enough fiber, either with or without a high carbohydrate content, improve the diabetic symptoms. That's because the dietary fiber is a sort of sponge containing the nutrients and is a nutrient that travels through the digestive tract from 8 meters to 10 meters and delivers the nutrients at a steady rate. It also plays an important role in adsorbing and excreting the waste products of the human body.

In other words, according to these studies, the intake of the dietary fiber did not only lower the insulin and the blood sugar, but, also, it recovered the abnormal lipid status. In particular, the type of the dietary fiber which was effective in the sugar metabolism was the guar [7].

As shown in Figure 5–9, a study of 25 foods showed a negative correlation between the total dietary fiber content and the blood glucose [8]. In other words, the intake of the dietary fiber–rich foods prevents the sugar concentration in the blood from rising sharply by appropriately controlling the absorption rate of the sugar components

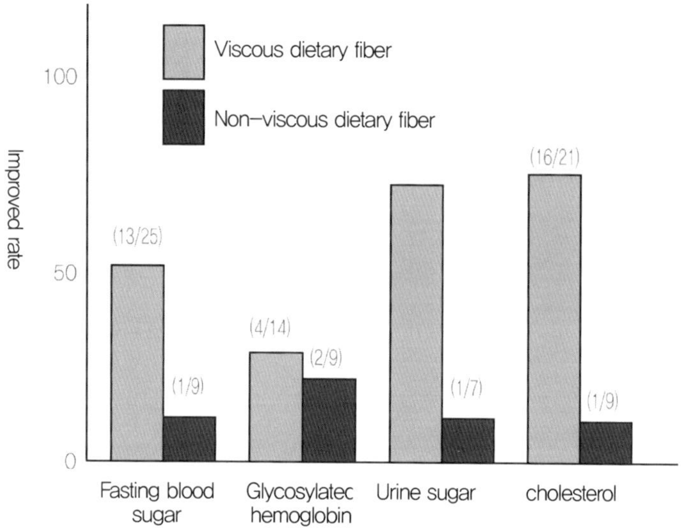

Figure 4–9. Diabetic healing effects of refined dietary fiber intake
The parentheses indicate significant improvements in the total number of experiments

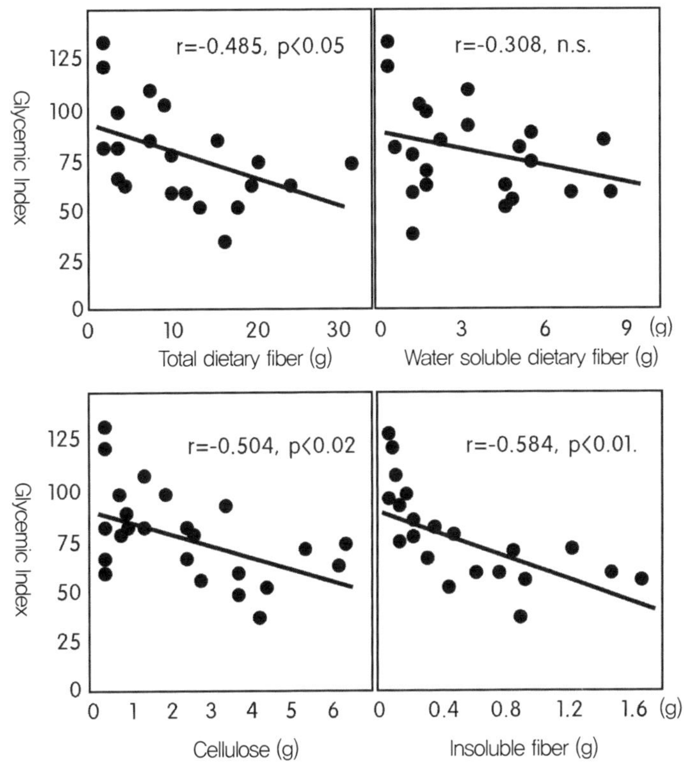

Figure 4-10. The relationship between glycemic index and total dietary fiber content of 25 foods(Content of dietary fiber g / carbohydrate 50 g).

The higher the intake of dietary fiber, the lower the glycemic index of foods, and when these foods are consumed, the sugar content is absorbed slowly so that the blood sugar does not rise excessively during a short period of time

4.7. Prevention of the cardiovascular disease involving the dietary fiber

Fiber lowers the serum cholesterol and the LDL cholesterol. Two effects are known. One is that the fiber blocks the cholesterol circulation, and the other is the action of the bacteria in the intestines.

First, the body synthesizes the bile from the liver to absorb the lipid, stores it in the gallbladder, and secretes the bile from the gallbladder when needed. The main ingredient of the bile is cholesterol. The dietary fiber is adsorbed by this cholesterol and leaves the feces. However, when there is a low fiber intake, the secreted cholesterol is reabsorbed in the ileum, which is the end of the small intestine. Second, the bacteria that ferment the cellulose in the field produce the acetic acid, the propianic acid, and the butyric acid, which inhibit the cholesterol synthesis. Are these fibers actually effective against heart disease? In 1986, a team had examined 43,757 healthy males aged from 40 years old to 75 years old regarding the 131 dietary items, and they had followed up for 6 years to investigate the 734 cases of the myocardial infarction.

According to the analysis published in 1996, the group with the highest fiber intake (the average of 28.9g), when quadrupled according to the degree of the fiber intake, had a higher, relative risk of myocardial infarction than the group with the lowest intake (12.4g) The risk was 0.59 (59%). They concluded that the dietary fiber is a very powerful factor in preventing myocardial infarction.

Another study in 1992 found that adding 15 grams of fiber a day lowers the serum cholesterol by 15 percent (Table 4–2). The results of these four–

Table 4-2. Calorie and absorption efficiency of whole wheat and white wheat

Kinds	Calorie intake	Absorbed calories	Fecal loss calorie	300g Intake time
Whole wheat food	2,470kcal	2,150kcal	320kcal	45 minutes
White wheat food	2,555kcal	2,455kcal	99kcal	35 minutes
Difference	85kcal	305kcal	221kcal	10 minutes

When the ingestion of whole wheat and white wheat lasts for one year, a weight difference of 13.6 kg will result.

Nutrition Today, 1976

week experiment showed that the serum cholesterol level had increased by 0.8% when the fake drugs were given, but had decreased by 5.6% for those with the 5g daily intake, 6.8% for 10g, and had decreased by 14.9% regarding the LDL-cholesterol for 15g. The recommended amount of the fiber is usually from 25g to 30g for adults and from 6g to 10g for water. The cellulose, the lignin, the pectin, the gum, the seaweed polysaccharides, and some hemicelluloses are abundant in the legumes, the nuts, the grains, the fruits, and the vegetables (Table 4-3).

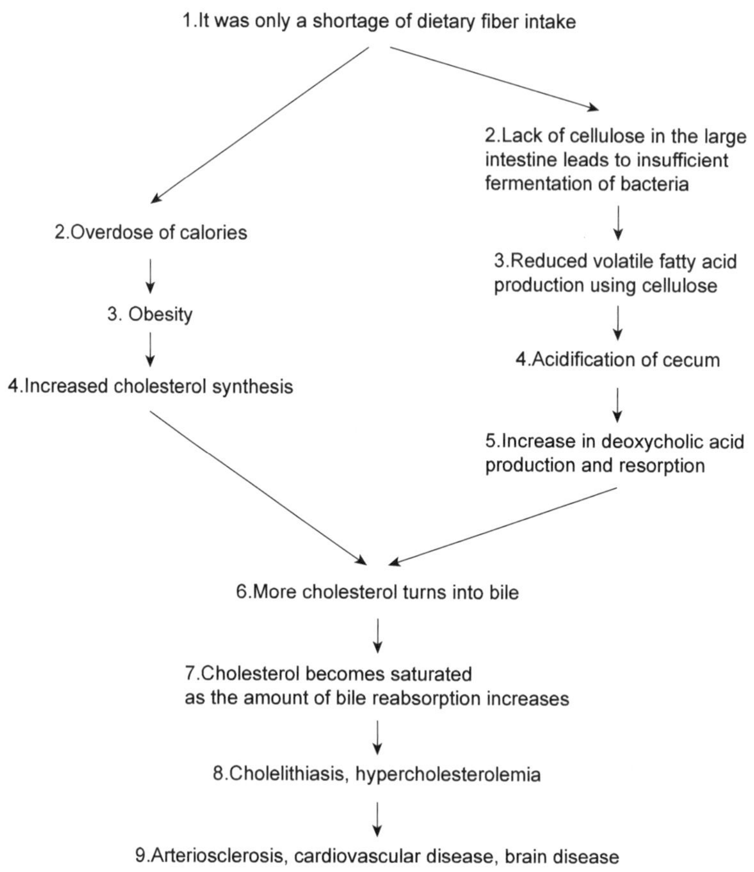

Figure 4–11. Mechanism of Reduction of Fiber Intake and Cardiovascular Disease

References : Song, SJ, Dietary therapy, SamYoung pub. 2001

4.8. The comparison of the nutrient uptake rate of the whole grains.

There is a simple feeling or argument that is not based on scientific evidence that the weed species are very low in nutrient uptake. The evidence-based research reports show that the nutritional intake of the whole grains is not significantly different from that of the grains.

In 1976, in the journal 'Nutrition Today' there was a study of the absorbed calories from the fiber-rich, whole-wheat flour food and the fiber-free, white flour food. As shown in Table 5-5, when the same 600g was consumed, the calories of the whole-grain food were 2555kcal, whereas the calories of the whole-meal food were 2470kcal, but the difference was only 85kcal. The actual amount of the absorbed heat was 2455kcal for the whole-grainfood and 305kcal for the whole-meal food. Therefore, it can be judged that the whole wheat provides enough nutrients.

The total amount of the calories in the feces was 99kcal, while that of the whole wheat was three times as high at 305kcal, but the rate of the nutrient uptake of the whole wheat was 87%. Although the rate of the absorption of the white-milled food was lower than 96%, it was rather desirable in terms of helping the diet naturally by providing the sufficient feeling of the fullness while providing a sufficient amount of the calories in view of the tendency of the chronic caloric excess consumption of the modern people. According to the above results, when we eat the wholegrain food, compared to when we eat the whole wheat food, the weight loss effect of 13.6kg is obtained per year.

Table 4-3. Comparison of intake of nutrients between vegetarians and non-vegetarians

nutrients	China	USA
Calories (kcal / day)	2641	1989
Total fat (calorie ratio)	14.5	34~38
plant based food fiber (g / day)	33	12
Total protein (g / day)	64	91
Animal protein (caloric ratio)	0.8	10~11
iron (mg / day)	34	18

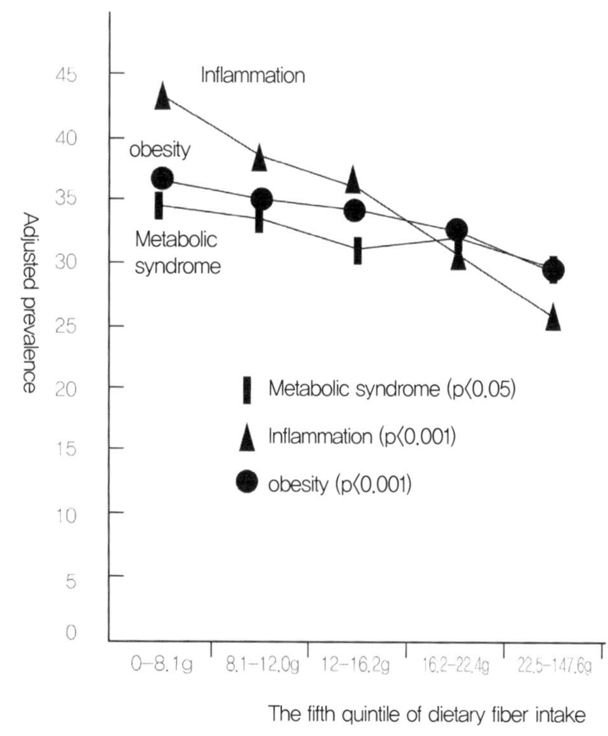

Figure 4-12. Dietary fiber intake and prevalence of metabolic syndrome

4.9. Constipation

The pathology of constipation: The physiological process often manifests itself as a colonic dysfunction or a colonic motility damage. The causes of constipation include the psychological and physiological factors as well as the movement disorders of the colon and the ankle dysfunction. The result of constipation is the increasing water absorption, and the stool will sustain the solids. At the same time, the toxins of the large intestine–the ammonia, the hydrogen sulfide, and the indole– are absorbed through the large barrier, and they enter the blood circulation system. Constipation causes an imbalance of the bacterial flora in the digestive tract, making the stool dry and making the constipation more severe. However, the constipation may be related to the body's active oxygen.

The radicals (OH), the other, free radicals (FRs), the single oxygen (O), the hydrogen peroxide (H_2O_2), and the other reactive oxygen species (ROS) damage the body's normal DNAs, proteins, enzymes, cell membranes, polyunsaturated fatty acids, other lipids, and lipid–containing organisms. In addition, the lipid peroxidation, which is produced by the oxidation of the lipid exposed to the free radicals, is, itself, a source of the free radicals that cause cancer, the inflammatory diseases, atherosclerosis, and the aging. Therefore, the human body protects itself from this active oxygen through the important, antioxidant enzymes, such as the vitamins

Table 4-4. Biochemical indicators of healthy children and chronic constipation children

group (70 people each)	plasma		Red blood cells		
	vitamin C (μmol/L)	vitamin E (μmol/L)	SOD (U/gHb)	CAT (K/gHb)	LPO (nmol/gHb)
Constipated children	46.59	20.65	1,943	269.3	25.22
Healthy children	58.35	27.15	2,206	327.3	19.18

World J Gastroenterol 2005, 11(3):368-371

C and E, the superoxide dismutase (SOD), and the catalase (CAT).

However, the large amounts of the radicals and the reactive oxygen species can be produced by the gut flora, which is in balance with the digestive tract and the excessive ammonia in the blood. And they act directly with the DNAs, thereby, destroying them, inhibiting the replication, and oxidizing the many organic substances and causing them to lose the function. Vitamin C, Vitamin E, the SOD, and the CAT eliminate the destructive actions of these toxic substances. The plasma vitamin E inhibits the lipid peroxidation.

70 children out of 132 children with the chronic constipation who were aged from 7 years old to 14 years old and 70 healthy children out of 137 healthy children were randomly selected to compare the biochemical indicators between these two groups. The blood pressure, the hemoglobin, and the albumin were not significantly different between the two groups. However, compared with the

healthy children, the constipated group had the significantly lower plasma, vitamins C and E, red blood cell SODs, and CATs. On the other hand, the LPO (lipid peroxidation) was very high in the children with the chronic constipation (Table 4–6).

Most (72.86%) of the chronically constipated children liked the fried foods, such as meat, pie, pork ribs, bread, and potato chips, but did not like the foods that were rich in vitamins and the fiber. This phenomenon not only maintains the solidification of the stool, but, also, slows the rate of the bowel movements and impairs the function of the anus rectum, thereby causing the constipation

4.10. The difference of the intestinal flora between the vegetarians and the non–vegetarians

Although the nutrients of the foods are absorbed and directly affect the health of the human body, they affect the human body by changing the type, ratio and activity of the microorganisms living in the digestive organs of the human body. In other words, the type of the diets changes the type and activity of the microorganisms by changing the survival environment of the microorganisms living in the human digestive tract, and the changed intestinal microflora, again, affects the carcinogens and the toxic substances in the digestive tract.

In 2004, Kassie and colleagues had examined the extents of the damages to the cellular genes by the dietary patterns. Eight patients, who were four healthy men, and four healthy women, who did not take a drug before, were recruited and the experiment was conducted. Four were vegetarians and the other four were the ordinary non–vegetarians, consuming 100 grams of meat a day. The feces were placed in a plastic bag in the absence of air. A total of 32 sterile rats were inoculated with the human feces. The mice inoculated with the vegetarian feces were fed a vegetarian diet, and the rats fed with the non – vegetarians' feces were fed a non–vegetarian diet.

The calorie and protein levels of the rats in both groups were the same. Four weeks after the inoculation of the feces, the

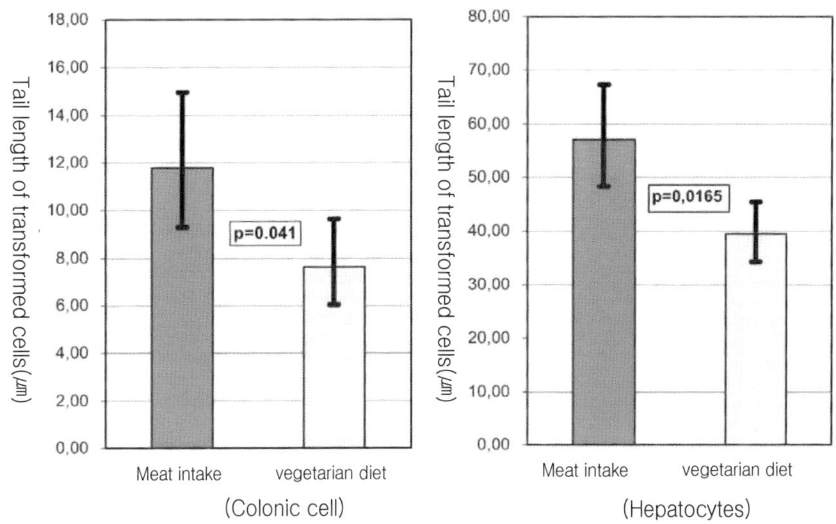

Figure 4-13. Gene strains in the colon and liver in vegetarian and non-vegetarian rats

There are few mutations in the genes in the vegetarian fed rats than in the meat-fed rats

carcinogens imidazoquinoline (IQ) was weighed 90 mg per 1 kg of the body weight. After 4 hours, the cells of the liver and the colon were examined on the slides. The length of the tail was measured. That is, if the length of the tail was long, it meant that the genetic transformation was big. The aromatic amine, or the imidazoquinoline (IQ), is known to damage the genes of the colon and the hepatocyte cells of the mouse several times in many cases. It occurs when the meat is burned.

The experimental results showed that the mean tail length of the transformed cells was 30% longer than that of the group of the rats that had been fed the vegetarian diet (Figure 4–13). The anticancer effect of the vegetarian diets was the same regarding both the colon and the hepatocytes. The authors estimate that the lactic acid bacteria were detected more in the feces of the vegetarians than in the feces of the non–vegetarians, and that the lactobacilli bound to the carcinogens and had reduced the toxic effects, thereby, leading to the decreased genetic mutations and the decreased incidence of thecancers in the colon and the liver.

4.11 The Oxford Vegetarian Study on Colorectal Cancer

Colorectal cancer is the second most common form of breast cancer in women, followed by lung cancer and prostate cancer in men, in Europe, the US, and the industrialized countries. There are the genetic factors, but the most important determinant is the diet. The numerous studies have shown that reducing the risk of the colorectal cancer is the major effect of the fruits, the vegetables, and the fiber, and the reduction of the meat intake (Fig. 4-14). In fact, the vegetarians have a significantly lower risk of colorectal cancer than non-vegetarians do.

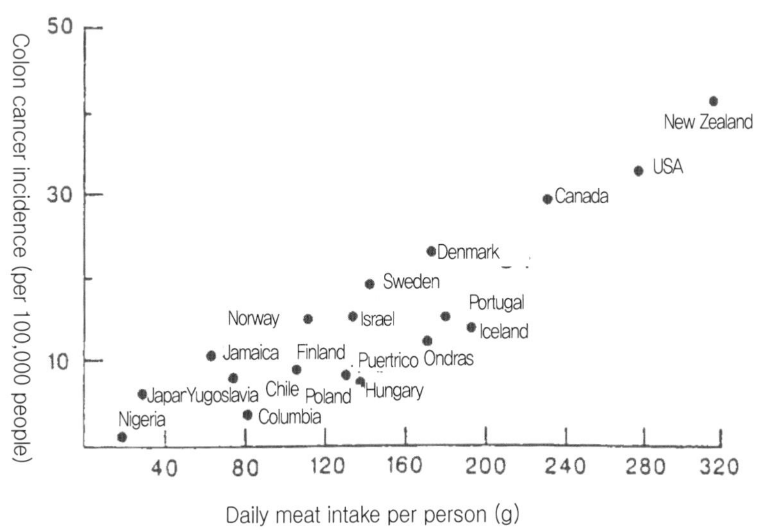

Figure 4-14. Proportion of meat intake and colorectal cancer incidence in the world

Table 4-5. The relative risk of cancer and the type of diet

Factor	Classification	Relative risk
sex	male	1.00
	female	0.85
Dietary Group	non-vegetarian	0.72
	vegetarian	1.00
meat	Do not eat	1.00
	Eat every day	1.34
fish	Do not eat	1.00
	Less than once per week	1.41
	More than once per week	1.38
egg	Less than once per week	1.00
	1-5 times / week	1.32
	More than 6 times / week	1.43
fruit	Less than 5 / week	1.00
	5-9 / week	0.58
	10 / week	0.57
Vegetable intake	low	1.00
	middle	0.52
	high	0.85
Whole wheat bread	5-9 piece/ week	1.00
	More than 15 pieces / week	0.86
White wheat bread	15 pieces or less / week	1.00
	More than 15 pieces / week	2.25
Dietary Fiber	low	1.00
	middle	1.03
	high	0.73
smoking	no smoking	1.00
	Currently smoking	1.88
alcohol drinking	Less than once / week	1.00
	1-7 times / week	1.69
exercise	Low	1.00
	plenty	0.82

The Oxford Vegetarian Study had been conducted in the UK regarding 11,140 vegetarians and non-vegetarians from 1980 to 1984. The participants recorded their diet patterns, dietary fiber intake, and lifestyle, such as smoking, alcohol consumption, and exercise,in a simple, food frequency questionnaire. A total of 10,998 participants had been followed for an average of 17 years, and the relationship between the diet and the colorectal cancer was analyzed. Among the 95 cases of the colorectal cancer, 39 cases involved the vegetarians and 56 cases involved the non-vegetarians. The relative risk was 0.85 for the non-vegetarians (1.00).

The unusual point was that, the more the white breads were consumed, the higher the risk of developing colon cancer was. The risk of developing colon cancer in a group 15 or less times per week was 1.25 or more. On the other hand, in the case of the whole wheat bread intake, which was not steadfast, the relative risk was low at 0.86 in the case of consuming 15 times or more a week. The fruit intake and the vegetable intake were significantly lower in terms of the risk of the outbreaks. Smoking and drinking were, also,the important factors in increasing the risk of the colorectal cancer. Exercise had reduced the risk of colon cancer. As a result, the following conclusions can be drawn:

1) Eating a lot of red meat produces the unhealthy results. On the other hand, the vegetarian diet represents the health benefits.

2) Be careful not to over-ingest the harmful foods, but it is more

important to maintain the good health by eating the fruits, the vegetables, the whole grains, and the other non−hydrops of the plant oils that are beneficial to the diet.

3) The excessive intake of the trans fats, the low linolenic acid intake, and the favorite pizza, ice cream, and cola are not healthy.

4) More extensive information is needed regarding the vegetarian and non−vegetarian diets. (3rd International Conference on Vegetarian Nutrition, 1999) (Am J Clin Nutr (1999) 70: 43S−8S)

4.12. The anticancer effect of the fresh vegetables

Vegetables have been shown to be effective in reducing the risk of developing the various cancers, but, in particular, the consumption of the green vegetables is more effective in preventing the cancer than ingesting the cooked vegetables. Lilly and John had analyzed

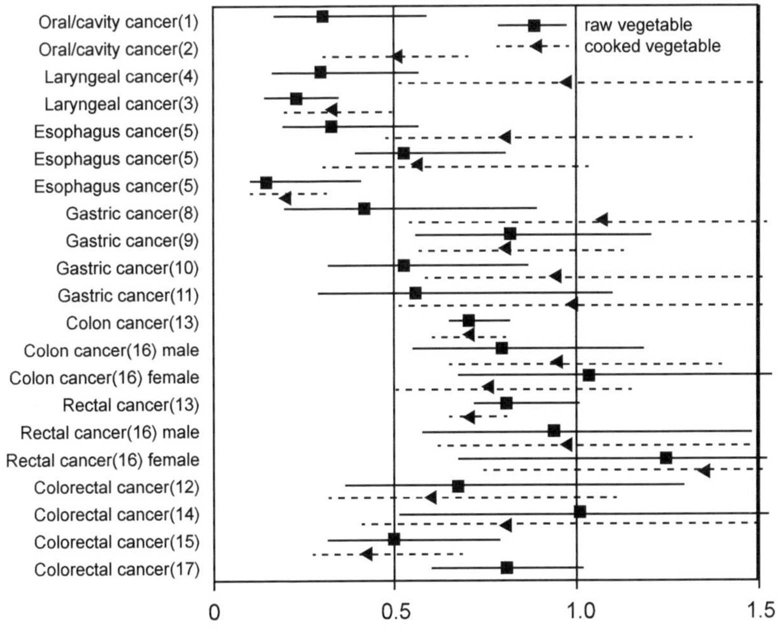

Figure 4-15. The relative risk of cancer occurrence according to the intake of raw vegetables and cooked vegetables

the 28 studies related to the cancer development of the raw and vegetarian diet from 1994 to 2003 and found the effect of the green vegetables on all of the digestive system that was related to the cancers, such as oral cancer, parietal cancer, larynx cancer, esophageal cancer, lung cancer, and gastric cancer. (Fig. 4-15, Table 4-8).

The cooked vegetables, with vitamin C, dissolve in water and reduce the heat-sensitive nutrients. The content of the carotenoids, which reduce the risk of cancer, changes before and after the

Table 4-6. vegetable intake and reduced cancer risk

Author (country)		vegetable	OR (hazard rate)	Comparison of intake
Levy (Swiss)	Oral cancer Esophagus cancer	raw	0.3	〉8.5 times: 〈 5.0times/week
		cook	0.14	〉8.6 times : 〈5.2 times/week
Francese (Italy)	Oral cancer Esophagus cancer	raw	0.4	〉14.1 times: 〈5 times/week
		cook	0.5	〉4.5 times : 〈1.5 times/week
Stephanie (Uruguay)	Laryngeal cancer (male)	raw	0.29	〉31g : 〈8.6g/day
		cook	0.96	〉87.7g : 〈35.5g/day
Connie (France)	Gastric cancer	raw	0.41	-
		cook	1.06	-
Botevek (Netherlands)	Gastric cancer	raw	0.81	74g : 8g/day
		cook	0.79	213g : 79g/day
Kim (Korea)	Gastric cancer	raw	0.55	-
		cook	0.98	-
Sentonje (Italy)	Colon cancer Rectal cancer	raw	0.67	〉76g : 〈46g/day
		cook	0.59	〉267g : 〈183g/day
Francese (Italy)	직장암	raw	0.8	12회이상 : 4.0회이하/주
		cook	0.7	7.3회이상 : 2.9회/주

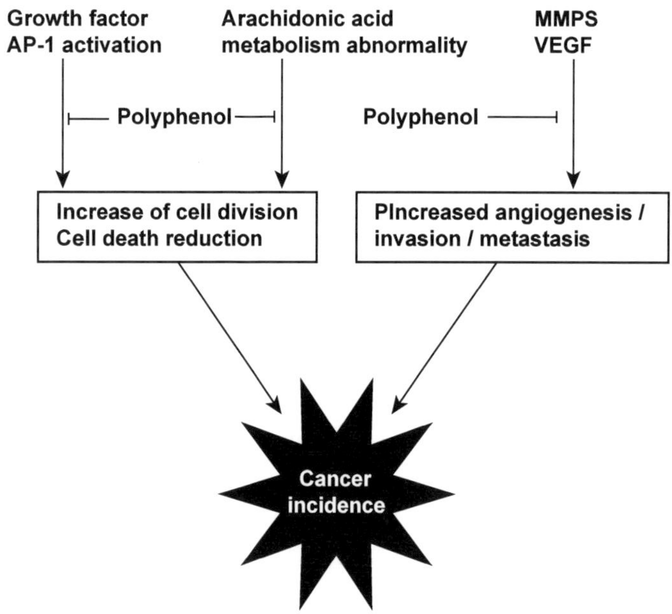

Figure 4–16. A schematic diagram of the effects of dietary polyphenols on the carcinogenicity..

heating in a microwave oven. In the case of kale, from 19% to 57% of the xanthophylls, which are the oxidized forms of the carotenoids after heating with a microwave oven, are lost. On the other hand, some nutrients, such as the tomato lycopene, increase after heating.

The enzymes play an important role in the original position in which the phytochemicals are produced and are easily destroyed by heat. The cruciferous vegetables and the garlic contain the anticancer phytochemicals and anticancer enzymes. The cruciferous vegetables contain the glucuronic acid in their cytoplasms, and these substances detoxify and release the urine when the alcohol or a toxic substance enters the cell.

In rats, the ingestion of the Brussels sprouts, a kind of cabbage, is inhibited by the proliferation of the cancer cells, the increased cell death, and the aberrant crypt foci. The allynace contained in the garlic converts the Alyne to Alicin, which is activated when crushing or cutting the garlic. However, heating in a microwave oven for 60 seconds is completely inactivating. In the case of mice, the production of the DNA byproducts after the addition of the carcinogens had decreased by 64% when the fresh garlic was added.

4.13. Heat affects the food structure and the digestibility

The main function differs for each fiber type. For example, the soluble fibrin helps reduce the insulin level. And insoluble fiber accelerates the speeds of the movements of the sides and combines with the carcinogens to increase the emission. Applying heat in the same way as steaming or tipping in water affects the physical structure of the food and affects the digestion and the physical properties. For example, the cooked vegetables increase the soluble fiber and reduce the insoluble fiber.

Heat causes the Myelin Reaction to increase the binding of the reducing sugars, the amino acids, the peptides, and the proteins, which can improve the color, taste, and flavor of the food. At the same time, however, the large amounts of the essential amino acids are destroyed. In addition, the binding of the protein to the sugar may make it harder to digest. For this reason, some products that are produced after the heat treatment are difficult to digest with the human digestive enzymes, such as trypsin. In addition, some of the products resulting from the excessive heat treatment may increase the levels of the inflammatory mediators and may even turn into the carcinogens. Most vegetables have fewer proteins, but myel can be easily caused by the heat applied to the sweet vegetables, such as the carrots and the tomatoes, along with the vegetables, beans, and fruits.

The overgrowth of the colon epithelial cells is known to be

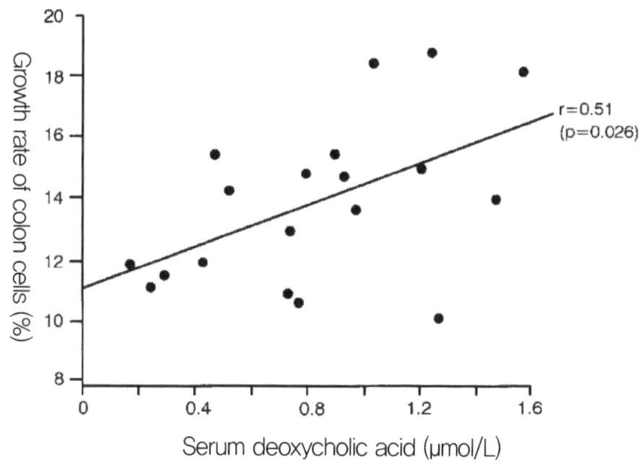

Figure 4-17. Proportion of Proliferation Rate of Deoxycholic Acid and Colonic Cell in Serum

the first stage of colorectal cancer. The over-proliferating cells initially begin in the form of a small benign adenoma, which enters the adenoma-dysplasia-carcinoma stage, and the overgrowth progresses very rapidly. In the case of the animals, the proliferation of the colon and rectum mucosa is promoted by the bile acid. The deoxycholic acid is the secondary bile acid, which has the most important effect on the proliferation. When the human cells had been cultured, the deoxycholic acid had rapidly increased the proliferative activity.

The epidemiologic studies, also, showed a higher risk of colorectal cancer when the secondary bile acids were increased. In a study of 19 patients, the higher the concentration of the deoxycholic acid in the serum, the faster the proliferation rate of the colon epithelial cells was, which meant that the risk of developing colon cancer was higher (Fig. 4-17).

The higher the intake of fat and meat, the higher the intake of cholesterol was and the higher the concentration of the bile acid was. In addition, when the meat intake is high, the fiber intake tends to be low. When the fiber intake is low, the fecal rate is slowed down in the digestive tract, a large amount of bacteria grow, and the amount of the bile acid to be reabsorbed is increased.

These factors cause a large amount of the bile to be released into the bowel, and the primary bile has a higher conversion rate than that of the secondary bile. That is, it stimulates the proliferation of the epithelial cells. And this promotes the cancer development.

Red meat has raised a lot of the scientific interest in the recent years regarding the fact that it increases the risks of the various cancers. Sandhu and his colleagues had analyzed 13 studies that were published until 1999, saying that the risk of developing colorectal cancer increases by 49 percent when more than 25 grams of meat are consumed. Several possible biological mechanisms have been described between the meat consumption and the development of colorectal cancer. The initial hypothesis was that the saturated fat increases the secretion of the secondary bile acids in the large intestine and shows an overgrowth effect, but, later, a more detailed analysis found some specific mutagenic carcinogens.

When meat is consumed as a source of protein, it is mostly

absorbed in the small intestine, but the rest is not absorbed and reaches the large intestine. There are many proteolytic bacteria in the large intestine, which decompose the proteins through the fermentation and the deamination. The metabolic substances, such as the ammonia, the amines, and the amides, which are produced during this process play an important role in the development of colorectal cancer. In rats, the ammonia had increased the proliferation rate of the colon epithelial cells.

4.14. The carcinogenic substances of meat.

The nitroso compound

In 2015, the International Agency for Research on Cancer (IARC), under the World Health Organization (WHO), designated the processed meats and the red meats, such as sausage, ham, bacon, and hot dogs, as Group 1 Carcinogens, together with tobacco, asbestos, and the arsenic. If you eat 50g of the processed meat every day, the incidence of cancer is increased by 18%. The

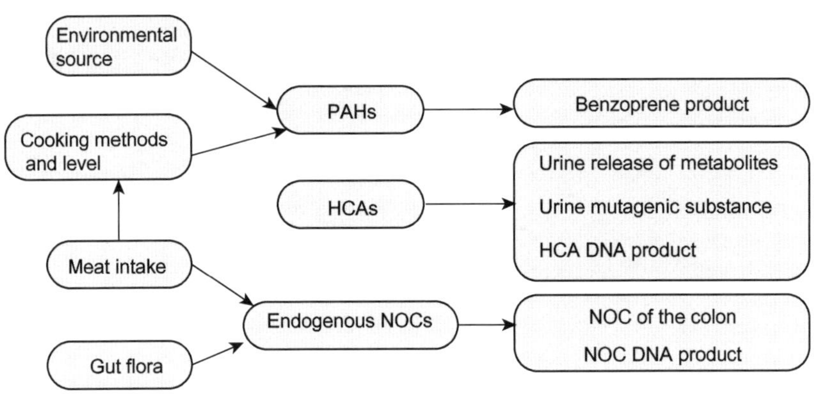

Figure 4-18. Generation process of meat-related mutants

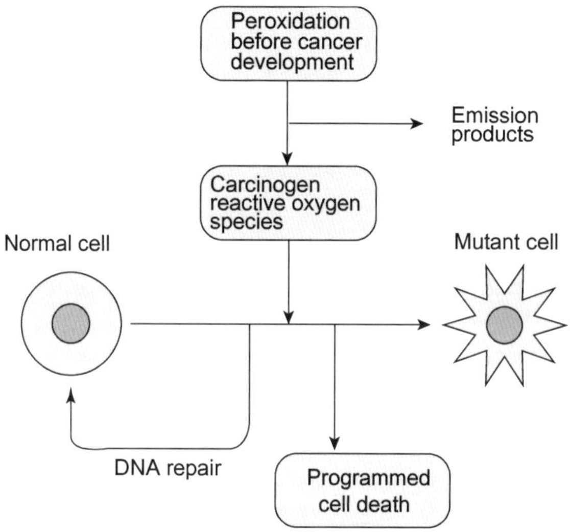

Figure 4-19. Early stages of mutation.

N-nitroso compounds (NOCs), which are a major carcinogen in meat, are produced by smokingthe meat, but the nitrogen compounds contained in meat are changed by heat. When from 60g to 600g of meat was consumed, the average amount of the feces per day was from 40g to 113g, which was more than three times higher when the meat consumption was high.

In recent years, it has been found that the heme iron promotes the production of the N-nitrosamine in the red meat. The dietary iron and the colorectal cancer risk are proportional. Bacon increases the production of the apparent, total N-nitroso compounds (ATNC) in the colon by from 10 times to 20 times.

Heterocycle amine

The heterocycle amines (HCAs), another major carcinogen in meat, are produced by the reactions of the creatine, the creatinine, the ammonia, and the sugar at the high temperatures. The HCAs production increases with the rising temperature and the longer cooking time. Cooked meat is known to be a major factor in the absorption of the HCAs. Most HCAs are the mutagenic substances that promote the development of cancer, especially the development of colon cancer.

There are more than 100 kinds of the polycyclic, aromatic hydrocarbons, and the benzopyran (BaP) is widely known as

Table 4-7. Dietary and abnormal follicle development

	diet	Diet's heme	adding	Number of mutations
A	CD	0	basa	324
	LH	0.25	small hemin	565
	MH	0.5	middle hemin	1233
	HH	1.5	many hemin	1901
	HG	1.5	hemoglobin	518
	TG	3.0	hemoglobin	457
B	HH	1.5	–	1901
	HHCA	1.5	Calcium addition	359
	HHAO	1.5	antioxidant	406
	HHOO	1.5	olive oil	389

A: Influence of hemin and hemoglobin B: Effect of inhibitor

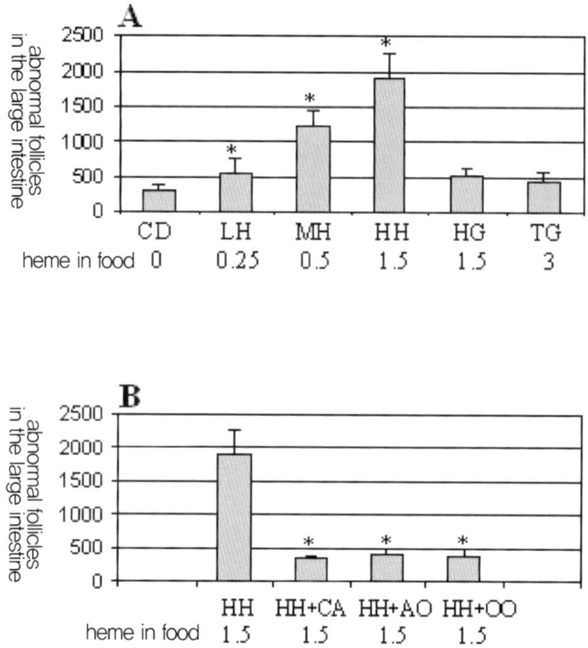

Figure 4-20. Number of abnormal follicular glands in the large intestine according to the type of food for 100 days.

a carcinogen. The benzopyran (BaP) is known to come from cigarettes, but a lot of benzopyrene is produced by the heat generated by burning meat.

According to one study in Sweden, the good-to-eat, brown meat had increased the risk of developing colorectal cancer by 2.8-fold and the incidence of colorectal cancer by six-fold. And it could reduce the cancer development by more than 70% through a dietary control. According to the epidemiological survey, the intake of the red meat had been higher in the cases of colorectal cancer, while the fishes had not shown any correlation. This difference is one of the causes of the heme iron that contains the iron.

Red meat contains 10 times more hemp meat than fish. The heat applied to the meat promotes the production of the carcinogens. Hem is a heme protein contained in the myoglobin and the like that are contained in the animal's muscle. The heme structure containing iron is converted to the carcinogenic substance called "hemin" by binding with the chlorine. In other words, the hemin is one of the main causes of colon cancer because the chlorine is bound to the heme iron by the lipid peroxide and the active oxygen. Four hypotheses have been proposed in relation to this: 1) Helmin promotes cancer development. The greater the dose, the more the cancer is promoted. 2) Free heme does not have the same effect as the heme bound to protein. 3) The inhibition of the lipid peroxidation inhibits the stimulation by the hemin. 4) High calcium intake reduces the carcinogenic effects of the hemin.

4.15. The meat-processed foods are even more dangerous

Various studies have shown that the processed meats, such as ham, jerky, and sausage,are more dangerous to the human body because the processed meats contain more nitrite, which is a source of the carcinogenic nitrosamines.

A research team at the Lausanne University Hospital in Switzerland had examined the risk of developing cancer according to the intake of the processed meat by comparing 660 patients with gastrointestinal cancer and the laryngeal carcinoma, such as oral cancer, pharyngeal cancer, and esophagus cancer, from 1992 to 2002.

As the intake of the processed meat was increased, the incidence of the upper, digestive tract cancer was higher. In particular, oral cancer and pharyngeal cancer were more prone to cancer. The risk of cancer in the men who had ingested a processed meat 0.8 times

Table 4-8. Age-specific cancer risk according to the intake of processed meat

consumption amount	ORs (Odds Ratios)	
	Under 60 years	60 years old or older
1	1	1
2	1.67 (0.79–3.55)	0.89 (0.39–2.01)
3	3.50 (1.64–7.47)	1.20 (0.56–2.60)
4	4.28 (2.03–9.06)	2.85 (1.29–6.27)

Annals of Oncology (2004) 15:346–349

Table 4-9. Cancer incidence according to processed meat intake

Cancer type	Meat intake (times / week)	Cancer incidenceORs	95% confidence interval
Oral cancer Pharyngeal cancer	〈 0.8	1	
	0.8-1.5	1.18	0.70-1.97
	1.6-3.2	2.74	1.70-4.42
	〉3.2	6.05	3.82-9.56
Esophagus cancer	〈 0.8	1	
	0.8-1.5	1.54	0.76-3.11
	1.6-3.2	2.64	1.35-5.09
	〉3.2	6.16	3.27-11.58
Laryngeal cancer	〈 0.8	1	
	0.8-1.5	1.19	0.51-2.78
	1.6-3.2	1.91	0.86-4.23
	〉3.2	4.38	2.09-9.20
Total	〈 0.8	1	
	0.8-1.5	1.28	0.85-1.93
	1.6-3.2	2.55	1.72-3.76
	〉3.2	5.78	3.96-8.42
Colon, rectal cancer	〈 0.8	1	
	0.8-1.5	1.23	0.74-2.04
	1.6-3.9	2.28	1.45-3.56
	〉4	3.37	2.15-5.29

Annals of Oncology (2004) 15:346-349

per week was 1, and those who ingested 3.2 times or more had a risk of six times or more. Similarly, for esophageal cancer, it was 6.16, for laryngeal cancer, it was 4.38, and, for colorectal cancer, it was 3.37 (Table 4-11).

The risk of the cancer caused by sausage, ham, etc. was analyzed at the age of 60 years old.The risk of the cancer from ingesting the processed meat was higher for those aged 60 years old. In the group above 60 years old, the risk of developing cancer in the lowest intake group was 1 and the risk of developing cancer in the highest intake group was 2.85., But, it was 4.28 in the group that was below 60 years old.

4.16. Diet, obesity, reflux, esophageal cancer, and the pathogenesis of gastric cancer

From 1976 to 1994, the incidence of adenocarcinoma in the United States had increased by 350%. This is an increase of 20.6% per year on the average, which was, also, seen in the UK, Australia, and the Netherlands. Epidemiological studies have shown that the incidence of esophageal adenocarcinoma is from six to eight times higher in the males than in the females. Adenocarcinoma of the gastrointestinal tract, also, occurred from three time to five times more frequently in the males than the females. The esophagus and the upper stomach are anatomically contiguous, and they share a pathologically shared part.

Studies of esophageal and gastric adenocarcinoma in Sweden and the United States in the mid-1990s showed that obesity and chronic, esophageal reflux were the major causes of esophageal cancer and gastrointestinal cancer.

Chow and colleagues found that obesity was easily determined by the body mass index (BMI), with the upper 25% of the BMI being four times more likely to develop esophageal adenocarcinoma than the lower 25% of the BMI, regarding which the incidence of adenocarcinoma was twice as high.

Lagergren and colleagues found similar results in a Swedish study where the upper 25% of the BMIs were 8 times more likely to have esophageal adenocarcinoma than the lower 25%.

In a US study, the upper 25% group was 2.3 times higher than the lower 25% group, and the BMI of 30 or higher was 4.3 times higher than the BMI of 22 of the lower risk group regarding the upper gastric adenocarcinoma.

4.17. Immigrants research

Since the 1970s, the dietary patterns in the Western society have been associated with the increased intake of the animal foods, the saturated fats, the sugars, as well as the increased incidences of colorectal cancer, breast cancer, and prostate cancer. At the time, however, the developing countries had still consumed one or two starchy foods, the fewer animal foods, the fats, and sugars. And there had been the lessWesternized cancers.

Immigrants research has shown the dramatic results in the research on the relationship between the diet and the disease. People who migrate from one country to another change to the local diet, and the incidence of cancer, also, tends to be local.

Table 4-10. Comparison of cancer incidence among Japanese immigrants (per 100,000 population, female)

Types of cancer	Japanese in Japan	Hawaiian immigrant Japanese	Hawaiian local white
Colon cancer	78	371	368
Rectal cancer	95	297	204
Prostate cancer	14	154	343
Breast cancer	335	1,221	1,869
Uterine cancer	32	407	714
Ovarian cancer	51	160	274
Lung cancer	237	379	962
Gastric cancer	1,331	397	217
Esophagus cancer	150	46	75
Cervical cancer	329	149	243

One of the most well–known examples is the case of the Japanese immigrants in the United States researched by Stone and Pero [14]. They had over 110 pages of the massive footpaths that had culminated in cancer and the prescription in the United States. They had compared the cancer incidence rates among the Japanese, Hawaiian, and Caucasian residents in Hawaii, where the incidence

Table 4–11. Comparisons of cancer incidence among Nigerians and US blacks and whites

Primary site of cancer	sex	Annual incidence per million		
		Nigeria Ibadan City	USA	
			Black	White
Colon cancer	male	34	349	294
	female		353	335
Rectal cancer	male	34	159	217
	female		248	232
Liver cancer	male	272	67	39
	female		86	32
Pancreatic cancer	male	55	200	126
	female		250	122
Laryngeal cancer	male	37	236	141
	female		149	141
Lung cancer	male	27	1,546	983
	female		1,517	979
Prostate cancer	male	134	724	318
Breast cancer	female	337	1,268	1,828
Cervical cancer	female	559	507	249
Uterine cancer	female	42	235	695
Lymph cancer (under 15yrs)	male	133	10	4
	female		5	3

of cancer was similar when the same area had been resided in regardless of the race (Table 4–12). For example, the number of the colon cancer was 78 per 100,000 Japanese in Japan, while it was 371 for the Japanese migrants in Hawaii and 368 for the Whites in Hawaii. On the other hand, regarding stomach cancer, it was 1,331 Japanese in Japan, while 397 Japanese in Hawaii was similar to 217 Whites in Hawaii.

A comparative analysis of cancer incidence shows that there is no difference in race between the cancer cases in the United States and the Nigerians in Africa. In the case of colon cancer, the Nigerians had 34 people per million inhabitants, but 349 people in the United States were nearly ten times as likely than the blacks. In the case of the lymphoma of those who were under 15 years old, there were 10 blacks in the United States, compared with 133 in Nigeria (Table 4–13).

They, then, analyzed the causes of the cancer deaths among the Americans, including lung cancer (24%), colon cancer (13 %), breast cancer (9%), prostate cancer (5%, and pancreatic cancer (5%)),which accounted for 60%. As a result of summarizing the causes of the various cancers, smoking was the main cause of lung cancer, and the incidence of colorectal cancer was positively correlated with the amount of the meat consumed per day through a straight line. They analyzed cancer and the cancer–inducing factors and concluded that 30% of all cancer deaths were due to smoking, 3% due to alcohol consumption, and 35% due to diet (Table 4–14)

Table 4-12. Percentage of Cancer Factors in the United States

factor	Percentage of all cancer deaths	
	Estimated rate (%)	An estimate of acceptable range (%)
tobacco	30	25~40
Alcohol	3	2~4
Diet	35	10~70
Food Additives	〈1	-5~2
Sexual activity	7	1~13
job	4	2~8
pollution	2	〈1~5
Industrial product	〈1	〈1~2
medicine & drug	1	0.5~3
Geographic physical factors	3	2~4
infection	10?	1~?
Unknown factors	?	?

4.18. Causes of the high stomach cancer incidence among the Koreans

Compared to the developed countries, there are many stomach cancer patients in the developing countries. A large amount of salt intake causes gastritis at an early stage and, later, increases the risk of gastric cancer. It is presumed that many gastric cancer patients in the developing countries eat a lot of the salted foods. In Australia, the incidence of gastric cancer had declined sharply from 25.9 per 100,000 in 1950 to 6.7 per 100,000 in 1994. This is largely attributable to the availability of the refrigerators and the ability to

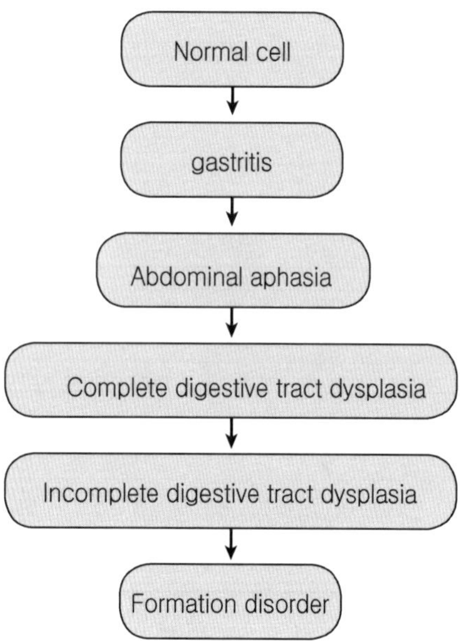

Figure 4-21. Progression before gastric cancer

consume the fresh vegetables during the entire 4 seasons. On the other hand, in Japan, the use of the salt-pickled foods continues to reduce the stomach cancer.

It is known that there are various, successive changes in the gastric mucosa before invasive tumors develop. The process is gastritis → incompetence → digestive tract → dysplasia. In various parts, asthmatic gastritis is often present and the other digestive tract dysplasia progresses (Fig. 4-21).

Numerous studies conclude that the ingestion of the salted foods increases the gastric cancer incidence. On the other hand, the higher the intake of the fresh vegetables and fruits, the lower the

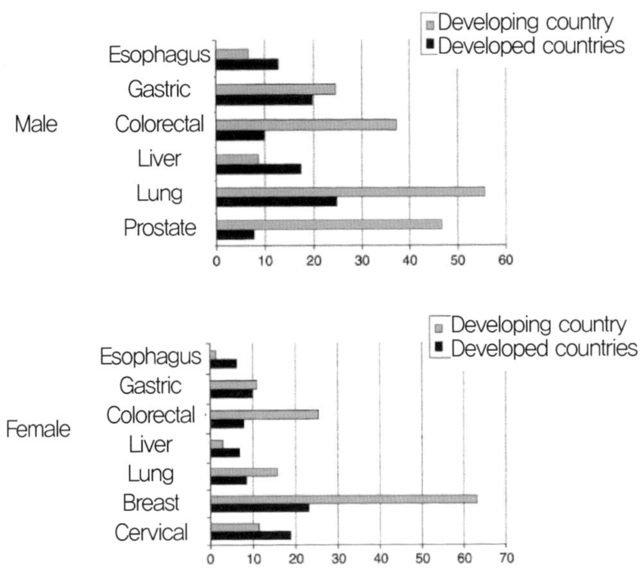

Figure 4-22. Incidence of age - adjusted cancer

Table 4-13. Food and Diet to Prevent Cancer

1	BMI should remain between 18.5 and 25. For adults, avoid weight gain.
2	Do regular physical activity.
3	It is not recommended to drink alcoholic beverages. If you drink it, do not take more than 20g.
4	This amount is within a beer or a glass of wine.
5	Do not expose food to aflatoxin.
6	Minimize the consumption of salted fish.
7	Especially children care. Take salt and salt appropriately.
8	Eat at least 400 grams of fruits and vegetables daily.
	Minimize meat intake. If you are not a vegetarian, reduce the consumption of preserved meat, sausages, jerky, bacon, ham, red meat (beef, pork, mutton).
	Do not eat foods or drinks that are extremely hot.

incidence of gastric cancer was.

60% of the cancers in the developing countries are the oral cancer, the pharyngeal cancer, and the esophageal cancer, which are associated with the trace element deficiencies that are mainly caused by a low intake of the fresh vegetables and fruits. Fresh fruits and vegetables defend against stomach cancer. Vitamin C, vitamin E, carotenoids, and selenium are the micronutrients that protect against gastric cancer. According to experiments in China, regarding the beta carotene, the selenium, and the vitamin E supplementation, the incidence of stomach cancer is very low.

Riboflavin, folic acid, vitamin C, and zinc are important in preventing these cancers. In addition, the habit of eating or drinking hot when eating food or drinking increases the risk of these cancers. The nitroso compounds are known as a carcinogen. The nitrates and the nitrites ingested in the body make it easy to get stomach cancer. An important source of these chemicals is the meat that has been preserved for a long time. The nitrate is, also, added to beverages

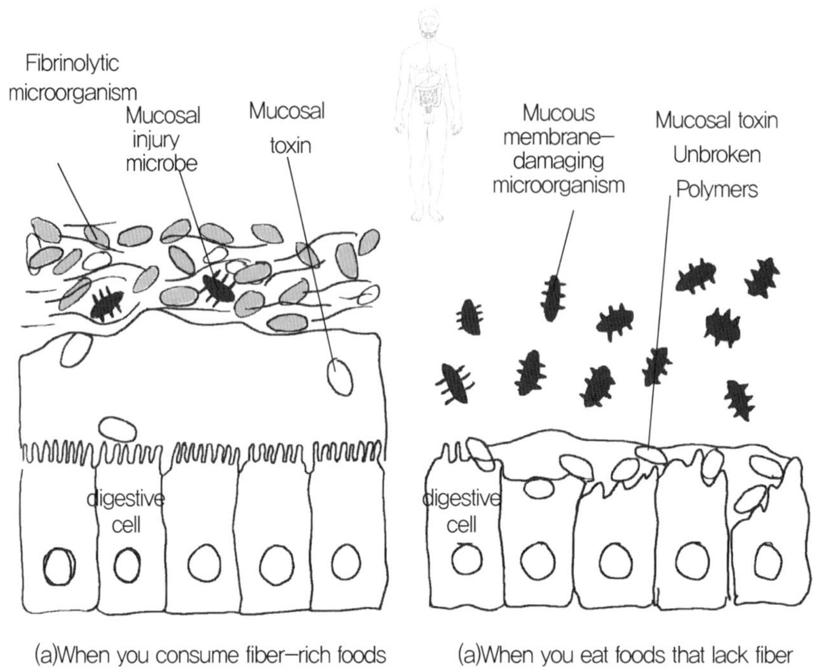

Figure 4-23. When the fiber-rich foods and deficient foods are consumed,

If you continue to eat flax-deficient food, the harmful microorganisms can create gaps between the intestinal cells, and the birds that cause various immune diseases as the cells pass through the cells can cause intestinal syndrome.

4.20. The comparison of the vegetarian and non–vegetarian fiber intakes

What is the difference between the vegetarian and non–vegetarian fiber consumptions? There is a slight difference between the studies, but the general tendency is similar. In Table 4–5, which is a comparison of more than 13,000 people described above, the vegetarian diet has the higher energy intake, the higher total fat intake, the higher saturated fat, and the higher cholesterol level than the non–vegetarian diet. The amount of the fiber was high. The vegetarian diet group had a fiber intake of 16 grams per day, while for the diet oyster, it was 14.3 grams. Compared to the non–dieters, the difference is even greater. The vegetarian group consumes an average of 23.4g of fiber, while the ovine consumes 15.6g of fiber, which is a statistically significant difference.

These results have the same pattern for the groups that are dieting to lose weight or for the vegetarians. Compared to thenon–vegetarians, the vegetarians had more than twice the intake of the whole grains and had consumed more beans or nuts.

Another example of the beneficial effects of the fiber–based, dietary patterns on the dietary fiber is in Colin Campbell's 'China Study'. A large–scale study of the diseases, the eating habits, and the patterns of life throughout China, which began in the early 1970s with the cancer of Ji Eun–rae, the former Chinese Prime Minister, had attracted the attention of the United States. This is because the cancer incidence rates were up to 100 times different in the regions of China. Under the auspices of the US government and the Chinese government, Campbell had been able to obtain the vast amounts of the data from 48 diseases and 367 factors through the blood and a questionnaire regarding 6500 people in 65 regions of China. Surprisingly, the intake of calories was higher for the Chinese, while it was the same for the fats and the protein. And there was a big difference in the intake of the vegetable fiber, which was 33 grams per day for the Chinese, while the average for the Americans was only 12 grams. And the cholesterol levels had the average of 127mg / dL for the Chinese people, but they were more than 215mg / dL for the Americans. The Chinese people had less cardiovascular diseases or diabetes than the Americans at the time and had no health problems. Indeed, in the southwestern regions of Sichuan and Guizhou, there were the hundreds of thousands of people who died of coronary heart disease before the age of 64.

4.21. The brown rice healing

The vegetarian healing period to be introduced here is an excerpt from Dr. Jeong, Sang-young's 'The Origin of Miracles' (Shijo Co., 2002). In the 1970s, Dr. Jeong Sang-young, a former Senator from Eunpyeong-gu, Seoul, recommended some patients to come to the clinic to get the experience of the natural remedies. This book has already been widely known to many people through the 17th edition in 2002. The content starts with the origins and the changes of brown rice and explains the advantages of brown rice and the treatment effect on the diseases, after the weather, the food issues, the hunger problems, and the experiences. Since the 1970s, the harmful effects of white rice have been increasing, so their experience is more important now. When you read these stories, you can see that, not only one disease, but, also, the various diseases are gradually healed at the same time. This proves that the basic condition of our body is health and that the natural healing power of the body progresses as a whole. Get the permission of your bereaved family and have some precious experiences.

(1) The dietary fiber effect on diabetes mellitus.

Recently, I have been feeling tired often, and I have been having the frequent urination, so I thought I would drink less water in the summer. But, especially, at night, because of the urination, I wake up several times, so there is a worry. So, I tried to drink less water on purpose. I do not think it is normal anyway. When I saw a doctor, the test result was diabetes. The doctor told me to eat barley rice. I tried to do it for a few days, but there was not much difference. Then, my wife was introduced to a counselor and she invited me to visit.

Now, I think I have become a diabetes patient. I've heard this. The lawmaker told me that diabetes treatment is by no means possible because diabetes comes from the diet and there is no dietary therapy. Brown rice contains a preventive and a remedy for diabetes in the eyes of the rice, so I emphasized that it is necessary to take the vegetable juice to clean the blood with brown rice.

I tried hard at the same time, and the number of the urinations had decreased and I was recovered from my fatigue. After 1 week, I came back to see that my diabetes was cured. I am so excited that diabetes will have the many kinds, but I am confident and I recommend you to try the cure. I have not been ill for a long time, but the diabetes will remain cured if I continue to have the rice cakes for a year. (Oodong River, Seongbuk-gu, Seoul)

(2) Recovery of cardiac asthma and hypertension

I have been suffering from hypertension for 14 years, suffering from shortness of breath, constipation, chest pain, weak eyesight, insomnia and severe headache. First of all, with the urgency of medication and continued to recommend the use of brown rice and non-salty foods, after two months, blood pressure near 200 without any medication was normalized and all symptoms disappeared. Now I'm almost convinced. I continued to suffer from brown rice and unpleasantness at first, but now I have become a habit and I am ready to die. Since then, normal activities have not been a problem. (Seoul, Republic of Korea)

(3) Vertebral disc prolapse and diabetes are recovered at once.

Seven years ago, he was diagnosed with severe diabetes because he had frequent coughs and urine and was not feeling well. I continued eating because I had to eat rice cooked here, but I did not see any effect. Then, unexpectedly two years ago, my back was so sick that I had a nervous breakdown after a long period of diabetes. If you have diabetes, then the neuralgia will be better. Your legs are stiff and your senses become dull, and you think that it is not so bad. I have been diagnosed with neurosurgery, but it is called spinal disc prolapse. I have a plaster bandage on my leg and I have to hold it for 10 years anyway.

I did not have money and I could not do it. I heard that I should also take vegetables and fruit juice, but I could not do it because of my condition, so I continued to eat the soy sauce in the rice cakes. After two years of testing, my diabetes was totally gone and my waist did not feel any abnormality even with hard manual labor. So my mission is to devote my time and energy to the enlightenment movement so that we can publicize the natural beauty of brown rice and help others. (70 years old Kim Won-dong, Ui-dong, Dobong-gu, Seoul)

4.22. The importance of fruit, vegetables, and whole grains

Traditionally, the method of classifying carbohydrates has been divided into simple or complex carbohydrates based on the number of simple sugars. Simple carbohydrates include monosaccharides and disaccharides. Monosaccharides include glucose, fruit sugars and galactose, and disaccharides include sugar, lactose, maltose, and the like. Complex carbohydrates are composed of longer polysaccharides with carbohydrate molecules such as starch. Jenkins et al. [1] pointed out that the carbohydrate exchange table does not reflect the effects of food on human physiology at all. First, factors such as dietary fiber, natural state of carbohydrates, and postprandial blood sugar are important factors. That is, even though it is said to be the same complex carbohydrate, white wheat bread, cakes, pastries and whole wheat or brown rice food made from refined white wheat flour can have different effects on the metabolism in the human body. In recognition of this difference, the concept of glycemic index (GI) was proposed in the early 1980s to more accurately measure the effects of carbohydrates on blood sugar. Glycemic index refers to the quality of carbohydrates [21], which measures the elevated blood glucose and insulin levels every 2 hours when ingesting 50 g of a food based on either white or glucose. For example, peeled potatoes have a sugar index of 94 and sweet potatoes of 44.

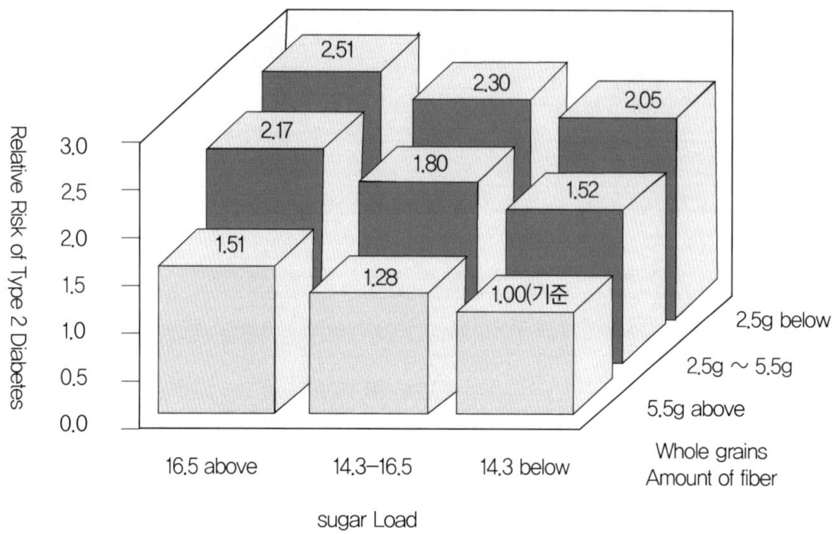

Figure 4–24. The risk of type 2 diabetes is low as the food is rich in fiber and low in sugar

Therefore, calorie intake and GI are different [22]. Thus, a more accurate concept emerged, glycemic load (GL) [23]. In 1997, Salmeron et al. Reported that, in various clinical trials in previous diabetic patients, the glycemic index concept does not reflect the fact that fibrin is improving diabetes, while fat is negative, such as increasing insulin resistance. And proposed a new concept to reflect this [3]. It is calculated by multiplying the per capita index by the amount of carbohydrate ingested when eating food on a daily basis. Therefore, fibrin or watery foods actually contain less carbohydrates, so the index is lower. If you know how quickly your blood glucose and insulin are increased without taking into account the actual intake of the food, the index includes the concept of a dose that can be taken at once to better predict blood glucose and insulin elevation do. For example, watermelon's sugar index is high at 72, but most watermelons are moisture, so the amount of sugar in the actual eating amount is not so high, so it is 4, which is low. Generally, fruits are high in water, so they belong to the very low part of the diet, even though the sugar index is high. In this respect, carbohydrates can be divided into relatively high carbohydrate sugars for refined carbohydrates and low carbohydrate sugars rich in moisture and fibrin.

Studies have shown that the higher the intake of refined carbohydrates, snacks, and desserts, the higher the tendency to gain weight [25], while the fruit or vegetables are beneficial for weight loss. And a low-carbohydrate diet is reported to be more effective in weight loss than a low-fat diet [26, 27], which is due to refined carbohydrates, not carbohydrates with enough fiber. The World Health Organization (WHO) has proposed guidelines to reduce the added sugar intake to 5% of energy intake [28], and various policies have been implemented worldwide to reduce sugar consumption [29, 30] Is that many foods that are currently commercially available remove and simplify the natural fiber and moisture to increase the density of carbohydrates. Even the same food may be affected by various factors such as cooking method,

Table 4-14. The sugar index and sugar load of various foods [31]

Food	Glycemic Index(White bread = 100)	Intake (g)	Carbohydrate per serving (g)	Glycemic load (Per serving)
Cup cake	104	38	26	19
Apple muffin	63	60	29	13
Coca-Cola (USA)	90	250ml	26	16
Carrot juice	61	250ml	23	10
Gatorade (Australia)	111	250ml	15	12
Bagels (Canada)	103±5	70	35	25
oat bran bread (Australia)	63±10	30	18	8
Rice bread (Carlos)	103±10	30	12	8
Corn Flakes (Kellogg)	130	30	26	24
Mousseli (Canada)	94	30	24	17
Rice (Bangladesh)	53±7	150	39	14
Rice (Japonica species)	68	150	38	18
Rice (brown rice, India)	43	65	38	11
Soy milk (Australia)	63	250ml	17	8
Apple	46	120	13	4
Banana (Canada)	66	120	25	12
Kiwi (New Zealand)	68	120	12	5
Mango (Philippines)	59	120	20	8
Orange (Canada)	73	120	11	6
Orange juice (Canada)	66	250ml	26	12
Peach (Canada)	40	120	13	4
Pear (Italy)	60±2	120	11	4
Plums (Canada)	34	120	14	3
kidney beans	19±5	150	25	3
Lentil beans	25	150	18	3
Soya beans	21	150	6	1
Spaghetti (tomato)	97	220	27	19

* If you ask less than 10, low, 10-20 usually 20 belongs to the higher side.

processing method, moisture content, cooking time, and variety.

4.23. Conclusion

In 2015, 280,000 new cancer cases were reported in only one year. This is one out of 183 people, and one out of three people in the world have cancer once in a lifetime. Cancer is known to be more painful in the treatment process. Medical bankruptcy due to the treatment costs leads to a national, fiscal crisis. The saturated fats and the cholesterol in meat and the carcinogenic substances produced during cooking are the important factors in the cancer development. On the other hand, the antioxidants and the various phytochemical-containing plant foods help prevent cancer. This is why the policy interventions are needed regarding the dietary patterns.

Healthy vegetarian diet includes eating whole grains. In the North American nutrition science, at least a half of the present grain intake is recommended, which will include the whole grains. The insoluble fiber, which is abundant in the whole grains, acts as a sponge to control the rates of the absorptions of the nutrients and to smooth the removals of the waste products

References

1. Klinks M: Paleodietetics: a review of the role of dietary fiber in preagricultureal human diets. In Topics in Dietary Fiber Research. Edited by Spiller GA, Amen RJ. New York: Plenum Press; 1978: 181

2. Burkitt DP: Epidemiology of cancer of the colon and rectum. Cancer 1971, 28:3–13.

3. Burkitt DP, Trowell HC: Refined Carbohydrate Foods and Disease. New York: Academic Press; 1975.

4. Heller SN, Hackler LR, Rivers JM, Van Soest PJ, Roe DA, Lewis BA, Robertson J: Dietary fiber: the effect of particle size of wheat bran on colonic function in young adult men. Am J Clin Nutr 1980, 33:1734–1744.

5. Painter NS, Burkitt DP: Diverticular disease of the colon: a deficiency disease of Western civilization. Br Med J 1971, 2:450–454.

6. Painter NS: Diverticular disease of the colon. The first of the Western diseases shown to be due to a deficiency of dietary fibre. S Afr Med J 1982, 61:1016–1020.

7. Jenkins DJ, Wolever TM, Jenkins AL, Josse RG, Wong GS: The glycaemic response to carbohydrate foods. Lancet 1984, 2:388–391.

8. Wolever TM: Relationship between dietary fiber content and composition in foods and the glycemic index. Am J Clin Nutr 1990, 51:72–75.

9. Zhou JF, Lou JG, Zhou SL, Wang JY: Potential oxidative stress in children with chronic constipation. World J Gastroenterol 2005, 11:368–371.

10. Kassie F, Lhoste EF, Bruneau A, Zsivkovits M, Ferk F, Uhl M, Zidek T, Knasmuller S: Effect of intestinal microfloras from vegetarians and meat eaters on the genotoxicity of 2–amino–3–methylimidazo[4,5–f]quinoline, a carcinogenic heterocyclic amine. J Chromatogr B Analyt Technol Biomed Life Sci 2004, 802:211–215.

11. Armstrong B, Doll R: Environmental factors and cancer incidence and mortality in different countries, with special References to dietary practices. Int J Cancer 1975, 15:617–631.

12. Sanjoaquin MA, Appleby PN, Thorogood M, Mann JI, Key TJ: Nutrition, lifestyle and colorectal cancer incidence: a prospective investigation of 10998 vegetarians and non–vegetarians in the United Kingdom. Br J Cancer 2004, 90:118–121.

13. Link LB, Potter JD: Raw versus cooked vegetables and cancer risk. Cancer Epidemiol Biomarkers Prev 2004, 13:1422–1435.

14. Ochsenkuhn T, Bayerdorffer E, Meining A, Schinkel M, Thiede C, Nussler V, Sackmann M, Hatz R, Neubauer A, Paumgartner G: Colonic mucosal proliferation is related to serum deoxycholic acid levels. Cancer 1999, 85:1664–1669.

15. Pierre F, Tache S, Petit CR, Van der Meer R, Corpet DE: Meat and cancer: haemoglobin and haemin in a low-calcium diet promote colorectal carcinogenesis at the aberrant crypt stage in rats. Carcinogenesis 2003, 24:1683–1690.

16. Levi F, Pasche C, Lucchini F, Bosetti C, La Vecchia C: Processed meat and the risk of selected digestive tract and laryngeal neoplasms in Switzerland. Ann Oncol 2004, 15:346–349.

17. Parkin DM, Bray FI, Devesa SS: Cancer burden in the year 2000. The global picture. Eur J Cancer 2001, 37 Suppl 8:S4–66.

18. Key TJ, Schatzkin A, Willett WC, Allen NE, Spencer EA, Travis RC: Diet, nutrition and the prevention of cancer. Public Health Nutr 2004, 7:187–200.

19. Doll R, Peto R: The causes of cancer: quantitative estimates of avoidable risks of cancer in the United States today. J Natl Cancer Inst 1981, 66:1191–1308.

20. Correa P, Piazuelo MB, Camargo MC: The future of gastric cancer prevention. Gastric Cancer 2004, 7:9–16.

21. Jenkins, D., et al., Glycemic index of foods: a physiological basis for carbohydrate exchange. The American journal of clinical nutrition, 1981. 34(3): p. 362–366.

22. Liu, S. and W.C. Willett, Dietary glycemic load and atherothrombotic risk. Current atherosclerosis reports, 2002. 4(6): p. 454–461.

23. Salmeron, J., et al., Dietary fiber, glycemic load, and risk of non-insulin-dependent diabetes mellitus in women. Jama, 1997. 277(6): p. 472–477.

24. Foster-Powell, K., S.H. Holt, and J.C. Brand-Miller, International table of glycemic index and glycemic load values: 2002. The American journal of clinical nutrition, 2002. 76(1): p. 5–56.

25. Fogelholm, M., et al., Dietary macronutrients and food consumption as determinants of long-term weight change in adult populations: a systematic literature review. Food & nutrition research, 2012. 56(1): p. 19103.

26. Cheung, B.M., The cardiovascular continuum in Asia–a new paradigm for the metabolic syndrome. 2005, LWW.

27. Zuniga, Y.L., et al., Rice and noodle consumption is associated with insulin resistance and hyperglycaemia in an Asian population. British Journal of Nutrition, 2014. 111(6): p. 1118–1128.

28. Guideline, W., Sugars intake for adults and children. Geneva: World Health Organization, 2015.

29. Lustig, R.H., L.A. Schmidt, and C.D. Brindis, Public health: the toxic truth about sugar. Nature, 2012. 482(7383): p. 27.

30. Malik, V.S., W.C. Willett, and F.B. Hu, Global obesity: trends, risk factors and policy implications. Nature Reviews Endocrinology, 2013. 9(1): p. 13.

31. Foster-Powell, K., S.H. Holt, and J.C. Brand-Miller, International table of glycemic index and glycemic load values: 2002. The American journal of clinical nutrition, 2002. 76(1): p. 5-56.

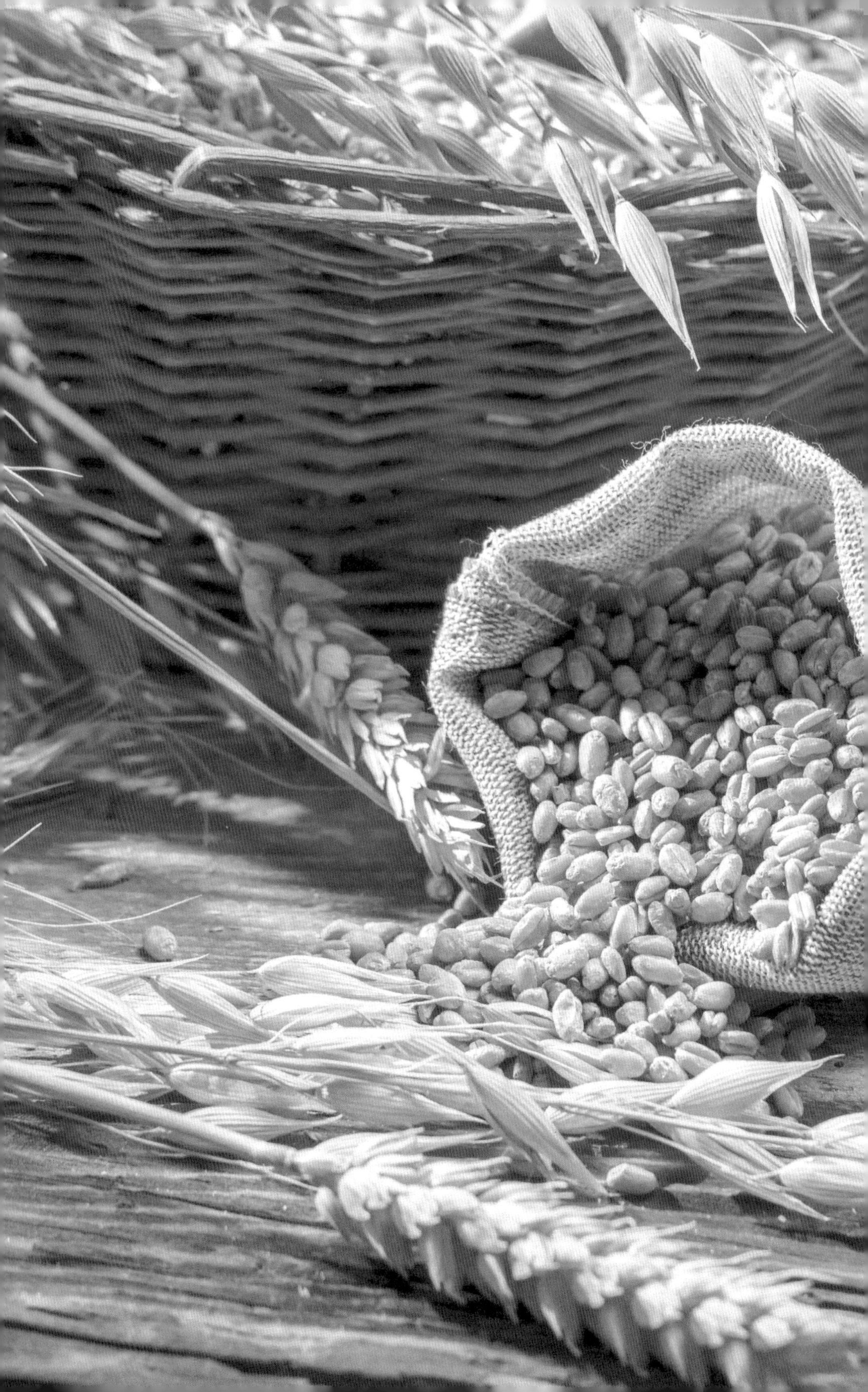

Chapter 5. Nervous System and Vegetarian Diet

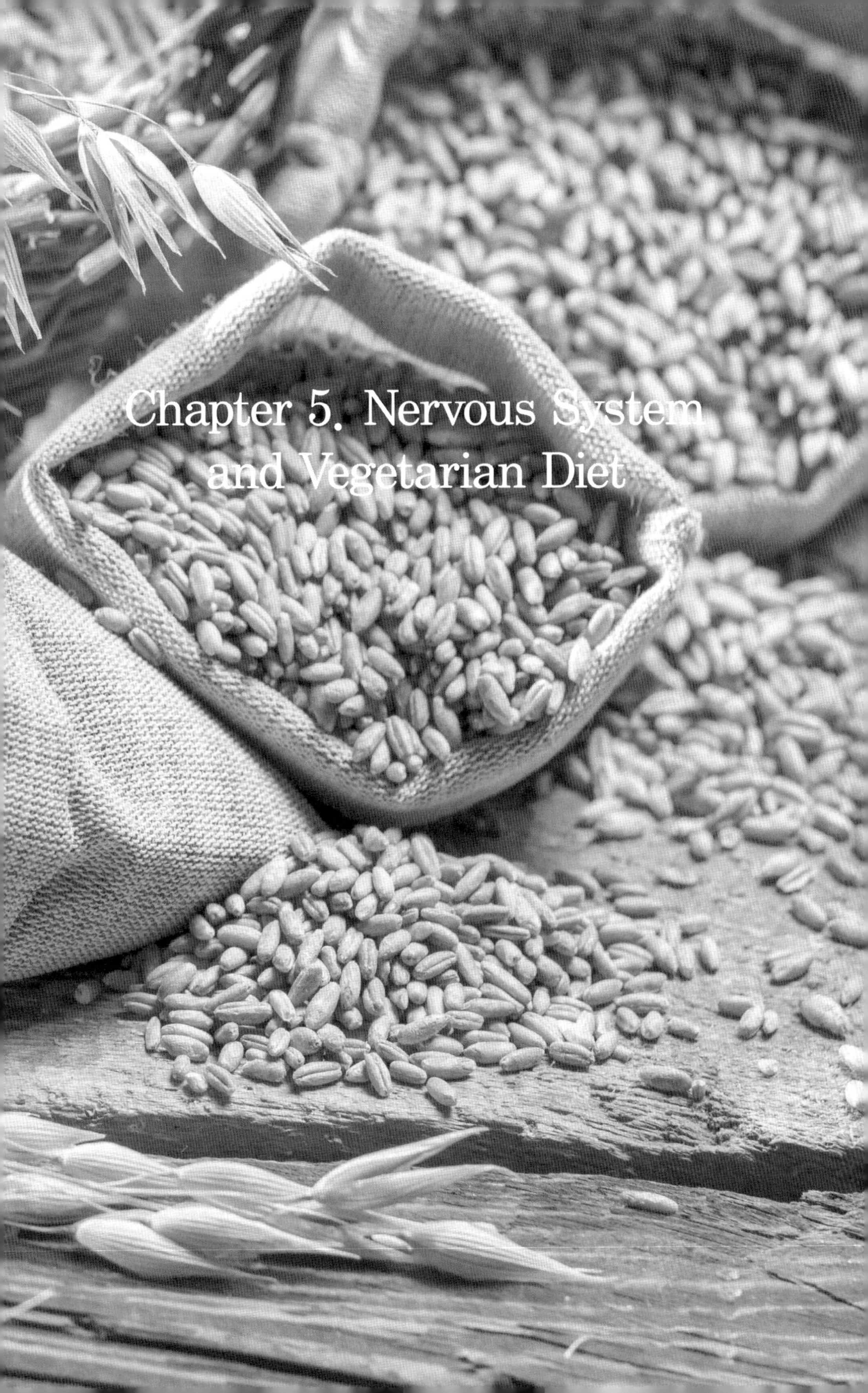

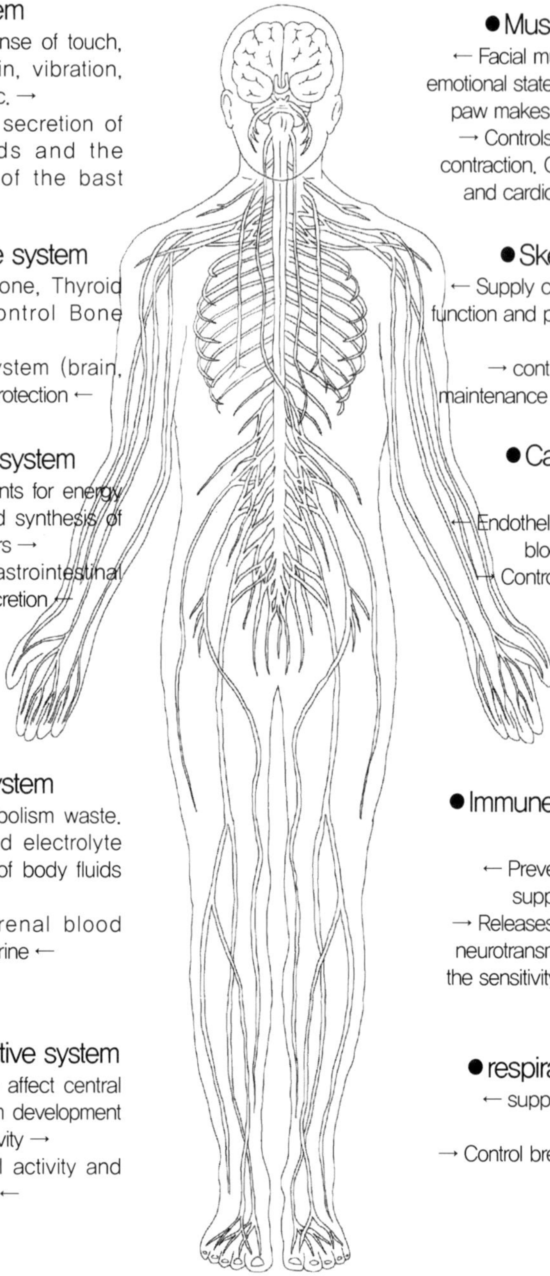

● Skin system

Provides a sense of touch, pressure, pain, vibration, temperature, etc. →
Controls the secretion of sweat glands and the contraction of the bast muscles ←

● Endocrine system

Growth Hormone, Thyroid Hormone Control Bone Growth →
Endocrine system (brain, chest, pelvis) protection ←

● Digestive system

Provides nutrients for energy generation and synthesis of neurotransmitters →
Controlling Gastrointestinal Motility and Secretion ←

● Urinary system

Remove metabolism waste. Adjust pH and electrolyte concentration of body fluids →
Controlling renal blood pressure and urine ←

● Reproductive system

Sex hormones affect central nervous system development and sexual activity →
Control sexual activity and sexual function ←

● Muscular system

← Facial muscles represent emotional state. The inner hind paw makes communication.
→ Controls skeletal muscle contraction. Control breathing and cardiovascular activity

● Skeletal system

← Supply calcium for nerve function and protect brain and spine
→ control bone growth, maintenance and positioning.

● Cardiovascular system

← Endothelial cells maintain blood–brain barrier
→ Control heart rate and blood pressure

● Immune / lymphatic system

← Prevent infection and support tissue repair
→ Releases hormones and neurotransmitters that affect the sensitivity of the immune response

● respiratory system

← supplies oxygen and removes CO_2
→ Control breathing rate and depth

Chapter.5 The nervous system and the vegetarian diet.

5.1. The structure and the role of the nervous system

In the nervous system, the cell that receives a signal from the outside of, or the inside of, the living organism is called the"sensory cell". The nervous system consists of the cells that can generate the action potentials and the cells that deliver the electrical signals are the neurons. Depending on the level of the structure in which the information is transferred from the sensory to the reactor, the animals can be divided into the following three categories:

The first is the animals with the simple structures, such as the sea anemone. They transmit the signals directly from the sensory to the effector through the neurons. The second is the animals that, like the squid, need the more active movements to find the food and the spouse. The neurons form the densely-packed ganglia to process more signals. The third is the vertebrate animals, which are in an advanced stage in which they memorize, organize, compare, and learn the signals. They are located at the center of

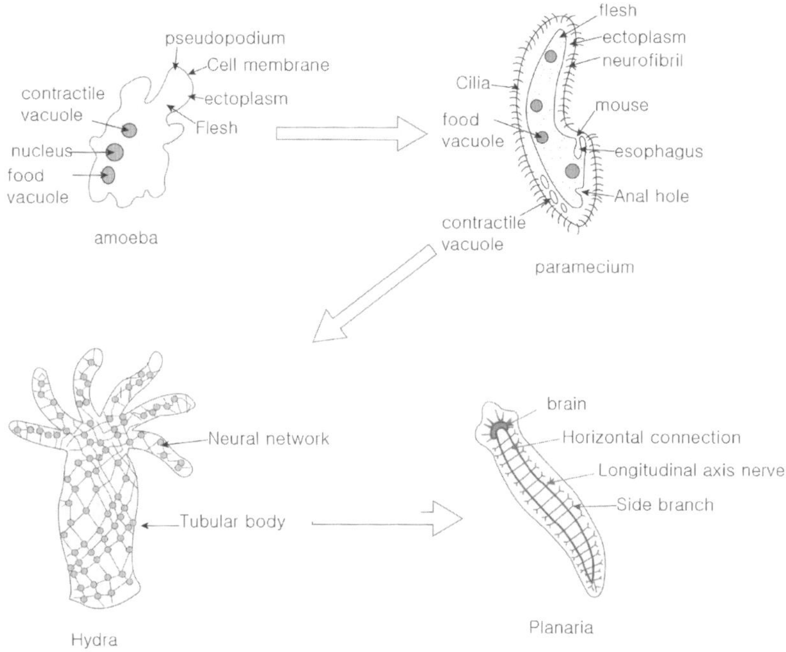

Figure 5–1. Developmental process of early nervous system

the ganglion, which is called the "brain". The brain, together with the spinal cord, constitutes the central nervous system (CNS). The neurons connected to the central nervous system, the sensory and the effector form the peripheral nervous system (PNS).

There are two types of the cells that constitute the central nervous system: The neurons and the glial cells. In the humans, the number of the neurons is 100 billion, and the glycopeptide is one trillion times ten times that number. If the total number of

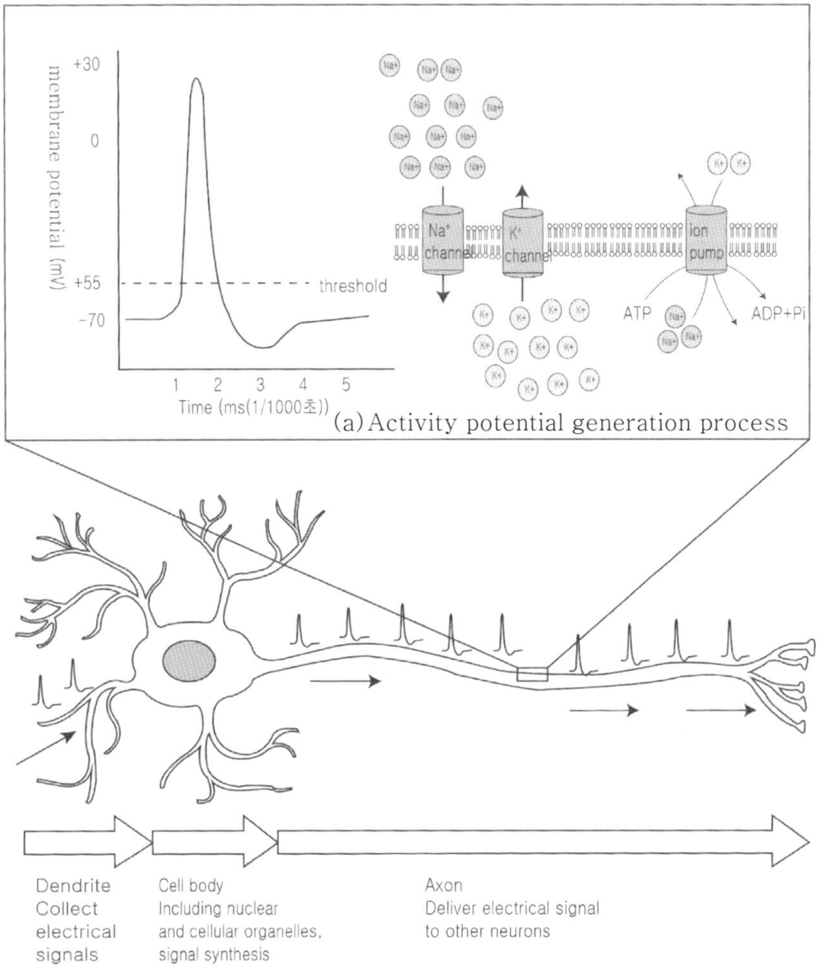

(a) Activity potential generation process

(b) Signaling process

Figure 5-2. The process of generating the voltage of the nerve cell

(a) In the resting state, the sodium cation outside the neuron cell has a high potassium concentration in the cell, and when the cell outside is 0, the inside of the cell has a negative voltage of −70 mM (polarization). When an external stimulus opens the sodium channel in the cell membrane of the neuron, the high concentration of sodium cation outside the neuron cell migrates into the cell. At this time, the inside of the cell is changed to the voltage of +30 mV compared to the outside of the cell (depolarization). As soon as the potassium cation channel is opened, the potassium cations inside the cell move out of the cell, and the inside of the cell returns to −70 mV again (repolarization). (b) The nerve signal is transmitted in the direction of dendrites, cell bodies, and axons.

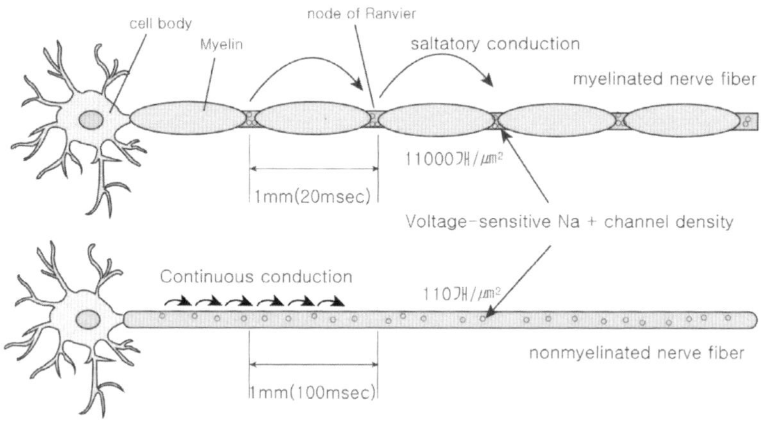

Figure 5-3. Differences between anhydrous and anterior nerves

((The anterior nerve is wrapped with myelin lipid, so the signaling rate is 100 times faster than anhydrosis))

Table 5-1. Characteristics of myelined nerve and non-myelined nerve

characteristic	Myelinated nerve	non-myelined nerves
Neurotransmission rate	100m/s	1m/s
Relative signal generation rate	34	1
The relative amount of information processing capacity	3000	1
Energetic mass required for neurotransmission	1	5000
Diameter of neurons required for signal transduction	1	400

the cells in the human body is about 50 clams, the central nervous system is about 2%. However, the energy used is 20%, which is the largest proportion for the animals.

The structure of the neurons can be divided into four parts: The cell body, the dendrites, the axons, and the axon terminals, and

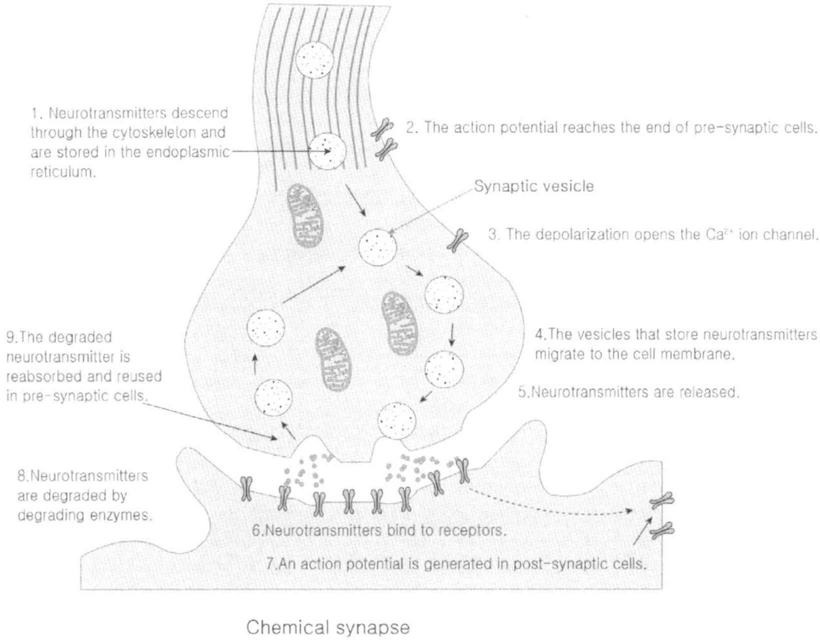

Figure 5–4. Signal transduction at synapses

each part has a characteristic function (Fig. 5–2). The dendrites are the protrusions like the branches that extend from the cell body and accept the information from the other neurons or sensory cells. Each type of neuron has the dendrites ranging from 4,000 to hundreds of thousands, making the connections with the other neurons. The cell body is the central part of the neuron with the nucleus and the cell organelles.

In the cell body, the information is synthesized to transmit the signals to the other neurons or motor cells, and the axons function. The thicker the axonal section, the faster the information transfer rate, the more the axon is insulated by the glial cells, and the faster the signal transmission. The coated portion wrapped around the lipids around the axon is called the "myelin", which is like a signal transmitted safely and accurately when the wire is coated with the PVC.

There are the nodule portions exposed between the myelinated portions, and the ion channels are dense. This causes the electrical signals of the neurons to be skipped over to the nodules. This is called "leaping", and the signaling rate is about 100 times faster than that of the anterior nerves that are not hydrated (Fig. 5–3).

The end of the axon is a small branch shape that is divided into the multiple strands from the axon, and the end is swollen. At this end, there are about 50 kinds of the neurotransmitters,which are the different kinds that are released to the other neurons to transmit the signals. The cells that send the neurotransmitters are called the "pre–synaptic cells", and the cells that receive the released chemical signal at the receptor are called the "post–synaptic cells". The distance between the neurons is called the "synaptic gap." (Fig. 5–4).

Glycopeptide is more than 10 billion times the number of the 100 billion neurons in the brain. Glycoproteins are the very important cells that do not receive or transmit any signals but play a crucial role in the survival and function of the neurons. There are many different types and functions of the glycoproteins, including the insulator function of the neurons, known as the myelin structure (low dendritic cells), the ability to receive the nutrients from the blood vessels to supply the nutrients to the neurons (glial cells), the ability to receive the foreign substances (small cells), and the function to protect the neurons by creating a barrier between the blood vessels and the brain (glial cells).

Glycopeptide is more than 10 billion times the number of 100 billion neurons in the brain. Glycoproteins are very important cells that do not receive or transmit signals but play a crucial role in the survival and function of neurons. There are many different types and functions of glycoproteins, including the insulator function of the neurons known as the myelin structure (low dendritic cells), the ability to receive nutrients from the blood vessels to supply nutrients to neurons (glial cells), foreign matter (Small cell), the function to protect the neurons by creating a barrier between the blood vessels and the brain (glial cells).

Central nervous system

The nervous system is divided into the central nervous system and the peripheral nervous system. The central nervous system is again composed of the brain and spinal cord. The brain is floating on a clear liquid called cerebrospinal fluid and is wrapped in a thin tissue like a spider web. The brain is divided into two parts, the left brain and the right brain, and it has the same size and shape as if it had its own two fists. 85% of the brain is water, and lipids account for more than 80% except water. The adult brain weighs about 1400 grams and weighs about 2% of the human body, but uses 20% energy. The main energy source is glucose, and in the case of fasting, a ketone body, which is made by converting lipids, is used as a main energy source. Even if the supply of oxygen is stopped

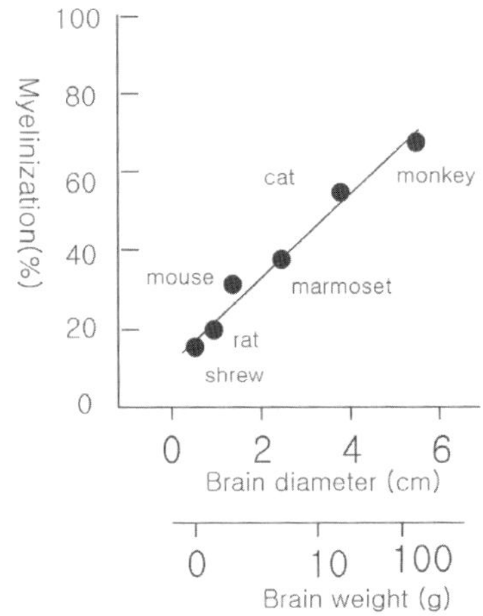

Figure 5-5. Comparison of myelinization of animals

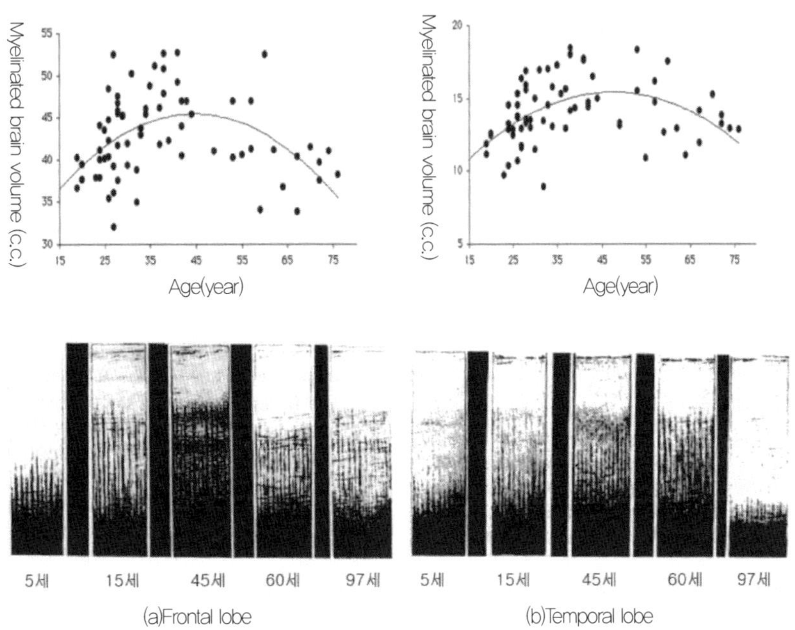

Figure 5-6. Myelination according to the age of a person

for only 4 to 5 minutes, the function is damaged. The brain has a variety of neurotransmitters that cause electrochemical reactions that can lead to an accident.

Brain consists of cerebrum, limbic system, gangrene, brain stem. The cerebrum accounts for 80% of the brain, the left is the general interpretation and the language center, the right is the sensory information analysis and the space interpretation, so it is also called the representational hemisphere. The cortex, which is about 4 mm thick, has a gray body (gray matter), but the amount of the brain is connected to the right and left brains. In reality, the gray matter is pink due to blood when it is alive. The brain has a lot of wrinkles and spreads to more than one sheet of newspaper, which can result in the placement of many neurons. The crest of the wrinkle is the ridge and the groove is the furrow. The cerebral cortex is divided into four parts: the frontal lobe (mystery, memory, and horse), temporal lobe (auditory sense, taste and smell), occipital lobe The main functions are divided and different.

The diencephalon is located inside and center of the cerebral hemisphere and consists of the thalamus, hypothalamus, and pituitary gland. The thalamus receives all sensory information from the body except the olfactory, and coordinates the flow of neural signals to connect to other parts of the brain. The hypothalamus has an "internal clock" and controls and receives signals about body temperature, body fluids, electrolytes, appetite, sleep,

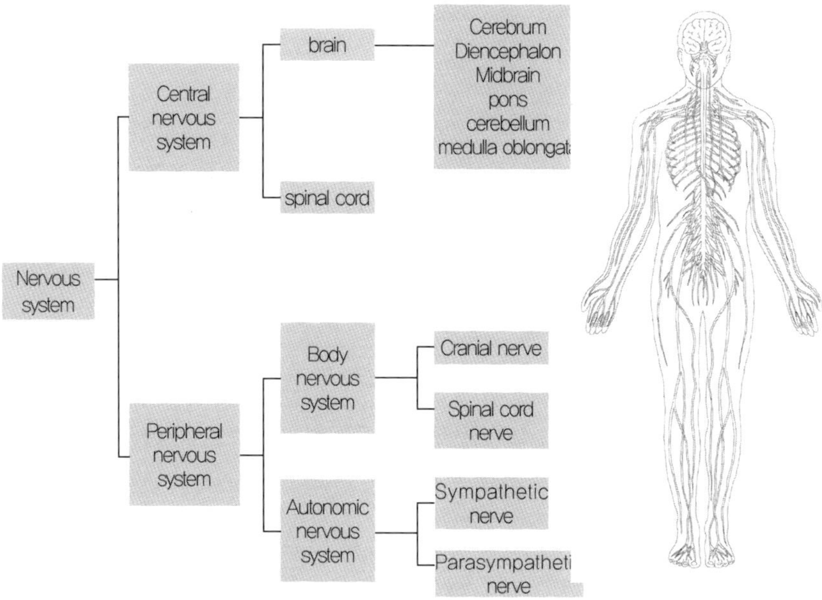

Figure 5-7. The nervous system of the human body

thirst, moisture, pulse, and blood pressure. The weight of the hypothalamus is not less than 1% of the brain weight, but it has the highest endocrine function and plays a key role in the homeostasis of the whole body by continuously controlling the lower hormone system. In other words, the nervous system and the endocrine system are integrated into the neuroendocrine system through the function of the hypothalamic neurons and endocrine cells.

The pituitary gland is in the form of a small pea at the front of the hypothalamus and amplifies by receiving electrical and chemical signals from the hypothalamic neurons. The pineal gland is a human body clock in the ventricle that releases melatonin to induce sleep.

The limbic system is developed from the mammalian stage and is responsible for emotions and motivation. Cerebral cortex, dentate gyrus, hippocampus, amygdala, brainstem, thalamus, hypothalamus, and brainstem. The hippocampus is related to the storage of memory contents, and the one way is associated with various emotions such as fear and anxiety, excitement, sadness, anger and so on. Behind the cerebrum is a cabbage-shaped cerebellum that is responsible for basic motor function.

The brain stem, also called the reptilian brain, connects the brain and spinal cord. In other words, all signals coming and going between the brain and the body should basically go through the brain stem. In reptiles such as lizards, the brainstem accounts for most of the brain. The basic functions of life such as breathing, pulse, blinking of the eye are covered by the brain stem. The brain stem can be divided into three parts: midbrain, pons, and training. The uppermost part of the brain stem receives signals from the eyes and ears to the midbrain and sends them to the thalamus. There are a lot of motor nerves, and it prevents other external stimuli from entering the brain during sleep. The pons is the leg brain and connects the cerebral cortex with the soft tissue. Pons leads to the sleeping phase of dreaming REM. The medulla oblongata is at the bottom of the brainstem and regulates respiration and heart rate. Coughing, swallowing, and vomiting.

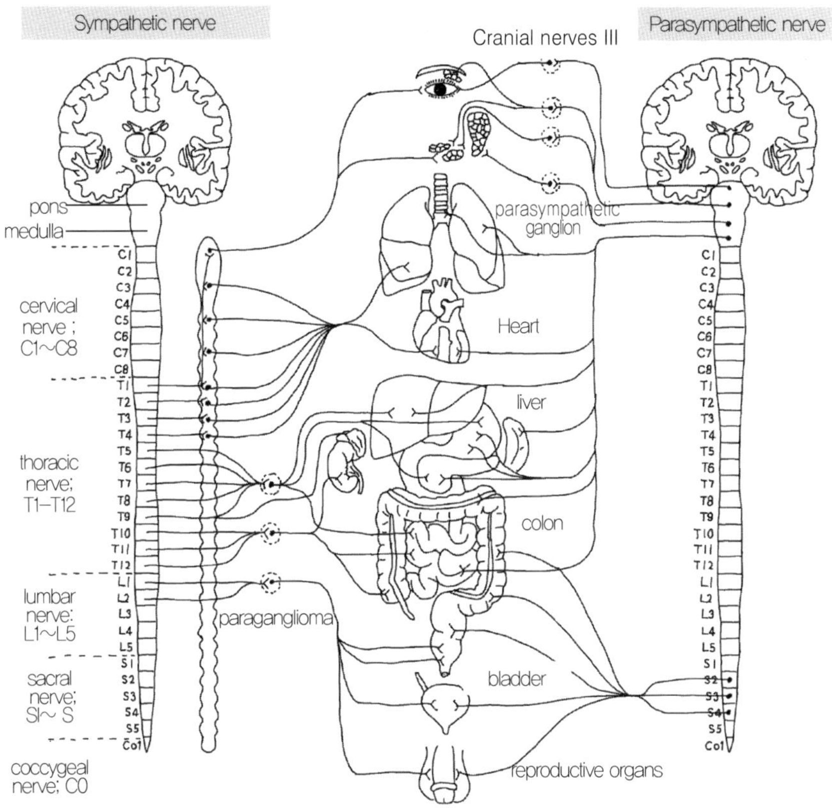

Figure 5–8. Sympathetic and parasympathetic nerves

The spinal cord is a bundle of nerves that connect the signal of the whole body to the brain and descend along the center of the spine.

Peripheral nervous system

The peripheral nervous system can be divided into the body nervous system and the autonomic nervous system to transmit and receive signals from the body terminal and the central nervous system. The body nerve is subdivided into two parts, cranial nerve and spinal nerve. Cranial nerves include twelve pairs of nerves connected directly to the brain, each with a unique name. Based on the function, the cranial nerves are sensory or sensory nerves, and Ⅲ, Ⅳ, Ⅵ, and VII cranial nerves are motor nerves, Ⅴ, Ⅶ, Ⅸ, It is classified as a mixed nerve.

The spinal nerve has 31 pairs of peripheral nerves entering and leaving the vertebral segments. There are 8 pairs of cervical nerves, 12 pairs of thoracic nerves, 5 pairs of lumbar nerves, 5 pairs of sacral nerves and 1 pair of coccygeal nerves. The nervous system controls the senses of skeletal muscles and senses that move according to the will, while the autonomic nervous system is distributed in the blood vessels, internal organs, glands, etc. to maintain the homeostasis of the human body unconsciously or reflexively. Because of this, the plant has the nickname of the nervous system. The autonomic nervous system can be divided into the sympathetic nervous system and the parasympathetic nervous system, both of which must be connected to other neurons in the ganglia to synapse in order for the axons starting from the brain and spinal cord to go into the corresponding organ. The preganglionic nerve fibers are called preganglionic fibers,

5.2. IQ examination of the vegetarian children

The American, vegetarian population is said to be over 7%. It is not hard to buy the vegetarian foods in a reasonable supermarket, and you can eat the vegetarian burgers conveniently at the fast food restaurants. The vegetarians organize the groups to spread the information on the benefits of the vegetarian diet, and, at the site of the animal protection group, there is a vegetarianism guide in the corner that emphasizes the vegetarian practice. The groups, such as the People for the Ethical Treatment of Animals (PETA), have more than one million members. However, until the 1970s and the 1980s, there had been the many suspicious views that the vegetarian diet could provide enough nutrition for the body. Of course, the main topic of the vegetarian papers published in the academic area since the 1990s is the findings on the prevention and treatment effects of the vegetarian diet.

Dwyer noted that, in the 1970s, he had been interested in the growth curve of the young vegetarians and that they would continue to be the vegetarians, including their children after they were married [1]. There have been the reports that the physical development and the mental abilities of many children in the Third World, which can only be vegetarian, nowadays, are much lower than the average. For example, in India, about 5% of all children had been in a depressed state, with the intelligence quotient (IQ) of 11. Therefore, this study was designed with the belief that the vegetarian children, also, lack the nutrition and, thus, their IQ may be lower than the average.

Thus, a growth and nutrition survey had been conducted for 28 vegetarian children living in the Boston area between 1974 and 1977, after receiving the parental consent. The children participating in the experiment were only from 2 years old to 8.4 years old, and the average age was only 4 years and 9 months old. All investigated children had been breastfed for an average of 10 months, and they began to eat the solids 6 months after their birth.

Seventeen children were the vegetarians who followed the vegetarian diet of Boston's East–West Organization, eight were the vegetarians who had their own diet, and three were the vegetarians who followed the dietary recommendations of the Seventh–day Adventist Church. Six of the healthy vegetarian children were the vegans. The nutrition survey was conducted by having a 24–hour recall, which recalled the memories within 24 hours of eating. The nutrition survey showed that all of the nutrients and calories intakes were enough to meet the recommended amounts, except for 23% protein, 13% lipid, 28% carbohydrate, and 64% total calories. However, the vitamin D and the vitamin B12 showed the particularly low intakes in the vegan children.

The IQ test was conducted under the guidance of a professional in a quiet room to avoid the distractions. The IQ is based on the average of the IQ according to the age, and the relative value is 100 (Figure 5–9). The survey results were in antithesis to the

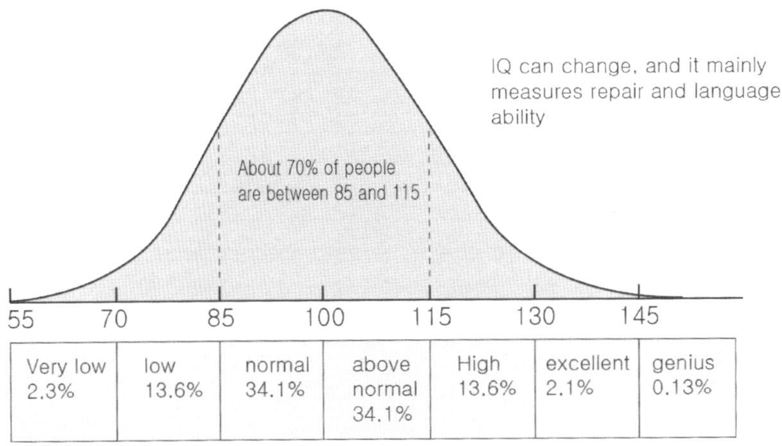

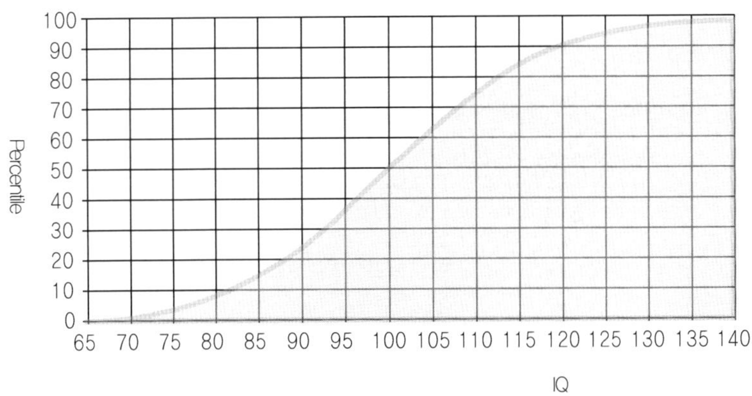

Figure 5-9. Distribution of IQ scores and intelligence level
The IQ of vegan is located in the top 90% of the average.

Table 5-2. The average IQ of vegetarian children [1]

Vegetarian form		Number of participants	Average IQ
Mactobiotic vegetarian	Vegan	6	119.3
	Lacto-ovo vegetarian	11	111.3
	Sum	17	114.1
General vegetarian		11	118.3
Total vegetarian average		28	115.8
Non-vegetarian			99

expectations of the researchers. The IQ of the vegetarian children surveyed was 116, which was much higher than the average of less than 100. The average IQ for the vegan girls, who were the 6 out of the 17 healthy and vegetarian children, was 119,and the average of the remaining 11 vegetarian children was 111. It was said that feeding the vegetarian diet to the children had shown the above-average, mental development. And the poor children in the Third World showed the lower scores regarding their mental development and their IQ testing, not because they were vegetarians, but because of the severe nutritional deficiencies, the very low levels of the education, the lack of medical care, and the exposure to the infectious diseases

There is another study about the relationship between vegetarian diet patterns and IQ. Although the reasons are not yet clear, intelligence is linked to health and survival potential. Several studies have shown that high IQ in childhood and adolescence is a lower risk of cardiovascular disease in adults. Gale and colleagues examined 8170 British men and women in their 30s who participated in a cohort study in the 1970s with their vegetarian diet and childhood IQs [2]. Children who were 10 years old at the time of 1970 were tested for intellectual competence over four categories: word definition, word similarity, numerical recall, and arithmetic. These scores are converted into IQs set to an average of 100 and 1Table sub-deviation of 15.

In their 30s, they were interviewed at home and asked if they were vegetarian and if they were vegetarian. A total of 366 respondents answered that they had a vegetarian diet, of which 123 were eating fish or chicken. Women (n=271, 74%) were more vegetarians than men (95, 26%) and those who answered that they were vegetarians had a high social status both during childhood and now. Had higher academic and language skills, but socioeconomic benefits did not reflect income. In the case of males, the average IQ was 106.1 for those in their teens who were vegetarians in their 30s, while the IQ for those not vegetarians was 100.6. In the case of women, the average IQ of women in their 30s was 104.0, while those of non-vegetarians were 99.0. That is, the IQ differences between male and female childhoods were 5.5 and 5.0, respectively, and these differences were statistically significant.

Their experiments have been related to knowing whether intelligence influences the choice of lifestyle that helps health. Before these studies, five studies have shown that the mortality

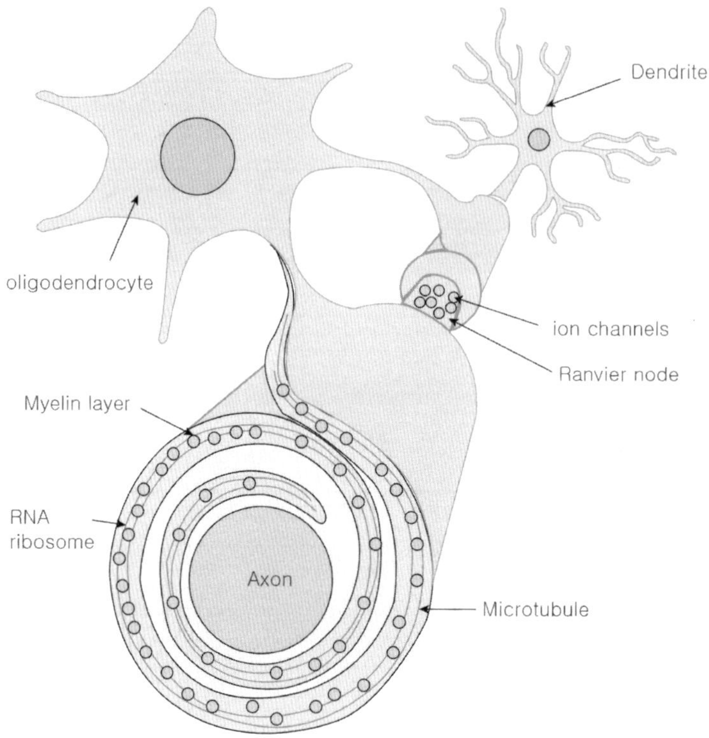

Figure 5-10. Structure and neurons of lipid myelin

rate of vegetarians is 76% lower than that of non–vegetarians even after adjusting for age, sex, and smoking. The vegetarians ate more vegetables, legumes, fruits, whole wheat bread, while less red meat. And the vegetarian patterns of life were lowering mortality from diseases such as cardiovascular disease and cancer. Another UK study of 1946 births found that children who ate a lot of fruit during their childhood grew up in the middle years, while children who ate fewer fruits during their childhood were eating small amounts of fruit in their growth. Positive nutrients that affect IQ include vitamin B, omega–3 fatty acids, and unsaturated fat. In addition to these, antioxidants and vitamins will be added. On the other hand, high levels of cholesterol, saturated fats, carcinogens in the carcasses, steroid hormones in the meat, and cellular waste will be negative nutrients for normal IQ development.

IQ is based on 100 for each age group. 1Table The semi–deviation is 15 points, and between 85 and 115, 68.2% people enter. And 95.4% of the 2Table semi–deviation range from 70 to 130. Meaning that the average of vegan children is 119 means that they are within the top 10%. Conversely, we can see how much the meat–centered daycare center and school meals are lowering our kids' IQs. IQ is mainly measured by repair and language ability. However, the effects of dietary patterns may affect the entire human body and overall intelligence?

5.3 The cranial protection against the antioxidants

The brain weighs about 2% of the whole body, but the calories used are from 20% to 30%. Thus, the brain is one of the most oxygen-intensive organs with the most calories among the body organs. A problem is that the free radicals that the nutrients in the brain make as a byproduct by burning the calories, also, increase.

The radical is a compound in which the two oxygen atoms, like the ordinary oxygen in the air, are not in a stable state but are either alone or in an unstable state by receiving the electrons. They try to give the extra electrons to another atom or molecule because the former is more or less than the normal one. When an electron is given to another substance, the substance that receives the electron becomes unstable and transmits it back to its surroundings. This chain reaction causes the active oxygen to have a very large, destructive power in the cell.

There are, also, the studies that say that the active oxygen is produced in one of the 25 oxygen molecules that are used in combustion and that more than 90% of all the diseases that occur are related to the reactive oxygen species. In other words, the active oxygen that is required to kill the bacteria is not properly regulated, and, if it is over-produced, the cells, the tissues, and the genes of the body are destroyed indiscriminately.

In particular, the brain is the most abundant organ among the body organs, and fat is very susceptible to the attack by the active oxygen. Therefore, the role of the antioxidants for the brain health is very important. The antioxidant activity in the human body is involved with the endogenous, antioxidant enzymes and the exogenous vitamins. Glutathione peroxidase, superoxide dismutase (SOD), catalase, and celluloplasmin are the endogenous, antioxidant enzymes. And the food ingredients are vitamin C, vitamin E, and the beta carotene.And the various phytochemicals are the exogenous antioxidants. In particular, vitamin C plays two roles in the formation of the aqueducts of the neurons that are important for the function of the brain. One is the cofactor of the myelin-forming enzyme that surrounds the neuron, and the other is the antioxidant that blocks the free radicals from forming in a few seconds. In the mycelial formation, the antioxidants function in a number of the mutually-independent ways, and, when one is present, it is a disorder.

The study of the importance of the antioxidants and vitamin C

Table 5-3. Vitamin C and vitamin E, the antioxidant effect of myelination [2]

Combination of compounds	Average myelination
vitamin C + vitamin E + antioxidant	18.80
vitamin C + antioxidant	12.46
vitamin E	0.00
vitamin C	0.625
vitamin C + vitamin E	8.00

GLIA 45:54-58(2004)

Table 5-4. Vitamin intake of Swedish and non-vegetarians [3]

Type	female			male		
	non-vegetarian	vegan	lacto-ovo vegetarian	non-vegetarian	vegan	lacto-ovo vegetarian
vitamin A (RE)	700	966	1,169	750	1,045	1,226
Thiamin (mg)	0.9	1.5	1.5	1.1	1.9	2.2
Riboflavin (mg)	1.1	1.1	1.9	1.4	1.2	2.8
niacin (NE)	12	26	32	15	34	48
vitamin B6 (mg)	1	2.1	2.0	1.3	2.7	2.8
vitamin B12 (μg)	1.4	0.0	5.0	1.4	0.1	5.9
folic acid (μg)	120	473	226	140	551	263
vitamin C (mg)	30	178	104	30	203	96
vitamin D (μg)	2.5	2.0	5.1	2.5	3.7	7.7
vitamin E (α-TE)	3.0	13	7.3	4.0	18	9.2

vitamin Refining and other supplements are excluded. vegan and lacto-ovo vegetarian are 15 each..
Am J Clin Nutr (2002) 76:100-6

in the formations of the herbaceous plants at the Mayo University School of Medicine in 2004 is noteworthy. The researchers excluded, one-by-one, the combination of the antioxidants, vitamin C, and vitamin E, and the nerve cells had been grown in the test tubes, and the rate of the formation of a few seconds in the brain cells was confirmed. The results showed that, when all three are included, the best growth in a few seconds is achieved(Table 5-3) [2]. Myelination is a very complex process to form the lipid membranes, so it can be assumed that the various forms of the antioxidants will work in a variety of the situations.

In other words, it is the easiest and most effective way to get the complex antioxidants through the natural foods rather than through some refined vitamin tablets. Vitamin E is an antioxidant that is especially important for the lipid oxidation and is rich in nuts and the like.

Most studies report that the vegetarians consume more fresh vegetables, fruits, and nuts than the non-vegetarians. One example had been in Sweden. In Sweden, roughly 5% of the students aged from 16 to 20 had received the school meals with the Uranus, vegetarian diet, and 0.1% had receivedthe fully vegetarian meals. In certain areas, such as the Northwest region of Sweden, the vegetarian meals had accounted for 2%. In Sweden, where the institutional, vegetarian meals had been well-established, they had been interested in increasing the student vegetarians and their vitamin intakes. As a result, the vegetarians had a higher intake of all the vitamins, except vitamin B12, than that of the non-vegetarians (Table 5-4) [3]. Perhaps, these results could be one of the explanations for the beneficial effects of vegetarian diet on the brain development.

5.4. The antioxidants and the Alzheimer's disease

The cause of dementia is not known precisely, but it is essentially related to brain cell damage. Alzheimer's disease and vascular dementia account for the majority of the dementia in the West, while, in Asia, there are many cases of stroke and vascular dementia.

The weight of the brain is only 2% of the body's weight, but it consumes a lot of oxygen, which is more than 20% of the total oxygen used by the body. The place to generate the energy by burning the fuel called "glucose" is the mitochondria, which are the organelles in the cell. About 1% of the oxygen used is not completely burned, and this produces the active oxygen and the free radicals. Thus, proper antioxidant supply is an important factor in

Table 5-5. Alzheimer's risk and antioxidant study summary [6]

Study	treatment	Results
Honululu Asian Aging Research (71-93 years old, 3,385 male)	vitamin C and E supplements	Vascular dementia lowered, Alzheimer's disease improved cognitive function
Nursing Health Research (70-79 years old, 14,968 female)	vitamin C and E supplements	Improve overall score than unused people
Rural group study (4,540 persons, 90% over 65 years old)	vitamin C and E supplements	Reduced risk of Alzheimer's disease, No effect when using vitamin alone
Chicago Health and Aging Project (2,889 communities, 65 to 102 years old)	In food, vitamin C, E, carotene	Vitamin E is effective in reducing cognition

Lancet Neurol 2004; 3:579-87

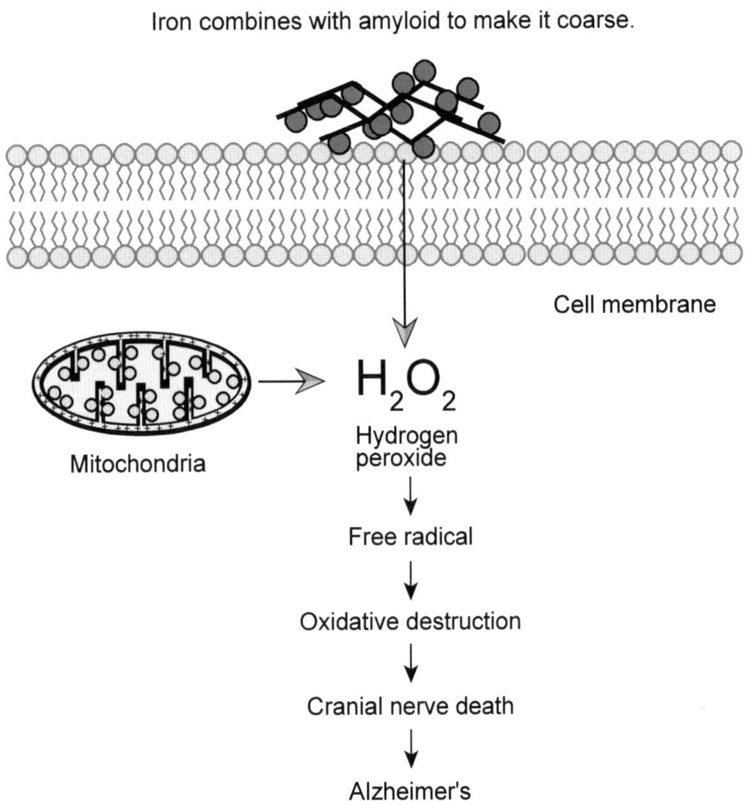

Figure 5-11. Oxidative stress process of Alzheimer's disease

maintaining the brain structure and function (Table 5-5).

Free radicals play an important role in the progression of the Alzheimer's disease, where the brain cells are destroyed. Research has shown that the process proceeds roughly as follows [4]:

First, if glutathione, an antioxidant enzyme, is not depleted or

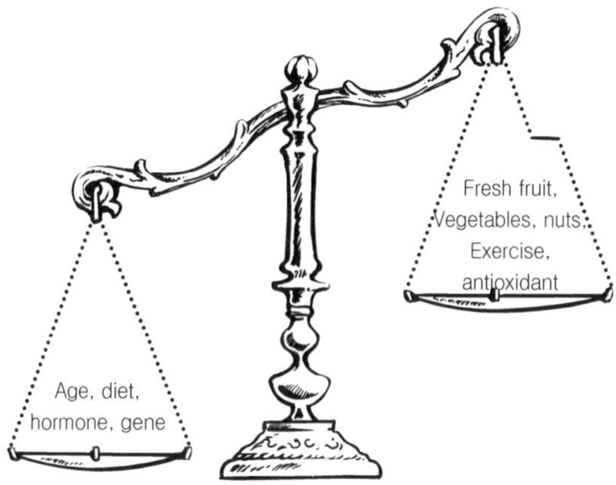

Figure 5-12. Risk factors for Alzheimer's disease and scales of therapeutic factors

reused for any reason, the free metal that does not bind to the protein accumulates in the brain tissue and starts to destroy the cranial nerve.

Second, the proteins are denatured to form the senescent plaques, which, in turn, increase the release of the inflammatory cytokines (Fig. 5-11).

Third, the iron binds to the modified proteins again, which, in turn, increases the free radicals. Eventually, the brain cells are gradually destroyed.

Notably, the metals, such as aluminum, iron, zinc, and copper, accelerate the aggregation of the specific proteins in the brain. Copper promotes the production of amylopectin beta in the pH range of from 7.4 to 6.8. It is necessary to remember that the animal food acidifies the human body.

Considering the above process, we can suggest the following several ways to prevent and slow down the progression of the Alzheimer's disease.

(1) Reducing the production of the free radicals to a stable level

(2) Increasing the antioxidants that can block the excess free radicals

(3) The supply of the omega-3 fatty acids that can block the inflammatory molecules. (Figure 5-12).

In fact, the concentration of the antioxidants in the blood of the Alzheimer's patients is lower than in the normal people. The antioxidant supplementation through food prevents the various diseases, including the central nervous system. In particular, vitamin C and vitamin E are known to be beneficial to the brain diseases. These vitamins are abundant in plants, including the nuts and the vegetables.

5.5. The excessive intake of the minerals and brain damage

Free metal ions play an important role in the brain damage process. In particular, an excessive increase in the iron in the blood increases the oxidation of the genes and the proteins in the cell, which, ultimately, contributes to the development of the brain diseases, such as the Alzheimer's disease and the Parkinson's disease. Iron is a typical transition metal because it facilitates the transfer of the electrons to catalyze the various chemical reactions.

From this viewpoint, the heme iron that is rich in the animal foods can cause an excessive iron uptake, which can be an important factor in the degenerative brain diseases. If you only look at the iron intake, the vegetarian diet has more of it than the animal-centered diet. However, the non-heme iron of the vegetarian diet has a very wide absorption spectrum, which varies ten times from 2.0% to 22.5% depending on the condition of the human body. On the other hand, the absorptivity of the hemp iron is doubled from 26% to 47%, and it has a narrower absorption rate than the vegetarian diet. This difference has a significant effect on the human body.

If the amount of the vegetable nonhemmetal consumed in a meal increases by four times from 1.5 mg to 6.0 mg, the portion absorbed by the human body is reduced by one third from 18% to 6%. Therefore, the total amounts of the iron that are actually absorbed are 1.5 mg × 0.18 = 0.27 mg and 6.0 × 0.06 = 0.36 mg, and a

Table 5-6. Degenerative brain diseases associated with metals [7]

disease	Related Metals	Metal protein, enzyme
Alzheimer's disease	cupper, iron, zinc	Amylopectin beta
Parkinson's disease	iron	Neuro melanin, etc.
Mad cow disease	cupper, iron	prion protein
Multiple sclerosis	iron	Not revealed
Down syndrome	cupper,iron,zinc	Amylopectin beta

L⊥Lancet Neurol 2004;3:431-34

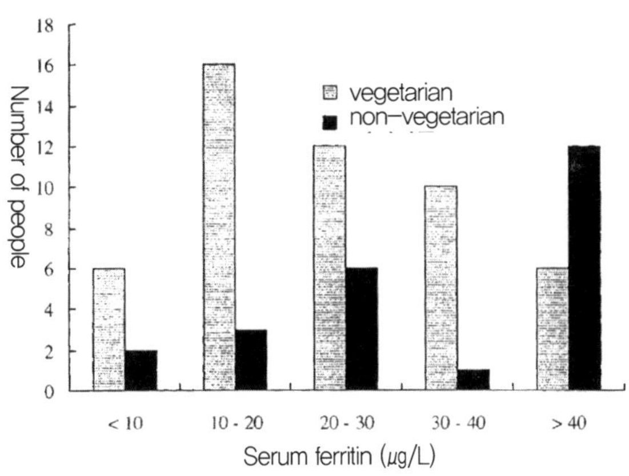

Figure 5-13. Serum ferritin comparison between vegetarian and non-vegetarian

certain amount of the iron enters the human body without any significant difference.

On the other hand, the heme iron absorbs 20% of the iron ingested, from 1.5mg to 6.0mg, into the human body, which is very different from0.3mg to 1.2mg. Thus, the amount of the hemolysis that is absorbed in the human body varies by 20 times depending on the situation.

The problem is that the excess iron in the hemp iron is used in the human body and accumulates in the cells and the tissues, which causes the oxidation and causes the various diseases. The list of these diseases includes the various brain diseases, including the Alzheimer's disease.

According to most reports, the vegetarians have the lower iron levels in their blood than the non-vegetarians. However, they are higher than the anemic standard. For example, there was a 1999 presentation on the iron intake and the body condition in the Australian, vegetarian women.

Ball and Bartlett had examined the amount of the iron ingested and the body retention on the part of 50 vegetarian women and 24 non-vegetarian women who were aged from 18 to 45 in Australia. The average daily intake of the iron among the vegetarians was 10.7 mg, which was slightly higher than that of the non-vegetarians, but the mean serum ferritin was lower among the vegetarians. However, there was no anemia in these patients (Figure 5-13) [7].

Ferritin is an iron storage protein that is used in the human body and stores the remaining iron. It can bind up to 4,000 irons per minute. The researchers pointed out that the abnormally high levels of the ferritin are harmful to the human body, although it can be a problem if an excessive iron loss occurs at the low ferritin levels. And the blood ferritin levels of the vegetarians are said to be within the stable range. Excessive accumulation of iron in the body is associated with the progression of the various degenerative diseases, such as cardiovascular disease and diabetes. In other words, the vegetarians will absorb the necessary amount of iron and prevent the unnecessary, excessive risks.

5.6. Vascular dementia.

Vascular dementia, which is common among Asians, is caused by a damage to the large blood vessels in the brain or a damage to the small blood vessels in the brain. In the central nervous system, 55 ml of the blood flows at a rate of 100 g per 1 minute. If the blood flow is slowed down, the normal function of the nerve cell is lost. If the blood flow is less than 10 ml, the brain tissue dies. This is called "the infarct of the brain tissue".

Ischemic stroke is often caused by thrombosis or embolism, especially when the blood flow is rapidly deteriorating. Thrombosis and embolism are the blood clots that are tangled with the cholesterol or the platelet aggregation, such as the plaque. When the blood clots block the blood vessels and a severe ischemia occurs, the energy initially stored in the nerve cells and the glycoproteins are depleted, followed by a destruction of the membrane potential process, which, in turn, leads to an excessive secretion of the excitatory neurotransmitters. This process destroys the neurons in a chain. Often,the large blood vessel injuries are caused by cerebral infarction, but the small blood vessel injuries are caused by hypertension or diabetes.

And the brain cells damage is a symptom of dementia, such as the delayed information processing, the memory impairment, the concentration deficiency, the depression, the weakening of the motor function, the Parkinson's disease, and the dysuria.

Thrombosis and embolism, which cause stroke, are from the same source as the cardiovascular disease that attacks. Therefore, it would be natural and effective to assume that a vegetarian diet that is beneficial to cardiovascular disease would be beneficial to stroke at the same time.

Several dietary factors have been shown to affect the vasculature, such as "Good for the heart is good for the head," which can be beneficial for the prevention of dementia.

In the fatty acid region, it is necessary to reduce the saturated fat and the cholesterol, to consume a lot of the unsaturated fatty acids, and to take the omega-3 and the omega-6 among the polyunsaturated fatty acids within the ratios of from 1:2 to 1:4. Several epidemiologic studies have shown that, the higher the intake of the omega-3, unsaturated, fatty acids, the lower the dementia. Omega-3 lowers the risk of a thrombus formation, thus, lowering the risk of a cardiovascular disease, lowering the risk of a cerebral infarction, and lowering the risk of vascular dementia. On the other hand, a high intake of the linoleic acid, belonging to the omega-6 family, increases the oxidation of the LDL-cholesterol, which causes more atherosclerosis and, eventually, worsens the cardiovascular disease, and damages the cerebral blood vessels.

The foods that are the most abundant with the omega-3 fats are the perilla and the flaxseed, followed by a variety of the nuts, seeds, and legumes.

5.7. Postpartum depression and the essential,fatty acids in mothers.

Increasingly,the depressed patients are increasing worldwide. In the United States, 60 years after 1945, thedepression had increased 20-fold. The World Health Organization (WHO) estimates that, by 2020, the most common illness will be depression.

However, psychological studies related to drugs or cognitive behavior are elaborately developed and prescribed, but, a considerable proportion of the depression patients do not improve their symptoms, and the depressive patients are increasing. The main reason is that the cause of depression has not yet been clearly identified, so, neither the prescription nor the treatment mechanism is clear. However, it is clear that depression is essentially related to the abnormalities in the neuronal function. Therefore, the maintenance of the healthy nerve cells is the first item to prevent and treat depression, and a nutritional approach, including the lipid, is needed.

In 2002, Dr. Hibbeln summarized the results of 41 studies from 23 countries that had already been published, and analyzed the relationship between the postpartum depression and the fish intake. He made two assumptions: One was that postpartum depression would be low in the countries with the high fish intakes, and the second hypothesis was that the high levels of the DHA in the maternal milk would have a low rate of the postpartum depression.

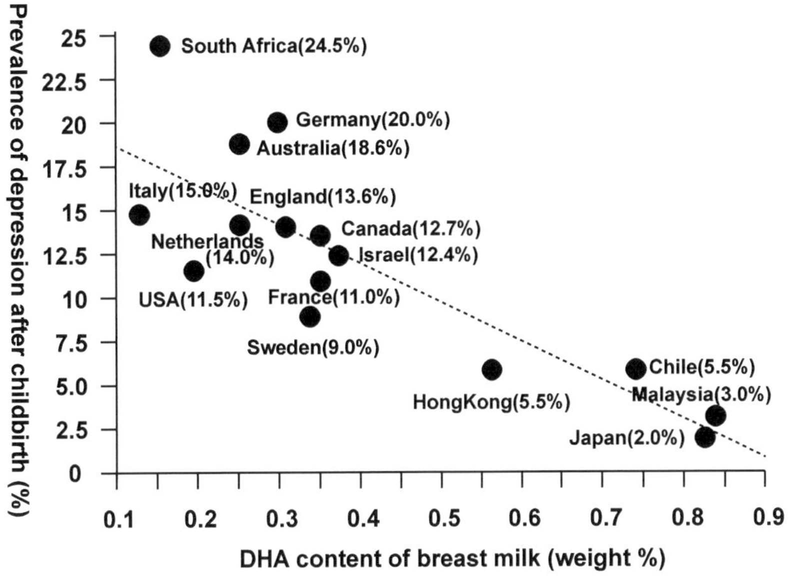

Figure 5-14. Relationship between DHA content of breast milk and depression after childbirth [8]

DHA in breast milk represents the maternal serum DHA level. The higher the DHA content of breast milk, the lower the prevalence of depression.

He calculated the EPA and DHA intakes based on the fish intake data that were reported. It is known that the composition of the fatty acid in the maternal milk is an index of the maternal, fatty acid composition. According to his research, when the breast milk was investigated in each country, the higher the DHA content of the breast milk, the lower the depression after the childbirth (Fig.

Table 5–7. polyunsaturated fatty acid intake of vegetarianfemale and non-vegetarianfemale

vegetarian diet	group	Linoleic acid (omega–6)	Linolenic acid (omega–3)
veganfemale	Non–lactating(10)	21.4±3.23	1.2±0.22
	lactating(19)	20.4±2.49	1.2±0.28
lacto–ovo vegetarianfemale	Non–lactating(18)	14.6±1.69	1.5±0.17
	lactating(21)	14.2±1.25	0.9±0.10
non–vegetarianfemale	Non–lactating(10)	9.1±1.07	1.1±0.15
	lactating(22)	11.8±1.22	1.0±0.08

J Pediatr (1992) 120:S71–7

5–14) [8].

These studies have shown that, when a diet lacking the essential fatty acids was supplied to the mother rats, the brain cells of the young rats had decreased the number of the dendrites, the length of the dendrites became shorter, and the cognition of the infants when the DHAs and the arachidonic acid had been properly supplied had developed.

The polyunsaturated fatty acids play an important role in the brain's actions, accounting for about 20% of the mass of the dried brain, excluding water, and about 30% of the central nervous system. Therefore, the lack of the essential fatty acids is the first concern in identifying the causes of the various neurological diseases. In particular, the depletion of the DHA and the EPA may cause the side effects that are related to the cranial nerves.

If so, can enough essential fatty acids be supplied to the vegetarians and their fetuses? The survey results of Sanders and Reddy in 1992 regarding the British veganv, the Ulan–vegetarians, and the non–vegetarian women are presented in Table 5–6.

As shown in Table 5–6, the non–vegetarian women have an average of 9.1 omega–6 fatty acids and 1.1 omega–3 fatty acids, compared with 21.4 omega–6 and omega–3 fatty acids. The fatty acid was 1.2. And,for the vegetarians, they were 14.6 and 1.5, respectively.

Comparing the absolute amount of omega–3, the vegetarian females had a higher proportion than the non–vegetarian females, but, the ratio of omega–6 was higher than that of the non–vegetarian females. This may be due to the vegetarian use of the omega–6–rich cooking oil. Especially, a cooking oil with a high omega–6 ratio is the corn oil. Therefore, if you use cooking oil, the omega–3 fatty acids rich in perilla oil or rape oil is recommended, and the soy is, also, recommended more than corn oil because the ratio of the omega–6 fatty acid and the omega–3 fatty acid is about 4: 1.

5.8. The dietary intake of the omega-3 fatty acids, the DHA and the EPA

There are two families of the polyunsaturated fatty acids: Omega-3 and omega-6. In the fatty acid structure below, the first double bond in the methyl group of the omega-3 fatty acid is at the third carbon position, the omega-6 fatty acid starts at the methyl group, and there is a double bond at the sixth carbon. The linoleic acid and the linolenic acid cannot be synthesized by the animals, but the plants synthesize.People must be supplied with food. This is why they are called the "essential fatty acids".

Linolenic acid, which is the main ingredient of the omega-3 fatty acids, is abundant in perilla, walnut, flaxseed oil, and rape oil. Linolenic acid is metabolized in the liver and is converted to the longer-chain, omega-3 fatty acids.The eicosapentaenoic acid (EPA),the docosahexaenoic acid (DHA), and the linoleic acid (omega-6) are converted to the arachidonic acid (Fig. 5-15). From

Table 5-8. Required fatty acid content of perilla

	Linoleic acid	Linolenic acid
Content (% by weight for total fat)	13.7	63.4

Source: Agricultural Development Administration,

** Perilla is one of the foods with the highest content of omega-3 fatty acids.*

It is recommended that adults consume two cookers as rice cooker, and children consume cookies as daily. Higher animals have higher levels of omega-3 in brain cells. Wash the perilla with water, steam it with steam, and dry it in the shade. Then grind it and keep it in the freezer. In the morning, put as much as two spoonfuls of fruit and perilla and then grind it in the mixer and use it as a morning substitute.

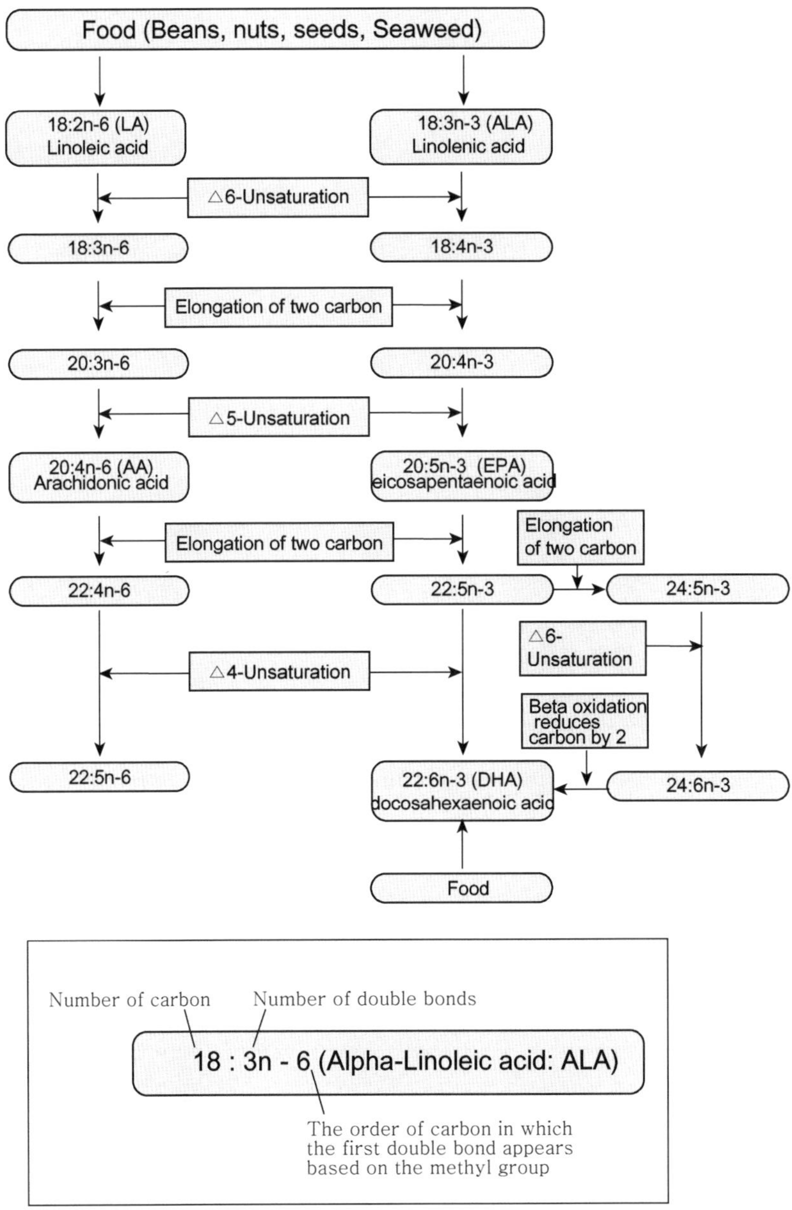

Figure 5–15. Unsaturation, extension and inversion of polyunsaturated fatty acids

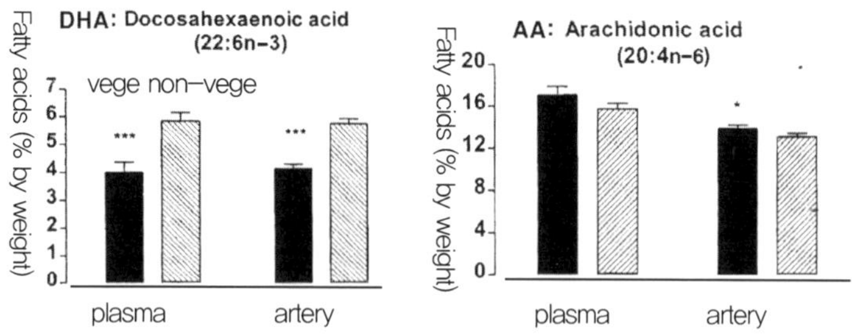

Figure 5-16. Comparison of fetal phospholipids in vegetarians and non-vegetarians

5% to 15% of the linolenic acid taken from the human body is finally converted to the DHA. In other words, the DHA required for the human body is consumed enough as the raw, linolenic acid, and it does not necessarily need to be consumed through fish. Excessive fish ingestion increases the risk of heavy metal contamination, especially in the case of the mothers, even in the presence of the trace amounts of the heavy metals, which can be very dangerous to the fetus.

So, are there any problems with the fetuses of the vegetarian mothers who do not receive the DHA and the EPA from the animal foods? Does the fetus grow well without any worry as the vegetarian, linolenic and linoleic acids are converted to the DHA, the EPA and the AA as needed in the human body?

According to a 1994 survey by Reddy and colleagues, they investigated the fetal plasma and arteries of the vegetarian and non-vegetarian mothers. According to the results, the vegetarian, maternal fetus had slightly less DHA and EPA than the non-vegetarian, maternal fetus. The omega-6 family AA was slightly higher in the vegetarian, fetal mothers (Fig. 5-16) [10].

The DHA and EPA synthesis is increased in proportion to the linolenic acid intake in the vegetarian mothers. Therefore, the use of the linoleic acid-rich perilla, the nuts, and the legumes is one of the important tips in a healthy, vegetarian diet pattern. One interesting fact is that only the vegetarian animals can synthesize the DHA and the EPA using the linolenic acid as a raw material, and the carnivores cannot convert them

5.9. The risk of the lipid peroxide.

Because it is an essential fatty acid, the polyunsaturated fatty acid,regarding which the attention should be paid to the ingestion, is very easy to oxidize in terms of the chemical structure. Therefore, it is very important to maintain the non–oxidized state. The lipid peroxidation in the blood can cause the various diseases, including cancer and diabetes, by making the immune cells excited and by making the various inflammations. In addition, the lipid peroxidation can, also, affect the nerve activity. A comparison of the relationship between the serum lipid peroxidation and the depressive symptoms showed that, the higher the concentration of the lipid peroxidation, the more severe the depressive symptoms (Fig. 5–17) [11].

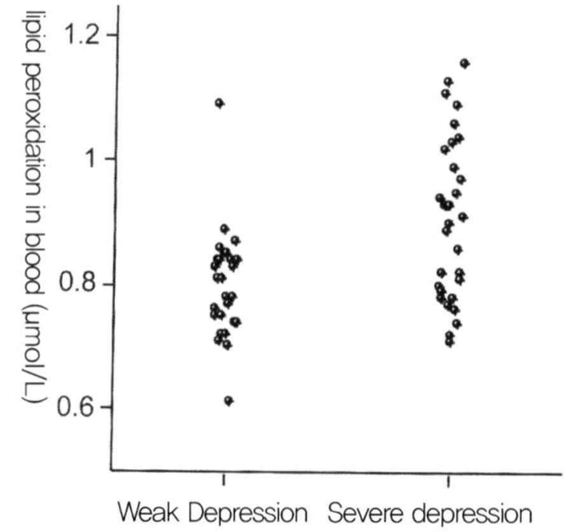

Figure 5–17. Lipid Peroxidation and Depression in the Blood

Therefore, when storing the edible oil, the nuts, and the seeds, minimize the contact with the oxygen at low temperatures, and pay particular attention to avoid direct sunlight. Especially, the vegetable cooking oil, which has a low boiling point and which can be easily oxidized because it has the many unsaturated fats, is recommended to be dressed and the frying is not recommended. Of course, maintaining the proper antioxidant function with the proper vegetable and fruit intake is, also, an important part. The supply of the vegetables and the fruits is, also, important for the acid–base balance

5.10. DHA deficiency and the suicide tendency.

The cerebral nerve damage caused by a deficiency of the nutrients, such as the essential fatty acids, is not only found in depression, but, also,in bipolar disorder, aggression, and schizophrenia. However, depression can lead to suicide. So, what is the relationship between suicide and the fatty acid intake?

From April 2002 to July 2002, a study was conducted at the Dalian Medical University in China. The authors examined the blood levels of the red blood cells in 100 patients who attempted suicide and 100 patients were admitted to a hospital with simple trauma. Here, the fatty acid composition of the red blood cells represents the total fatty acid level of the body. The degree of the suicidal tendency of the patient was measured by the 'Hamilton rating scale of depression' consisting of 24 items.

Studies have shown that the patients who attempted suicide

Table 5-9. Fatty acid levels of red blood cells

	% For total fatty acids		
	Suicide attempter	Normal	p value
EPA	0.74	1.06	〈0.0001
DHA	4.4	5.3	0.0003
Omega-6 Fatty Acids	28.4	27.8	0.25
ω-6/ω-3	3.6	3.0	〈0.0001

Biol Psychiatry 2004;56:490-496

Table 5–10. The relative risk of suicide attempts (Odds Ratios: OR)

Among fatty acids		Quartile				P
		1	2	3	4	
EPA	average (%)	0.35	0.58	0.94	1.57	<0.0001
	OR	1.00	0.38	0.32	0.12	
DHA	average (%)	2.71	4.18	5.36	6.86	0.0003
	OR	1.0	0.78	0.56	0.22	

Biol Psychiatry 2004;56:490–496

have the lower mean EPA, DHA, and total omega–3, fatty acids than normal people (Table 5–9). On the other hand, there was no significant difference in the saturated, fatty acid, the monounsaturated fatty acid, and the omega–6, polyunsaturated, fatty acid. However, the stearic acid was slightly higher in the suicide attempt group (Table 5–9) [12].

However, the authors suggest that the most important finding in the study is the EPA level of the red blood cells. That is, the EPA level of the lipids constituting the erythrocytes was 8 times lower than those of the lower group and the upper group when quadrupling the 100 subjects. The highest EPA content in the group with the highest fatty acid content was 0.12 (Table 5–10).

The authors have not been able to clarify the relationship between the lack of the DHA and the EPA that would make suicidal impulses stronger, but they suggest two hypotheses.

First, we considered the dysfunction of the serotonin system as an important suicide risk factor. Second, the lack of the omega–3, fatty acids in the body tissues can lead to a decline in the serotonin

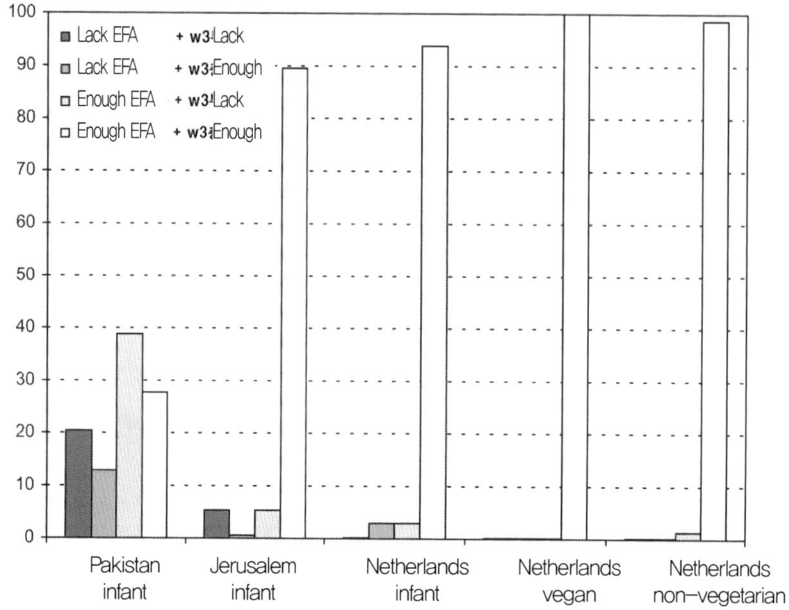

Figure 5-18. Comparison of Omega-3 fatty acid intake among vegetarians and non-vegetarians

production. In other words, the dysfunction of the serotonin-producing neurons is associated with depression and aggression, which can be caused by a deficiency of the omega-3 fatty acids. The high levels of the stearic acid, an 18-carbon, saturated, fatty acid, in the suicide attempt group will weaken the fluidity of the cell membranes, but the relationship with suicide has not yet been established.

If so, can the essential fatty acids, especially the DHA and the EPA, be supplied to the vegetarians? In 2002, a team of the Dutch medical researchers had examined the fatty acid status in omega-3 and in the healthy, non-vegetarian groups and 12 vegans, especially with regard to the long-chain, polyunsaturated, fatty acids, the DHA, and the EPA. At that time, the researchers noted that the omega-3 deficiency in the body did not appear symptomatically for long periods of time, and they were looking for a way to diagnose it before it became deficient.

The omega-3 deficiency causes the problems in the nervous system maintenance and the networking of the nervous system, but, in children, it is associated with the growth disorders, the skin lesions, the subsequent thirst, the increased susceptibility to infection, the decreased vision, the fatty liver, and the infertility. This can be a very serious problem. The survey showed that most children, except the Pakistani children, who had a difficulty in consuming the vegetable oil and the fish, had little problems. Especially, the vegans had been supplied with the 100% essential, fatty acids and the omega-3, fatty acids (Fig. 5-18) [13].

5.11 The Triune brain and the vegetarian

According to the evolutionary evidence based on the physical evidence, such as the fossils, the mammals had originated from the reptiles about 200 million years ago, resulting in the explosively diverse species. Some of the criteria that distinguish the mammals from the reptiles include the circulatory organs and the regulation of the body temperature, and there are, also, the distinctive features in the brain's structure, which leads to the mammalian behavior that is different from that of the reptiles.

In 1967, MacLean proposed the "triune brain" hypothesis, in which the human brain, which is seen as one, is actually composed of the three distinct "brains". In the evolutionary sequence, these brain names were named "the reptilian brain", "the former mammalian brain" (or limbic system), and "the new mammalian brain" (neocortex or primate brain) [15] (Figure 5–19).

According to the Triune brain hypothesis, the brain wings or the higher brain structures (limbic) are added to the basic reptilian brain to form a more evolved brain. Then, the neocortex is added on the axes of the reptilian brain and the early mammalian brain. At this time, the higher brain functions more highly, while the lower brain provides more animal and instinctive functions to the humans.

"Man inherently inherited three brains. The oldest brain is the brain of the

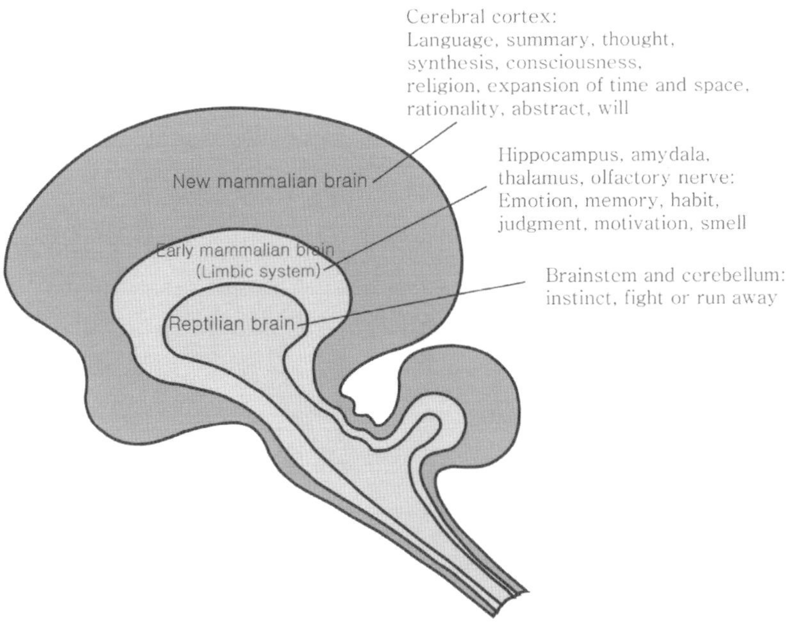

Figure 5–19. McLean's triune brain

reptile, the second is the sub–mammalian brain, and the third brain is the newest brain, developed in the late mammals and culminated in the humans. This third brain gave the humans the unique strength of using a symbolic language."

According to McLean's explanation, in the human brain, the instinctive reptilian brain works in the form of the basal ganglia. The early mammalian brain plays a role in the behaviors that appear in the everyday, social life. Indeed, a comparative study of the behaviors of the animals reveals the self-preservation and the survival of the species with the emergence of the limbic structures. It is, also, at this time that the formation of the care associated with the basic survival and the reduction of the cannibalization of the offspring are often seen in the reptiles

5.12. Personality, the self, and the prefrontal cortex

Harlow's report on the character Gage is widely known as the first example of the relationship between the brain and the personality. In 1848, Gage was a 25-year-old construction worker who had been sweating for the construction of a railway line. Fortunately, he recovered and regained almost the same physical health and mental abilities as before. But, he could not go back to work and had to spend the rest of his life wandering. Because his personality had changed dramatically, according to the literature, he had become indifferent to people, unable to control his impatience, fickle, unstable, and unable to control his instinctive desires [16].

His former employer refused to hire him because the change was too great. His friend said, "He was no longer Gage." Several cases have been reported related to the damage of the frontal lobe following the report of Hollow. EVR was 35 years old, and the

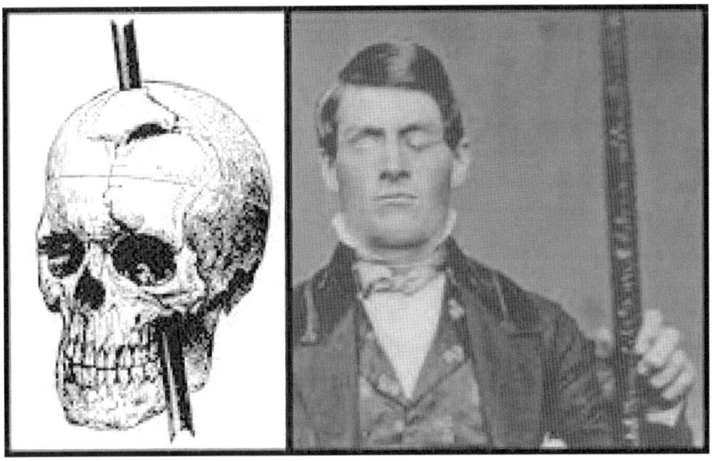

Figure 5-20. Phineas Gage

meninges were removed the orbital, frontal lobe. After the surgery, he appeared normal in the basic, psychological tests, but his social, occupational, and personal activities could not be continued. He was subjected to divorce and bankruptcy, and he was unable to perform the activities that were related to his daily work [16].

5.13. The dietary pattern,the ability to empathize, and the difference of the brain activity

Filippi et al. had investigated the brain's response to pain among the vegan, lacto-ovo vegetarian, and non-vegetarian to the people and animals through the functional MRIs.

When the subjects of study showed the pictures of the people suffering from the other people and the animals, the vegetarian group activated the cerebral cortex, associated with the empathy with the others, but the non-vegetarians were more active in terms of the instinctual anxiety and the limbic area, one-way relationship with the self-protection (Fig. 5-21) [17].

What is unusual is that the vegan showed the more active brain activity when they saw the suffering of the animals, rather than

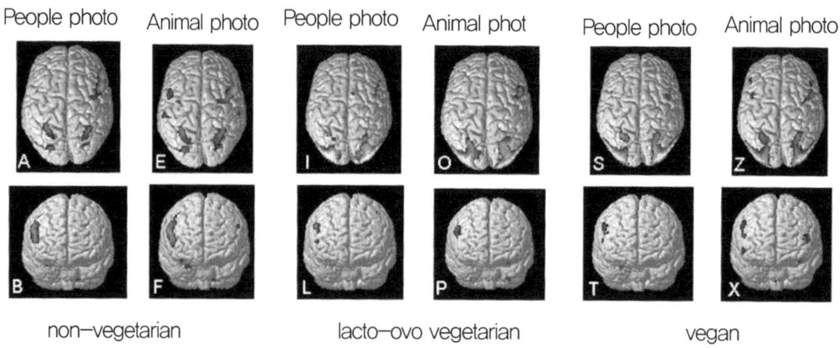

Figure 5-21. Differences in brain response sites between vegetarians and non-vegetarians for the pain of others and animals

seeing the human suffering. It can be a clue to the understanding of vexation sympathy of vegan. Because the ability to empathize can lead to the differences in the positions of the public, such as the social welfare, the vegetarian patterns can, also, be related to the social consciousness of the individuals and the society. Future research is expected

References

1. Dwyer JT, Miller LG, Arduino NL, Andrew EM, Dietz WH, Jr., Reed JC, Reed HB, Jr.: Mental age and I.Q. of predominantly vegetarian children. J Am Diet Assoc 1980, 76:142–147.

2. Gale, C. R., Deary, I. J., Schoon, I., Batty, G. D., & Batty, G. D. (2007). IQ in childhood and vegetarianism in adulthood: 1970 British cohort study. BMJ : British Medical Journal, 334(7587), 245.

3. Podratz JL, Rodriguez EH, Windebank AJ: Antioxidants are necessary for myelination of dorsal root ganglion neurons, in vitro. Glia 2004, 45:54–58.

4. Larsson CL, Johansson GK: Dietary intake and nutritional status of young vegans and omnivores in Sweden. Am J Clin Nutr 2002, 76:100–106.

5. Zhu X, Raina AK, Lee HG, Casadesus G, Smith MA, Perry G: Oxidative stress signalling in Alzheimer's disease. Brain Res 2004, 1000:32–39.

6. Luchsinger JA, Mayeux R: Dietary factors and Alzheimer's disease. Lancet Neurol 2004, 3:579–587.

7. Doraiswamy PM, Finefrock AE: Metals in our minds: therapeutic implications for neurodegenerative disorders. Lancet Neurol 2004, 3:431–434.

8. Ball MJ, Bartlett MA: Dietary intake and iron status of Australian vegetarian women. Am J Clin Nutr 1999, 70:353–358.

9. Hibbeln JR: Seafood consumption, the DHA content of mothers' milk and prevalence rates of postpartum depression: a cross–national, ecological analysis. J Affect Disord 2002, 69:15–29.

10. Sanders TA, Reddy S: The influence of a vegetarian diet on the fatty acid composition of human milk and the essential fatty acid status of the infant. J Pediatr 1992, 120:S71–77.

11. Reddy S, Sanders TA, Obeid O: The influence of maternal vegetarian diet on essential fatty acid status of the newborn. Eur J Clin Nutr 1994, 48:358–368.

12. Tsuboi H, Shimoi K, Kinae N, Oguni I, Hori R, Kobayashi F: Depressive symptoms are independently correlated with lipid peroxidation in a female population: comparison with vitamins and carotenoids. J Psychosom Res 2004, 56:53–58.

13. Huan M, Hamazaki K, Sun Y, Itomura M, Liu H, Kang W, Watanabe S, Terasawa K, Hamazaki T: Suicide attempt and n–3 fatty acid levels in red blood cells: a case control study in China. Biol Psychiatry 2004, 56:490–496.

14. Fokkema MR, Smit EN, Martini IA, Woltil HA, Boersma ER, Muskiet FA: Assessment of essential fatty acid and omega3–fatty acid status by measurement of erythrocyte 20:3omega9

(Mead acid), 22:5omega6/20:4omega6 and 22:5omega6/22:6omega3. Prostaglandins Leukot Essent Fatty Acids 2002, 67:345–356.

15. Fokkema MR, Smit EN, Martini IA, Woltil HA, Boersma ER, Muskiet FA: Assessment of essential fatty acid and omega3-fatty acid status by measurement of erythrocyte 20:3omega9 (Mead acid), 22:5omega6/20:4omega6 and 22:5omega6/22:6omega3. Prostaglandins Leukot Essent Fatty Acids 2002, 67:345–356.

16. MacLean PD: The Triune Brain in Evolution: Role in Paleocerebral Functions. Springer; 1990.

17. Baars BJ, Gage NM: Cognition, Brain, and Consciousness. MA, USA: Elsevier; 2010.

18. Massimo Filippi, Gianna Riccitelli, Andrea Falini, Francesco Di Salle, Patrik Vuilleumier, Giancarlo Comi, Rocca MA: The Brain Functional Networks Associated to Human and Animal Suffering Differ among Omnivores, Vegetarians and Vegans. Public Library Of Science 2010, 5:e20847.

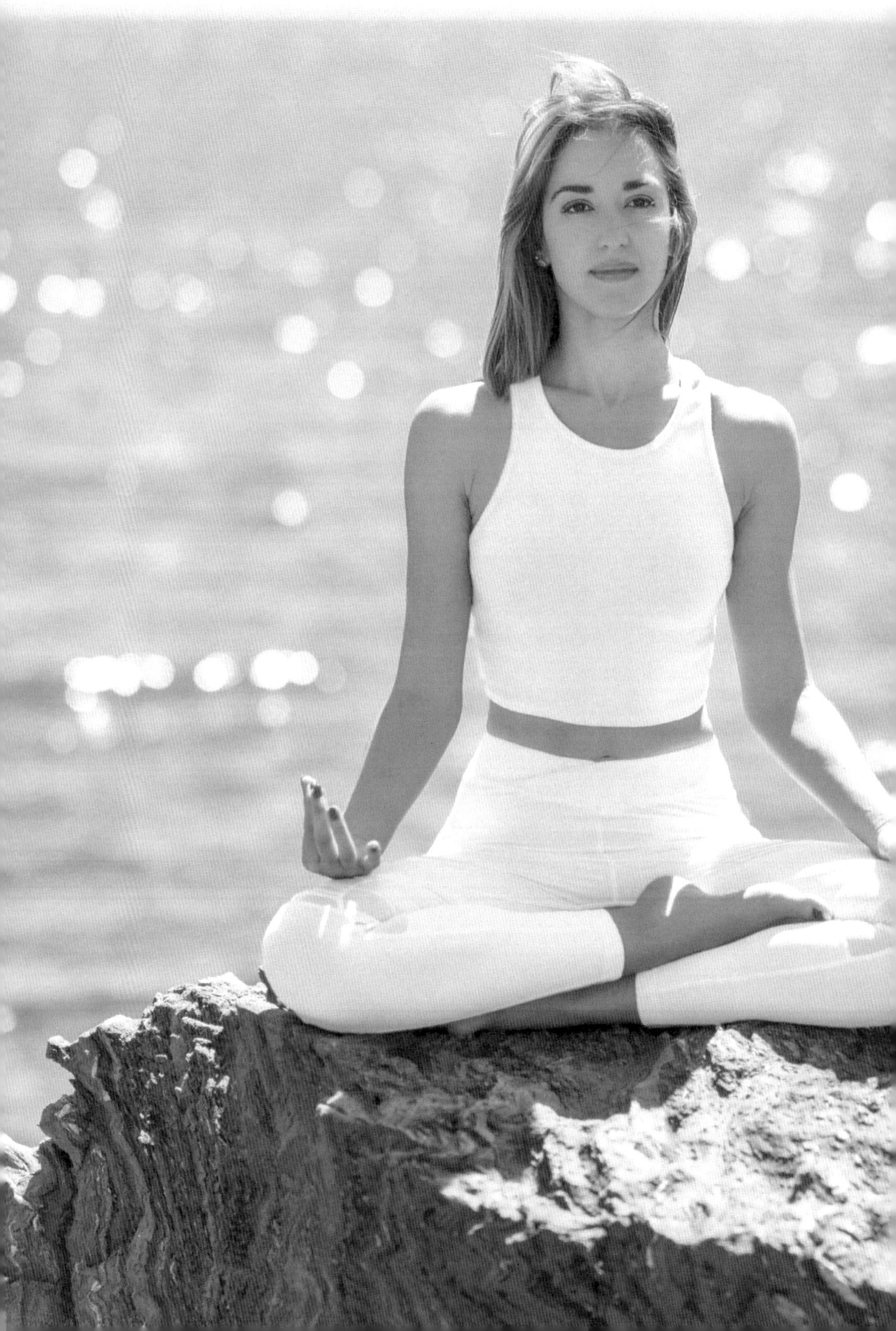

Chapter 6. Respiratory System and Vegetarian Diet

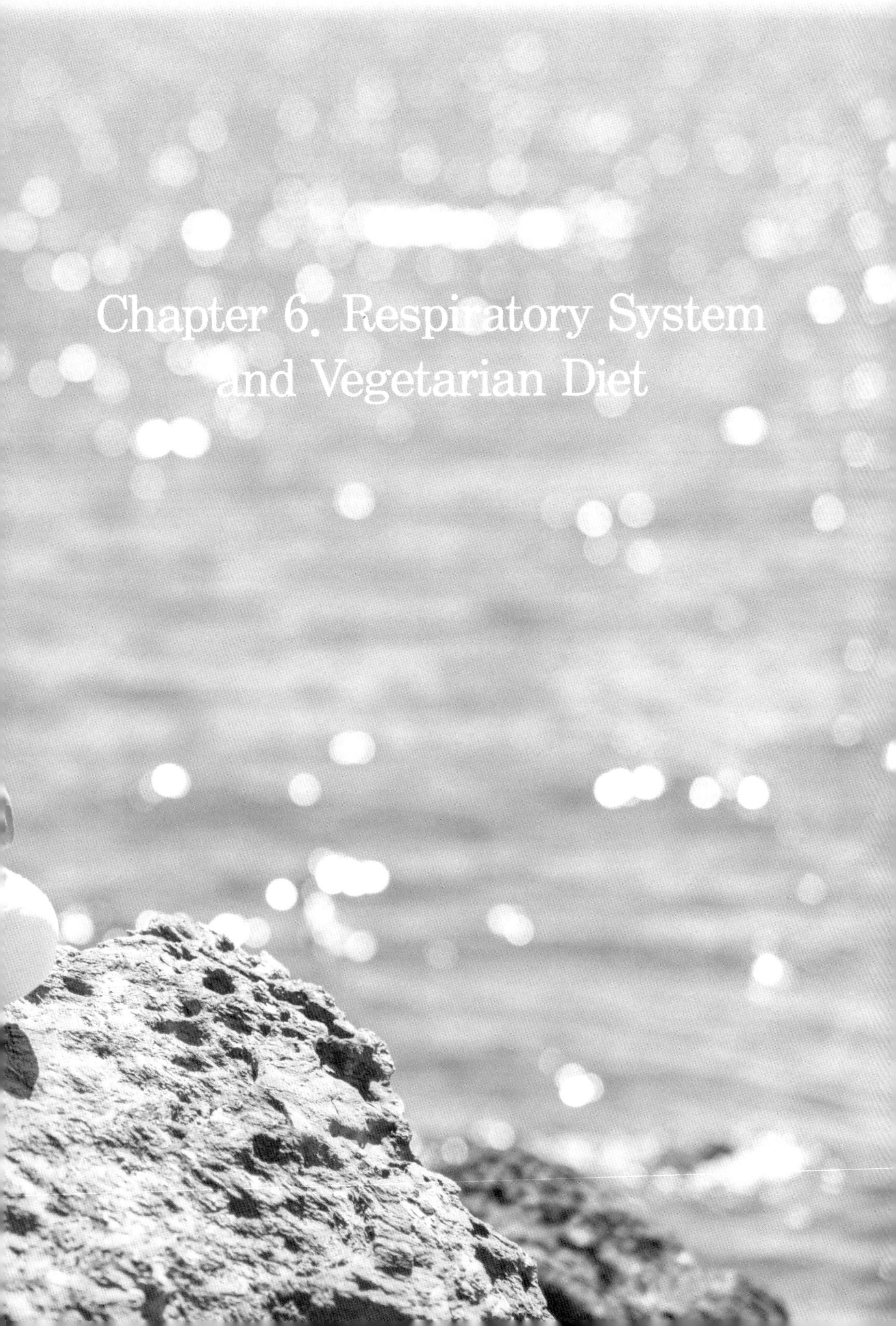

● Skin system

Protect upper respiratory system. The nose hair protects the external material from entering the nostrils →

● Muscular system

← Muscle activity produces CO_2, respiratory muscles fill the lungs with air and emptied. Other muscles also control the respiratory tract.

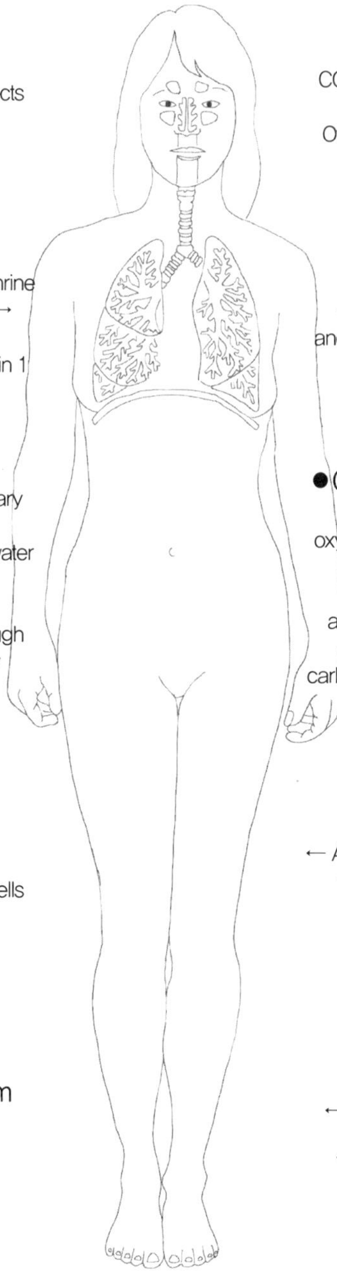

● Endocrine system

Epinephrine and norepinephrine regulate respiratory activity →
Conversion enzyme of lung capillary converts angiotensin 1 to angiotensin 2 ←

● Nervous system

← Check respiratory volume and blood gas level and adjust respiration rate and depth.

● Digestive system

Provide substances necessary for respiratory cells such as substrate, vitamin, mineral, water and ion →
Increased pressure of the pleura and peritoneum through contraction of the respiratory muscles makes defecation possible ←

● Cardiovascular system

← red blood cells move oxygen and CO_2 between lung and peripheral tissue
→ The activity of angiotensin 2 regulates blood pressure and volume, and carbonate ion contributes to the insect action of blood..

● Urinary system

Removing Organic Waste Generated by Respiratory Cells →
Allows adjustment of pH by removing CO_2. ←

● Immune / lymphatic system

← Amygdala prevents infections from entering the respiratory tract
→ Alveolar phloem cells present antigens to specific defense and respiratory defense systems

● Reproductive system

Control breathing speed and depth during sexual intercourse←

● Skeletal system

← Exercise of the rib enables breathing.
The skeleton surrounds and protects the lungs.

Chapter 6. The respiratory system and the vegetarian diet.

6.1. The structure and the function of the respiratory system

The energy required for all of the activities of the human body is obtained by burning oxygen. Unlike the aquatic organisms that use the skin or the gills, the terrestrial organisms use a structure called the "respiratory system" for the rapid diffusion of the gases. There are the three major types of the respiration in the human body: The cellular respiration, the organic respiration, and the bodily respiration. Obesity is the exchange of the gas between the lungs and the blood vessels, and the respiration is the transfer of the oxygen bound to the hemoglobin of the red blood cells to the peripheral cells. The cell respiration is the way in which the energy is obtained from the oxygen delivered into the cell by oxidizing the nutrients through the mitochondria.

The external respiratory system of the human body is largely divided into the above-mentioned higher system and lower system. The gauze consists of the nose, the nasal cavity, and the pharynx, and the following pharynx consists of the larynx, the trachea, the bronchus, and the alveoli. The meter filters the impurities of the air coming in from the outside into the lungs, warms them in a manner similar to the body temperature, and adjusts the humidity. By doing so, the subtle surface of the scale becomes dry or uncooled by the outside air. This conditioning of the air reaching the alveoli is primarily enabled by the respiratory mucosa. The following diagram is made up of a bronchial branch system and the alveoli, which are the moving passages of the gas. The alveoli is the basic unit for the gas exchanges with the capillaries.

The organs are divided into 19 successive sections starting from the branch of the trachea. The diameter of the bronchus is 0.5 mm. At the end of the bronchus, there is a breathing part, which shows no mucus and cilia, but the alveoli and the diffusive gas exchange take place. At this time, the total surface area of the alveoli is at least from 35 times to 140 times the surface area of the body surface. The alveoli are the air pockets of the lungs. There is an alveolar membrane between the inner space of the alveoli and the blood of the blood vessels, which is thinner than a hundredth of a centimeter or even 1 / 10,000th of a centimeter, allowing the gas exchange between the alveoli and the blood.

The alveolar epithelial cells are divided into the type 1 cells and the type 2 cells. The type 1 cells constitute from 90% to 95% of the alveolar surface, which is important for the maintenance of the alveolar capillary membrane and which is responsible for the diffusion exchange of the gas. The type 2 cells are the granular, alveolar cells, accounting for from 5% to 10% of the alveolar surface area. They produce the metabolic and enzymatic actions, such as the production, storage, and secretion of the surfactants that lower the surface tension of the alveoli. If a surfactant is not secreted, the small alveoli will collapse and damage the gas exchange function.

The respiratory tract protects against the bacteria through the macrophages of the mucous ciliates and the alveoli. The dust and the pathogens in the inhaled air adhere to the mucous layer above the ciliary layer. The ciliates move forward and backward at a rate of 2 cm per minute to allow the esophagus to swallow with the cough reflexes and the saliva.

The gas exchange in the alveoli

The pressure of the air is expressed as 1 atm or 760 mmHg because the mercury column has the pressure of up to 760 mm. The air is 80% nitrogen, 20% oxygen, and 0.03% carbon dioxide. The pressure shows that the oxygen pressure is 160 mmHg and the carbon

Table 6-1. gas pressure

gas	Venous blood	Arterial blood	Alveoli	atmosphere
Oxygen	40mmHg	100mmHg	105mmHg	160mmHg
carbon dioxide	46mmHg	40mmHg	40mmHg	0.3mmHg

dioxide pressure is 0.3 mmHg. On the other hand, the oxygen gas pressure in the alveoli is 105 mmHg and the pressure of the carbon dioxide in the alveoli is about 40 mmHg, so that the oxygen and the carbon dioxide diffuse in the opposite directions in the alveoli. The gas pressure is proportional to the concentration. The factors affecting the diffusion of the oxygen in the alveoli are the oxygen pressure in the atmosphere, the alveolar ventilation rate, and the oxygen consumption rate in the body.

Arteries are the blood vessels that pass out of the heart, and the veins are the blood vessels that circulate throughout the body. Therefore, the venous blood comes from the body tissues, has a high carbon dioxide concentration (46 mmHg), and has a low oxygen concentration (40 mmHg). The difference in the gas concentration in the alveoli and the capillaries causes the diffusion to continue until the gas concentrations are balanced on both sides. In the blood, the oxygen is either dissolved in the plasma or bound to the hemoglobin in the red blood cells. Since oxygen is not well-soluble in water, it is usually bound to the hemoglobin. The amount of the oxygen bound to the hemoglobin per liter of blood is 197 mL, and the dissolved amount is only 3 mL.

The hemoglobin molecules in the red blood cells are the four subunits bound to the proteins, and each subunit is a combination of the heme and the globin peptides. Each hemoglobin contains one iron ion (Fe^{2+}) and can bind to one oxygen molecule. In other words, the hemoglobin in the red blood cells binds to a total of four oxygen

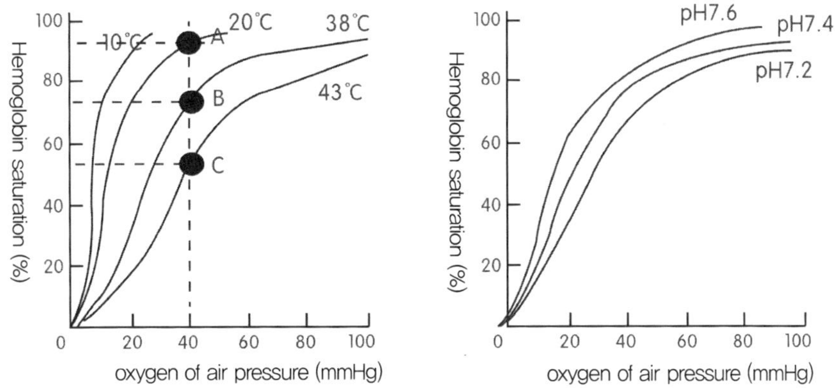

Figure 6-1. Oxygen dissociation curves with changes in temperature and pH

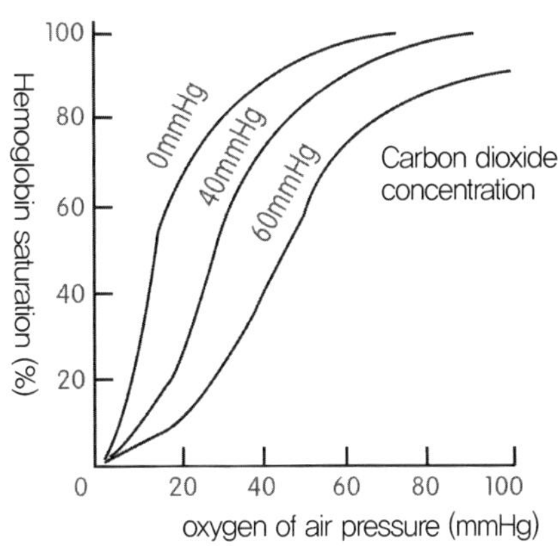

Figure 6-2. Oxygen dissociation curve change according to carbon dioxide concentration

molecules.

$$O2 + Hb \rightleftarrows HbO_2$$

The ratio of the binding of the hemoglobin to oxygen, that is, the saturation ratio (O_2 binding to the Hb) / (the maximum amount of the Hb that can bind to the O_2) × 100.

The most significant influence of the saturation rate of the hemoglobin is the oxygen concentration (pressure) in the blood, which has the oxygen–hemoglobin dissociation curve. The curves are the sigmoidal curves with the steep slopes at from 10 mmHg to 60 mmHg of the oxygen pressure and a gentle slope at from 70mmHg to 100 mmHg. When the partial, oxygen pressure is 60 mmHg at the room temperature, the bonding rate is 90%.And, when the oxygen concentration is higher than 60%, the bonding rate is gradually increased (Fig. 6–1).

The reason for drawing the sigmoid curve is that, when the oxygen molecule is first bonded to the heme, the bonds between the four globin subunits are separated from each other and the three–dimensional structure is easily deformed to bond with the oxygen. The oxygen pressure in the plasma and the red blood cells entering the lungs is 40 mmHg, which is about 75% of the hemoglobin saturation (Fig. 6–2).

In addition to the oxygen concentration, the hemoglobin saturation is influenced by the carbon dioxide concentration, the hydrogen ion

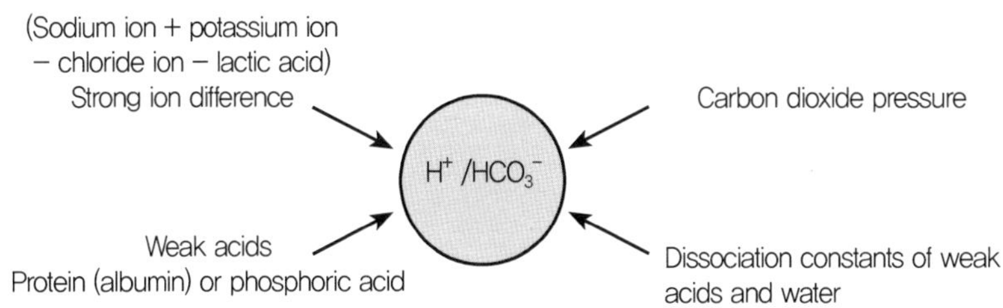

Figure 6–3. Factors affecting acid balance by Stuart hypothesis

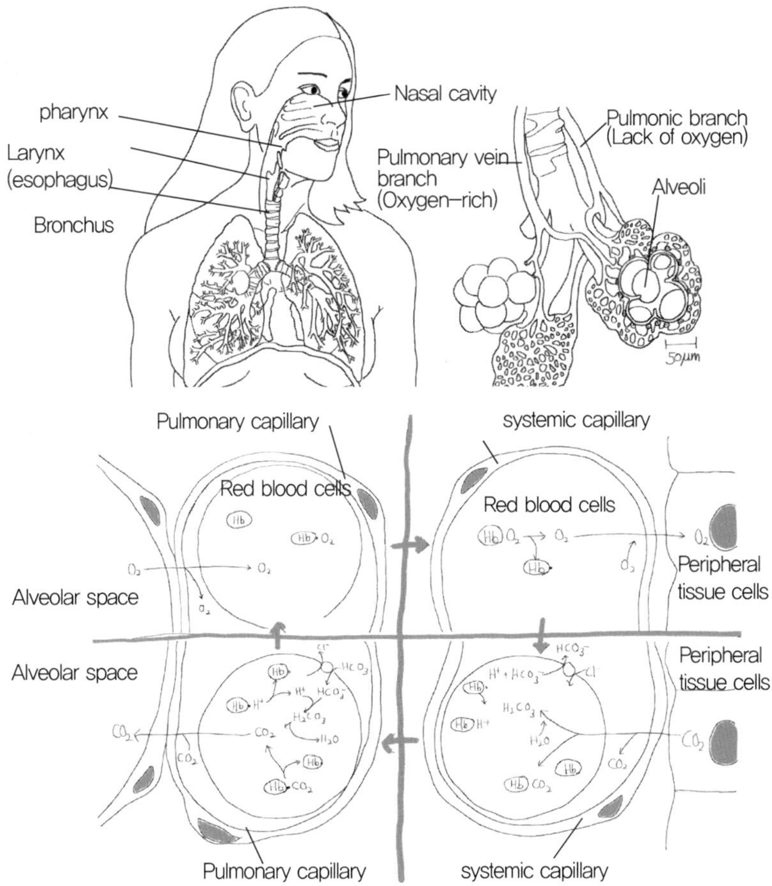

Figure 6–4. Controlling the acidity of carbon dioxide during the breathing process

concentration, the temperature, the 2,3–diphosphoglycerate, and its concentration or level is higher at the periphery than at the lungs. As it increases, the oxygen–hemoglobin dissociation curve shifts to the right, and the binding rate of the hemoglobin to the oxygen decreases, thereby, causing the oxygen to migrate to the tissue.

This allows the oxygen bound to the hemoglobin in the peripheral tissues to be easily removed and transferred to the tissue cells. That is, the metabolic activity is active in the peripheral tissues, so that the temperature is high, the concentration of the carbon dioxide is high, the acidity is high, and the concentration of the 2,3–diphosphoglyceric acid is high.

In the peripheral cells, the oxidized nutrients are released into the carbon dioxide (CO_2) and the water, where only 10% of the carbon dioxide is dissolved in the plasma, 30% is bound to the hemoglobin and migrates to the carbamino–hemoglobin, and 60% is bicarbonate. The blood is transferred to the lungs. This reaction can be written as:

$$CO_2 + H_2O \rightleftarrows H_2CO_3 \text{ (carbonate)} \rightleftarrows HCO_3^- \text{ (bicarbonate ion)} + H^+$$

$$CO_2 + H_2O \rightleftarrows H_2CO_3 \text{ (carbonate)} \rightleftarrows HCO_3^- \text{ (bicarbonate ion)} + H^+$$

After reaching the lungs, the deoxyhemoglobin releases the hydrogen and becomes the oxidized hemoglobin. At this time, the released hydrogen ions are converted into the carbonates and the

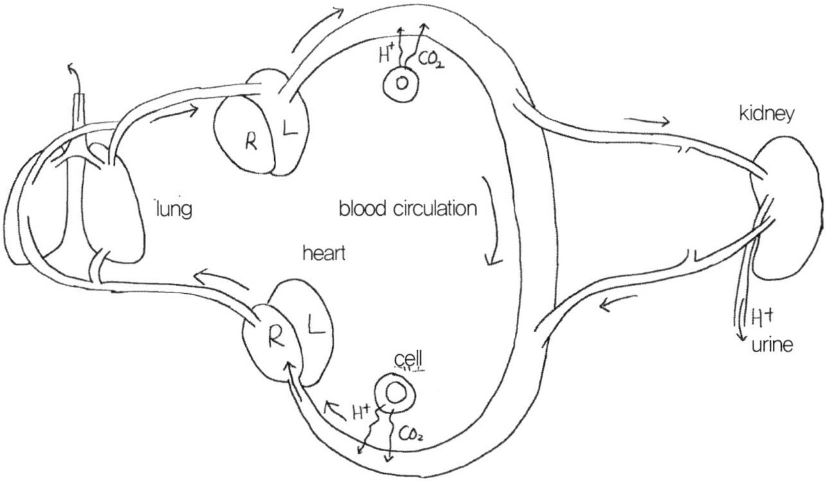

Figure 6–5. Acid base control in respiration and kidney

Table 6–2. The result of hypercholesterolemia and physiology of blood due to excessive meat intake[6]

Nutrition, metabolism effect	Acceleration of catabolism
	Anabolic inhibition
	Increased Insulin Resistance
Effect on bone	Physico–chemical dissolution of bone
	Increased osteoclast function
	Functional weakening of osteoblast
	Increased levels and effects of parathyroid hormone
	Reduced vitamin D synthesis
Effects on hormones	Decreased growth hormone secretion
	Reduction of IGF–1 response
	Insulin–mediated inhibition of glucose metabolism
	Thyroid hormone levels decreased
	Thyroid stimulating hormone increase
	Increased cortisol production
	Calcium changes and reduced parathyroid hormone sensitivity

bicarbonates. And the carbon dioxide that is generated at this time goes out through the respiratory system. Through this process, the body can maintain the constant, hydrogen ion concentration. If the ventilation is not done properly due to a lung disease or the like, the concentration of the carbon dioxide in the artery increases and the concentration of the hydrogen ions in the artery increases, thereby increasing the acidity (decreasing the pH). This is called a "respiratory acidosis".

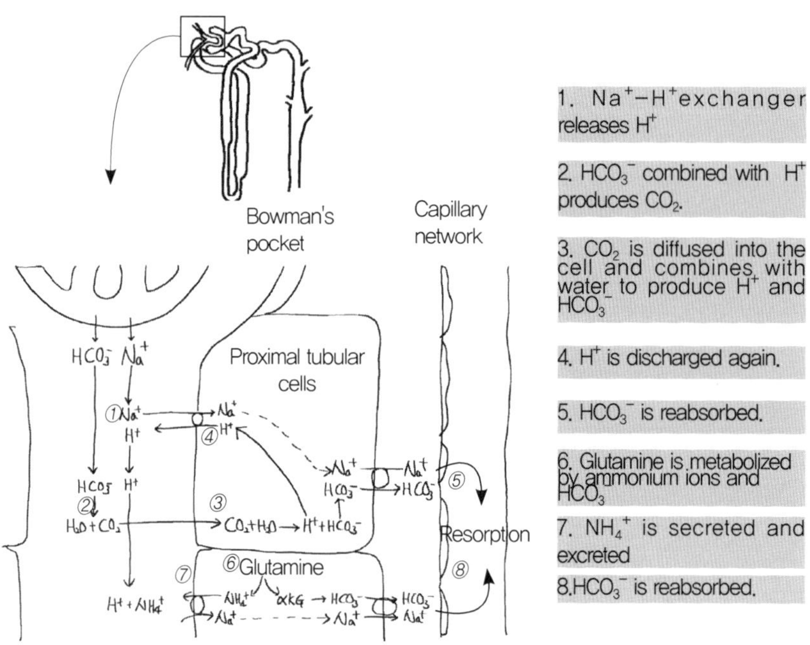

Figure 6-6. Controlling Acid Base with Sodium and Carbonic Acid in the Kidney

6.2. The acid–base balance and the vegetarian diet

Since almost all intracellular enzymes maintain their function in an acid–base balance state, the acid–base balance in the body is a very important factor in maintaining the normal function of the

Table 6–3. High protein diet and results[6]

	Daily protein intake			Result / increased risk
	A	B	C	
Control experiment				
normal adult	1.6			Increase insulin secretion
normal adult	1.7			Increase in renal net acid discharge (RNAE)
normal adult	2.4			Oxalic acid, glycosic acid Emission increase
normal adult	2.4			Increased calcium excretion
normal adult	2.5			Decreased insulin sensitivity, increased hepatic glucose release
normal adult	2.8			Increased bone resorption
normal adult	2.8			Increased glomerular filtration rate
normal adult	2.9			Plasma glutamine reduction
Epidemiological investigation				
normal adult		0.65		Increased glomerular filtration rate
normal adult		0.84		Increased non–bicarbonate production
50~75세			0.1	Microalbuminuria
9세이상			0.5	diabetes
20~79세			Quartile 4	Renal cell carcinoma (relative risk 1.9–fold increase)
70세			Quartile 3	Prostate cancer (odds ratio 13.5)
35~59세	〉1.8			Bone fracture (relative risk 1.22–fold increase)

A: Protein recommended intake divided by 0.75 g / kg body weight per day. 2, which means twice as much intake.

B: Correlation between protein intake and outcome C: Mean of the study group Mean protein intake

cells. In general, the pH of the human body is maintained within the range of 7.37 ~ 7.43, and there are two ways to regulate it– by exhaling the carbon dioxide through the respiration or the excretion of the nonvolatile acids or bases through the kidneys. The kidney reabsorbs most of the bicarbonate ions (HCO_3^-) that are filtered in the glomeruli.

Stewart noted a strong ion difference, the total concentration of the weak acids, and the partial pressure of the carbon dioxide (pCO_2) as the three major factors affecting the maintenance of the acid–base equilibrium in the human body. The strong ion difference is the difference between the strong acid and the strong base, which is calculated as "sodium ion + potassium ion – chloride ion – lactate". If the difference of the strong ions is increased, the hydrogen ion concentration is decreased to alkalize (increase the pH).

Usually, the strong ionic difference has a positive value. For this reason, the negative ions with a negative value and the carbon dioxide are injected to balance the body fluid. So, when one of these three factors changes, the acidity of the body fluid changes. If the CO_2 increases through respiration, the concentration of the hydrogen ions increases soon. And the other elements of the body work to buffer them.

The total concentration of the weak acids is usually affected by the protein (albumin) or the phosphoric acid. Thus, the changes in the nutrients through the ingested food affect the pH of the human body, which can be calculated as the potential, renal acid load

(PRAL) [2]. The 'potential kidney load' can be calculated from the nutrients in 100 g of food using the following formula [3].

Potential elongation load (mEq) = 0.49 × protein (g/100 g) + 0.037 × phosphoric acid (mg/100 g) − 0.021 × potassium (mg/100g) − 0.026 × magnesium (mg/100g) − 0.013 × calcium (mg/100g)

If the potential kidney load regarding a food has a negative value, it is alkalized, whereas, if it has a positive value, the blood is presumed to have been acidified. For example, the vegetables and the fruit that are rich in potassium, magnesium, and calcium and the potential elongation load value are negative and alkaline. On the other hand, when the protein, the cheese, and the grains are consumed, the protein and the phosphoric acid are abundant and the potential elongation load value becomes acidic.

For example, when 8.5 g of the food−borne, nutrient supplements had been consumed by 34 healthy men and women for 14 days, the pH of the urine had increased from 6.07 to 6.27 at first. This suggests a decrease in the acid load in the body [4]. Another study showed that the plasma had become more alkalinized, ie, the pH had become higher when the dietary protein (9.4%) and the high carbohydrate (65.5%) had been fed than when the high protein (25.3%) and the low carbohydrate (10.1%) had been fed for 4 days.

6.3. The maximum oxygen uptake and cancer

'Maximal oxygen uptake (VO_2 max)' means the maximum amount of the oxygen that can be consumed when exercising at sea level. Therefore, the maximum oxygen uptake is used not only as a cardiovascular action but, also, as an indicator of the function of the respiratory system. The maximum oxygen uptake is used to measure the risks of the various types of mortality, including the death by cardiovascular disease. Recently, it has been reported about its relationship with cancer. That is, a lower maximum oxygen uptake leads to an increased mortality from breast cancer.

According to Peel et al. [2009], the mortality was almost three times higher for the people with the maximum oxygen intake of less than 8 METS (28 mL/kg.min) [7]. In another study of 248 patients, the maximum oxygen uptake in the breast cancer patients was 32% lower than in the healthy controls [8]. Summaximal exercise testing can be used to measure the cardiopulmonary function in the patients with the congestive heart failure [9], stroke [10], as well as the patients with the various cancers [11].

The acid–base balance of the blood, also, affects the 'maximum oxygen uptake'. One study found that the low protein–high carbohydrate group had lasted longer with the 100% maximum oxygen uptake until the exhaustion during the cycle (345 sec. vs. 221 sec. in the low–protein intake group). The acid–base balance affects the skeleton and the muscles, thus affecting the physical

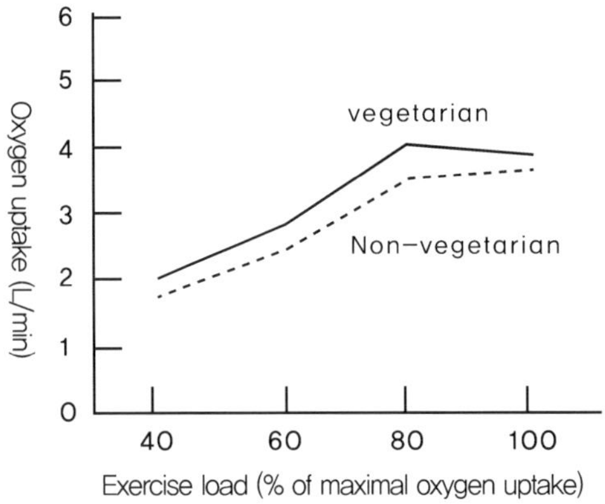

Figure 6–7. After non–vegetarian and low protein diet, measure your fitness with your bike

activity. The acidification in the muscle cells is associated with fatigue. When the extracellular fluid is alkalized, the fatigue is relieved by the rapid removal of the hydrogen ions from the muscle cells [12].

6.4. The low-protein diet and the increased oxygen consumption

To investigate whether nutrition affects the acid-base balance and, furthermore, the exercise capacity, Enni et al. had examined the difference between the low-protein diet and the normal diet. A total of 9 healthy adults (with the mean age of 23.5 years) were recruited. One group was fed a vegetarian diet for 4 days and the other group was fed a regular diet for 4 days. Before and after the experiment, the exercise ability was measured with a cycle ergometer. The blood was collected to confirm the acid-base balance. At 40%, 60%, 80%, and 100% of the maximum oxygen uptake (VO_2 max), they were measured three times for 10 minutes each.

There was no significant difference in the arterial blood, hydrogen ion concentration, the strong ion difference, the total concentration of the weak acid, the pressure of the carbon dioxide, and the concentration of the carbon dioxide between the two groups. There was no difference in the exercise time until the fatigue. However, the vegetarian group showed a significant increase in the strong ion difference in the resting state (38.6 vs 39.8, $p = 0.009$). The VO_2 was significantly higher in the vegetarian group at 40%, 60%, and 80% of the maximum oxygen uptake.

Acidosis lowers the binding rate of the oxygen to the hemoglobin and, thus, lowers the oxygen content in the blood. After the vegetarian diet, the participants were interpreted as having increased the oxygen transfer capacity in the blood. However, the other factors other than the strong acid differences were rapidly found by the acid−base balance mechanism of the human body. Although the amount of the energy consumed was 390 kcal less in the vegetarian diet, there was almost no difference in the exercise capacity compared to the non − vegetarian diet. The glycogen content of the muscles was not low in the vegetarian diet.

Changes to the vegetarian diet have increased the oxygen utilization, which causes the differences and the concerns in the various areas of the body. The list of the interests includes the diseases such as cancer.

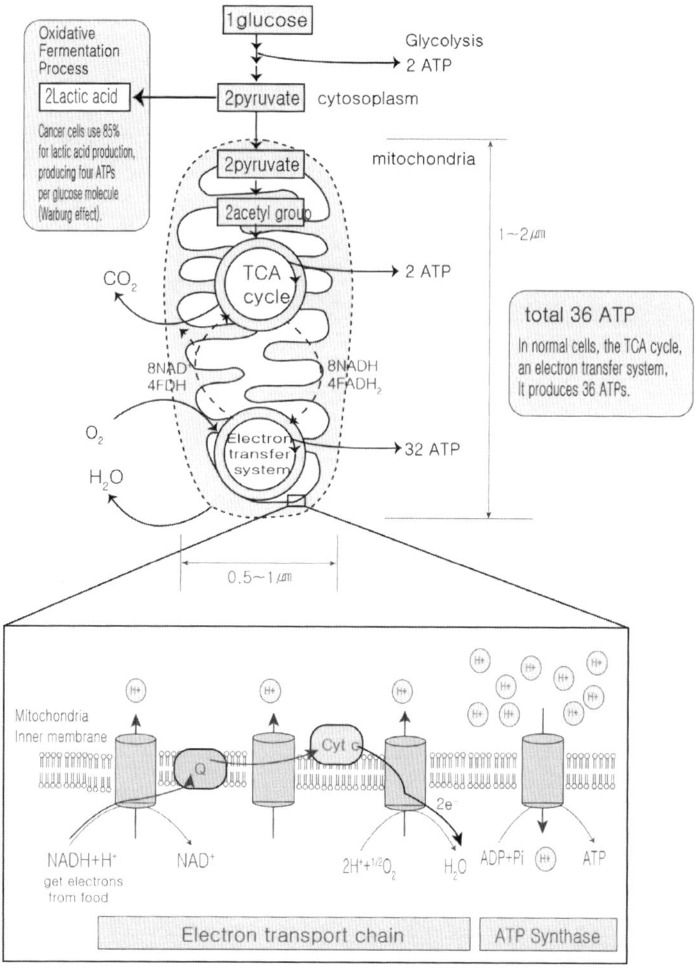

Figure 6-8. Aerobic respiration and anaerobic fermentation process in cytoplasm and mitochondria

Cancer cells are mostly damaged by mitochondria and can not use lipids as an energy source, and they need more carbohydrates as nutrients. Therefore, when the ketone type (lipid / (carbohydrate + protein) = 4) or fasting, cancer cells die because they can not use carbohydrates. Normal cells, however, become healthier by using mitochondria and using lipids and ketones as energy sources. For more information, please refer to 〈Cancer Healing Principle of Atopage and Fasting, by Aaron KJ Lee, 2018〉.

6.5. The anaerobic fermentation and cancer

The cellular respiration process of the human body is largely divided into two phases: The TCA circuit and the oxidative phosphorylation. The process involves the separation of one molecule of glucose into two molecules of the pyruvic acid without the oxygen, resulting in the two ATPs. The ATP is a chemical energy that is common to all living organisms.

The two pyruvic acids that are produced then combine with the oxygen in the mitochondria in the cell via the TCA circuitry and the oxidative phosphorylation to produce six carbon molecules and six molecules of water. In this process, the 36 ATPs are generated. That is, when there is no oxygen, only two ATPs are produced, but 18 times as many ATPs are produced as the oxygen is supplied.

However, if the oxygen is insufficient, the pyruvic acid produced in the process enters the TCA circuit and cannot be used, so it enters the fermentation process and turns into the lactic acid.

The cardiopulmonary function can be measured by the amount of the oxygen absorbed at the maximum oxygen uptake, which can be used to estimate the mortalities of a variety of the diseases, including cancer. Various studies have shown that the low values of the maximal oxygen uptake increase the cardiovascular disease and the breast cancer mortality [7, 13, and 14].

In 1956, Warburg insisted that cancer cells ferment without oxygen. That is, the motive power of cancer is the insufficient cell respiration by the damage of the mitochondria. He writes in the journal 'Science'in a paper entitled, 'The Origin of Cancer Cells', and explains [15]. There are two stages in the development of cancer. The first step is the irreversible damages of the cells by the ultraviolet rays, the tar, the pressure, the urethane, the toxic substances, etc., but their common features are the damage of the oxygen in the breathing process of the cells.

The second stage of cancer development is the process through which the oxygen–breathing process gets the energy through the fermentation to make the damaged cells survive. They develop the fermentations that do not require oxygen to survive abnormally. It is like the yeast, a lower organism. He claims that all cancer cells die when they are not supplied with all the nutrients for 24 hours at 38 degrees Celsius. However, even if only one–fifth of the energy is supplied, the cancer cells survive without dying, Just as the yeast cells, like the lower animals, can survive for a long period of time without the oxygen breathing or the fermentation and get packed tightly. In fact, the metabolic energy of the cancer cells is comparable to that of the yeast.

So, how can the cancer cells proliferate despite the low energy production rates? It becomes possible by changing the cancer cell metabolism so that the fermentation speed is faster. That is, the enzymes related to the fermentation are found more frequently in the cytoplasms of the cancer cells [15]. Gatenby et al. had examined the highly–malignant breast cancer cell lines called the "MCF–7"

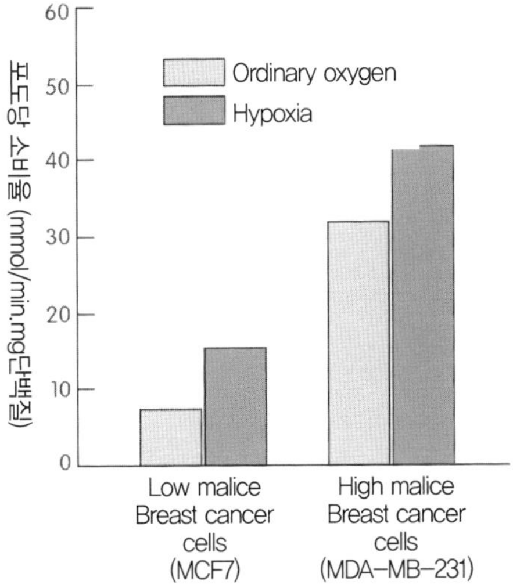

Figure 6–9. The glucose consumption rate of cancer in normal oxygen and hypoxic state

and the "MDA–MB–231", which are the lowly–malignant breast cancer cell lines, to confirm the glucose consumption rate. The experimental results showed that the glucose consumption was higher in the malignant cells, especially the glucose consumption in the hypoxic conditions [16].

6.6. Alveolar ventilation

Usually, breathing is done unconsciously. However, we can consciously control the speed and depth of breathing, which can help maintain the physiology and health of the body by changing the respiratory rate of the body. The concept to understand this process is the 'alveolar ventilation rate'.

For normal people, the breathing per minute is about 12 times, and the amount of breathing is about 500ml. Therefore, the ventilation rate per minute becomes 6,000 ml, which is the number of the times per 500 ml multiplied by 12 times. However, the gas exchange between the lungs and the capillaries occurs only in the alveoli. That is, the volume of 150 ml, which is the airway's volume, does not change. 150ml is left in the air when breathing. Thus, the amount of the gas actually reaching the alveoli is 500 ml − 350 ml = 150 ml. And, since the breathing is 12 times per minute, the respiration rate per minute would be 4,200 ml when multiplying the 350ml by 12 times (Table 6-4).

If you slow down your breathing rate and, instead, breathe deeper through double breathing, the amount of the air supplied to the alveoli becomes greater. Let's say that the respiration rate is six times that of the normal one, and let's say that the volume of one breath is 1,000 ml, instead. Then, subtracting the 150ml of the air space, which is an 'anatomically dead space', the actual amount of the ventilation becomes 1,000ml−150ml = 850ml. Multiplying the

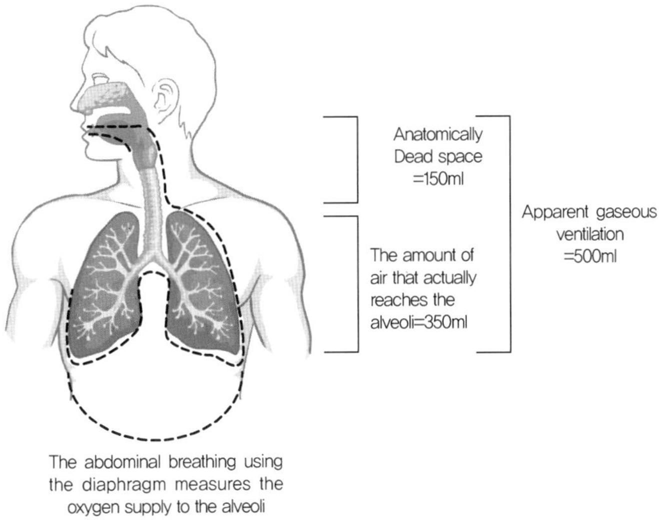

Figure 6-10. Apparent volume and alveolar volume

Table 6-4. Effects of respiratory pattern on alveolar ventilation

object	Tidal volume (ml)	Anatomically dead space (Airway volume, ml)	Volume of gas reaching the alveoli (ml)	Respiratory rate per minute	Alveolar ventilation rate per minute (ml / min)
A	150	150	0	40	0
B	500	150	350	12	4200
C	1,000	150	850	6	5,100

The slower you breathe, the more oxygen you get. One red blood cell has 250,000 hemoglobin, and one hemoglobin molecule binds to four molecules of oxygen. Therefore, one red blood cell can transport 1 million oxygen molecules. The erythrocytes of the human body have a nucleus disappearance and a concave shape, which broadens the Table area that can bind with oxygen. And the shape of the narrow blood vessels through the transformation. Therefore, as you slowly breathe, the red blood cells come into close contact with the capillary walls to be easily supplied with oxygen. In the process of doubling breathing, praying, meditation, and danson breathing, the breathing process is as slow as possible and the process of exhaling helps to provide more oxygen.

850ml by 6 times per minute becomes 5,100ml, which means 900ml more than the 4,200ml of the daily respiration

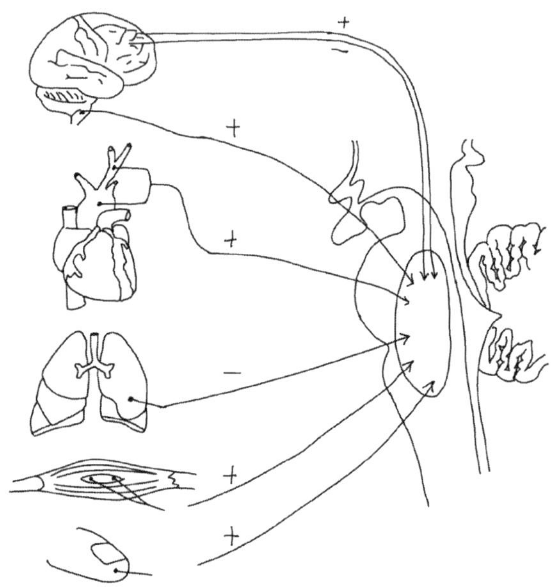

Figure 6–11. Factors Affecting Respiration

6.7. interaction between anxiety and respiration.

The exercise in the chest is accomplished by the periodic contractions of the inspiratory and expiratory muscles. The motion commands for the contraction of these muscles are made by a complex, neural network of the brain. There are two major paths to determine the command of the breathing: One is a physiological, metabolic demand and the other is a psychological state.

First, the central control of the metabolic breathing is the breathing and the pneumothorax. These autonomous breathings, also, respond to the changes of the emotions.

Second, the starting point for controlling the psychological breathing is in the cerebral cortex. Animal experiments with cats showed that the motor neurons associated with the rib muscles on the opposite side of the brain were activated when the primary motor cortex in the cortical cortex was stimulated with electricity. However, the final respiration signal is the result of the intricate interactions between the brain stem, the limbic system, and the cerebral cortex. Studies in animals and humans, for example, have shown that the respiration rates increase in the fear and anxiety states. In other words, the greater the degree of anxiety, the faster the respiration rate, and, as the respiration rate increases, the actual amount of the inhaled oxygen decreases. On the contrary, slowing the breathing rate slowly may lower the degree of anxiety. According to Masaoka et al., the anxiety index and the respiration

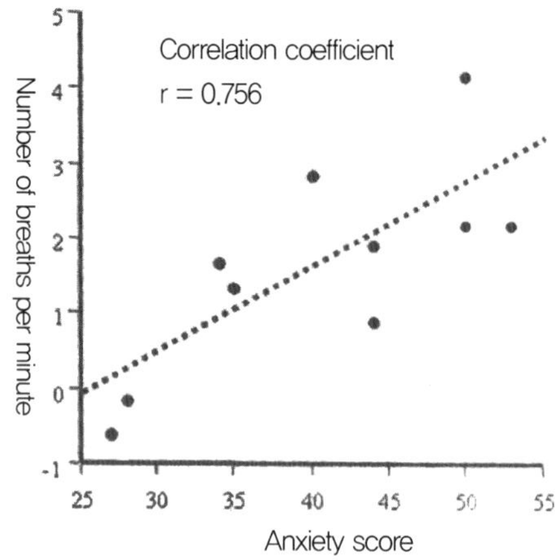

Since the correlation coefficient r is 0.756, the value of r^2 is 0.571. In other words, 57.1% of anxiety can be explained by the number of breaths per minute.

Figure 6–12. Correlation between respiratory frequency and subjective anxiety score
Anxiety scores were measured using Spielberger's State–Trait Anxiety Inventory.

rate were positively correlated. [17] (Fig. 6–8).

References

1. Lindinger MI: Origins of [H+] changes in exercising skeletal muscle. Can J Appl Physiol 1995, 20:357–368.

2. Remer T: Influence of nutrition on acid–base balance—metabolic aspects. Eur J Nutr 2001, 40:214–220.

3. Remer T, Dimitriou T, Manz F: Dietary potential renal acid load and renal net acid excretion in healthy, free–living children and adolescents. Am J Clin Nutr 2003, 77:1255–1260.

4. Berardi JM, Logan AC, Rao AV: Plant based dietary supplement increases urinary pH. J Int Soc Sports Nutr 2008, 5:20.

5. Greenhaff PL, Gleeson M, Maughan RJ: The effects of dietary manipulation on blood acid–base status and the performance of high intensity exercise. Eur J Appl Physiol Occup Physiol 1987, 56:331–337.

6. Metges CC, Barth CA: Metabolic consequences of a high dietary–protein intake in adulthood: assessment of the available evidence. J Nutr 2000, 130:886–889.

7. Peel JB, Sui X, Adams SA, Hebert JR, Hardin JW, Blair SN: A prospective study of cardiorespiratory fitness and breast cancer mortality. Med Sci Sports Exerc 2009, 41:742–748.

8. Jones LW, Courneya KS, Mackey JR, Muss HB, Pituskin EN, Scott JM, Hornsby WE, Coan AD, Herndon JE, 2nd, Douglas PS, Haykowsky M: Cardiopulmonary function and age–related decline across the breast cancer survivorship continuum. J Clin Oncol 2012, 30:2530–2537.

9. Kemps HM, Schep G, de Vries WR, Schmikli SL, Zonderland ML, Thijssen EJ, Wijn PF, Doevendans PA: Predicting effects of exercise training in patients with heart failure secondary to ischemic or idiopathic dilated cardiomyopathy. Am J Cardiol 2008, 102:1073–1078.

10. Eng JJ, Dawson AS, Chu KS: Submaximal exercise in persons with stroke: test–retest reliability and concurrent validity with maximal oxygen consumption. Arch Phys Med Rehabil 2004, 85:113–118.

11. Carlson LE, Smith D, Russell J, Fibich C, Whittaker T: Individualized exercise program for the treatment of severe fatigue in patients after allogeneic hematopoietic stem–cell transplant: a pilot study. Bone Marrow Transplant 2006, 37:945–954.

12. Robergs RA, Ghiasvand F, Parker D: Biochemistry of exercise–induced metabolic acidosis. Am J Physiol Regul Integr Comp Physiol 2004, 287:R502–516.

13. Blair SN, Kohl HW, 3rd, Paffenbarger RS, Jr., Clark DG, Cooper KH, Gibbons LW: Physical fitness and all-cause mortality. A prospective study of healthy men and women. JAMA 1989, 262:2395–2401.

14. Blair SN, Kampert JB, Kohl HW, 3rd, Barlow CE, Macera CA, Paffenbarger RS, Jr., Gibbons LW: Influences of cardiorespiratory fitness and other precursors on cardiovascular disease and all-cause mortality in men and women. JAMA 1996, 276:205–210.

15. Warburg O: On the origin of cancer cells. Science 1956, 123:309–314.

16. Gatenby RA, Gillies RJ: Why do cancers have high aerobic glycolysis? Nat Rev Cancer 2004, 4:891–899.

17. Masaoka Y, Homma I: The effect of anticipatory anxiety on breathing and metabolism in humans. Respir Physiol 2001, 128:171–177.

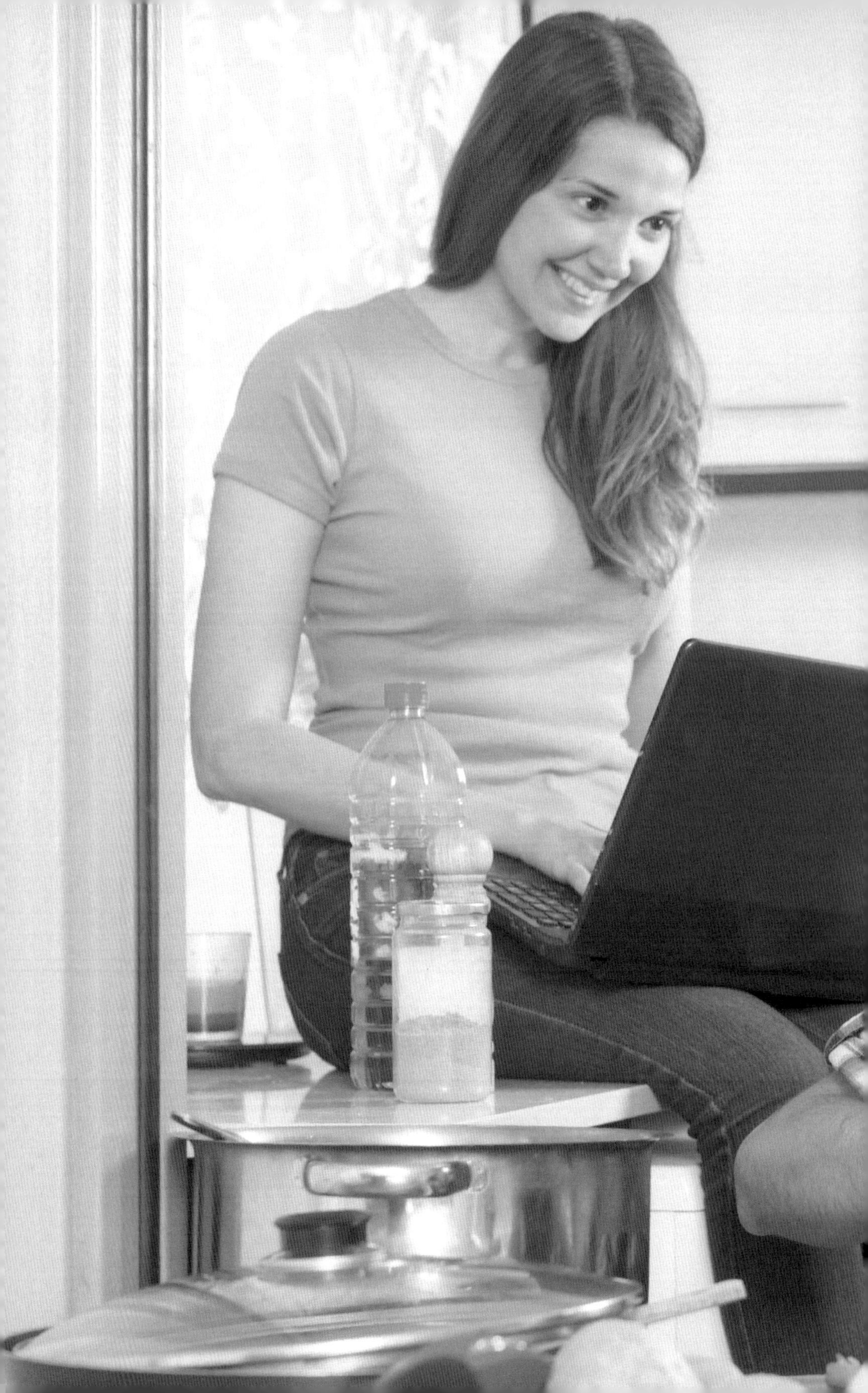

Chapter 7. Reproductive System and Vegetarian Diet

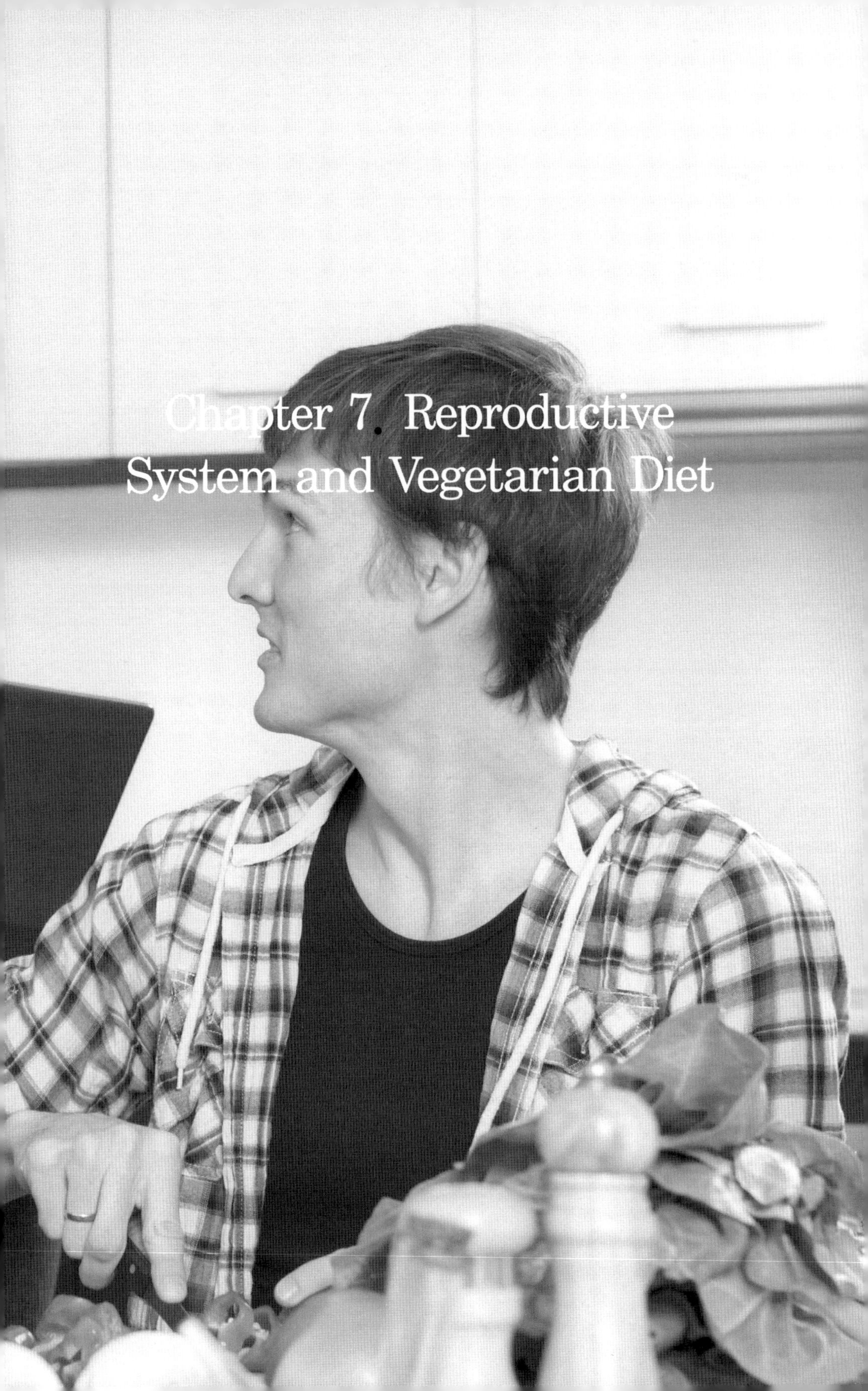

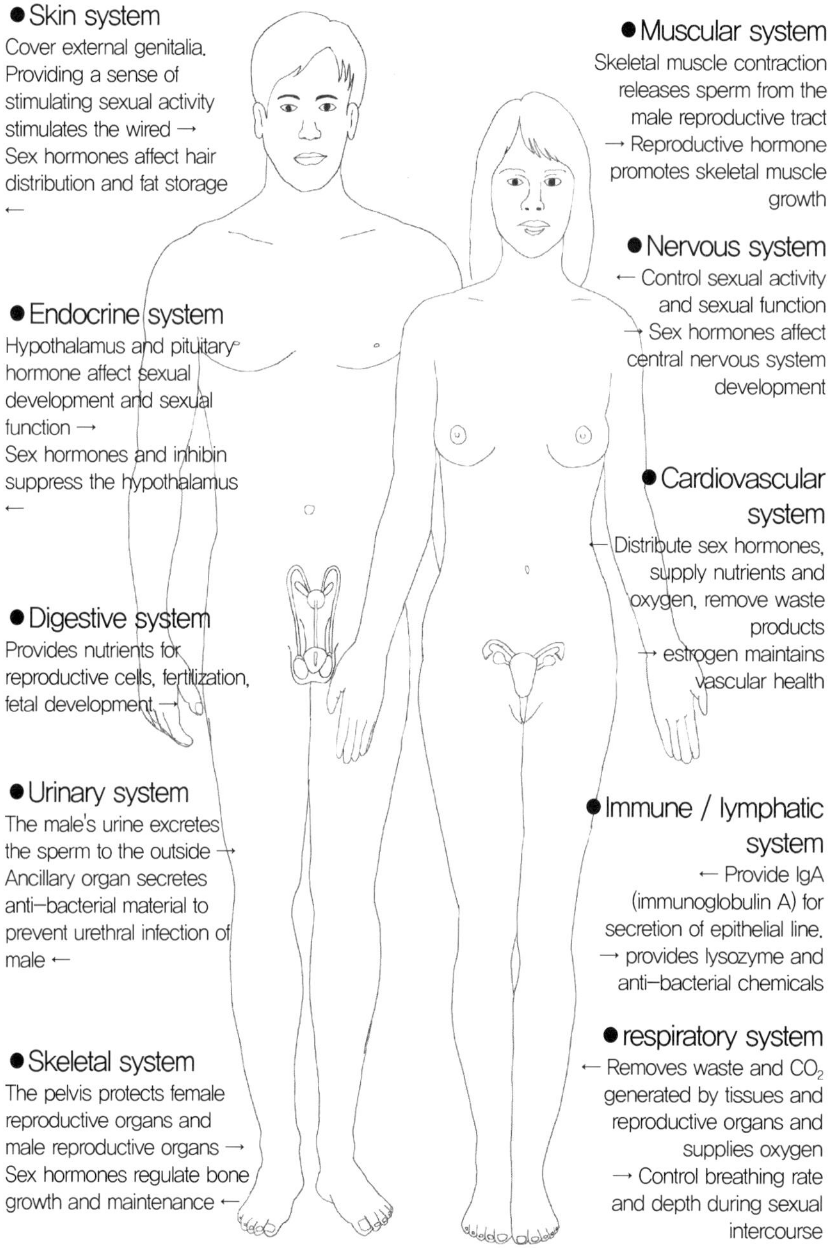
● Skin system
Cover external genitalia. Providing a sense of stimulating sexual activity stimulates the wired →
Sex hormones affect hair distribution and fat storage ←
● Endocrine system
Hypothalamus and pituitary hormone affect sexual development and sexual function →
Sex hormones and inhibin suppress the hypothalamus ←
● Digestive system
Provides nutrients for reproductive cells, fertilization, fetal development →
● Urinary system
The male's urine excretes the sperm to the outside →
Ancillary organ secretes anti–bacterial material to prevent urethral infection of male ←
● Skeletal system
The pelvis protects female reproductive organs and male reproductive organs →
Sex hormones regulate bone growth and maintenance ←
● Muscular system
Skeletal muscle contraction releases sperm from the male reproductive tract
→ Reproductive hormone promotes skeletal muscle growth
● Nervous system
← Control sexual activity and sexual function
→ Sex hormones affect central nervous system development
● Cardiovascular system
← Distribute sex hormones, supply nutrients and oxygen, remove waste products
→ estrogen maintains vascular health
● Immune / lymphatic system
← Provide IgA (immunoglobulin A) for secretion of epithelial line.
→ provides lysozyme and anti–bacterial chemicals
● respiratory system
← Removes waste and CO_2 generated by tissues and reproductive organs and supplies oxygen
→ Control breathing rate and depth during sexual intercourse

Chapter 7. The reproductive system and the vegetarian diet.

7.1. The structure and the function of the reproductive system

The reproductive system is not an organ that is concerned with the survival of the individual, but it is essential for the continued maintenance of the human species. Sexually, the mature males and the mature females produce the germ cells, respectively, and the fetus is fused into one by sexual intercourse.

The human reproductive system produces, stores, nourishes, and transports the germ cells. The reproductive cells of the mother and the father are combined and become a fertilized egg. After 15 to 20 years from the birth as the fetus, he or she becomes an adult. During this developmental period, the hormones emerge from the reproductive system and produce the sexually-specific patterns directly. The reproductive system consists of the gonads, the adjunct tubes, the ancillary organs, and the perineal structures, and they can be defined as follows:

(1) The gonads are the organs that produce the germ cells and the hormones.

(2) The tube receives and transports the germ cells.

(3) The associated tubes and the associated organs secrete a liquid into the reproductive system or the other secretory tubes.

(4) The perineal structure is known as 'external genitalia'. Both the male and female reproductive tracts are connected to the open passages outside the human body, but the male and female reproductive systems are functionally and structurally very different.

7.2. The male reproductive system

The basic structure of the male reproductive system is the testes, the nocturnes, the vas deferens, the ejaculatory ducts, and the urethra. The external genitalia consist of the scrotum surrounding the testes and the penis, the erectile organs associated with the urethra. The testis is flat and egg-shaped, and it is approximately 5 cm long, 3 cm wide, and 2.5 cm thick. Each weighs 10g ~ 15g and rests in the skin pocket.

The inside of the testis is a tightly-twisted tubule, in which the sperms are formed. The inside of each tube is made up of the several layers of the epithelial cells. The rounded germ cells, first, become mature as they move from the outer layer to the inner

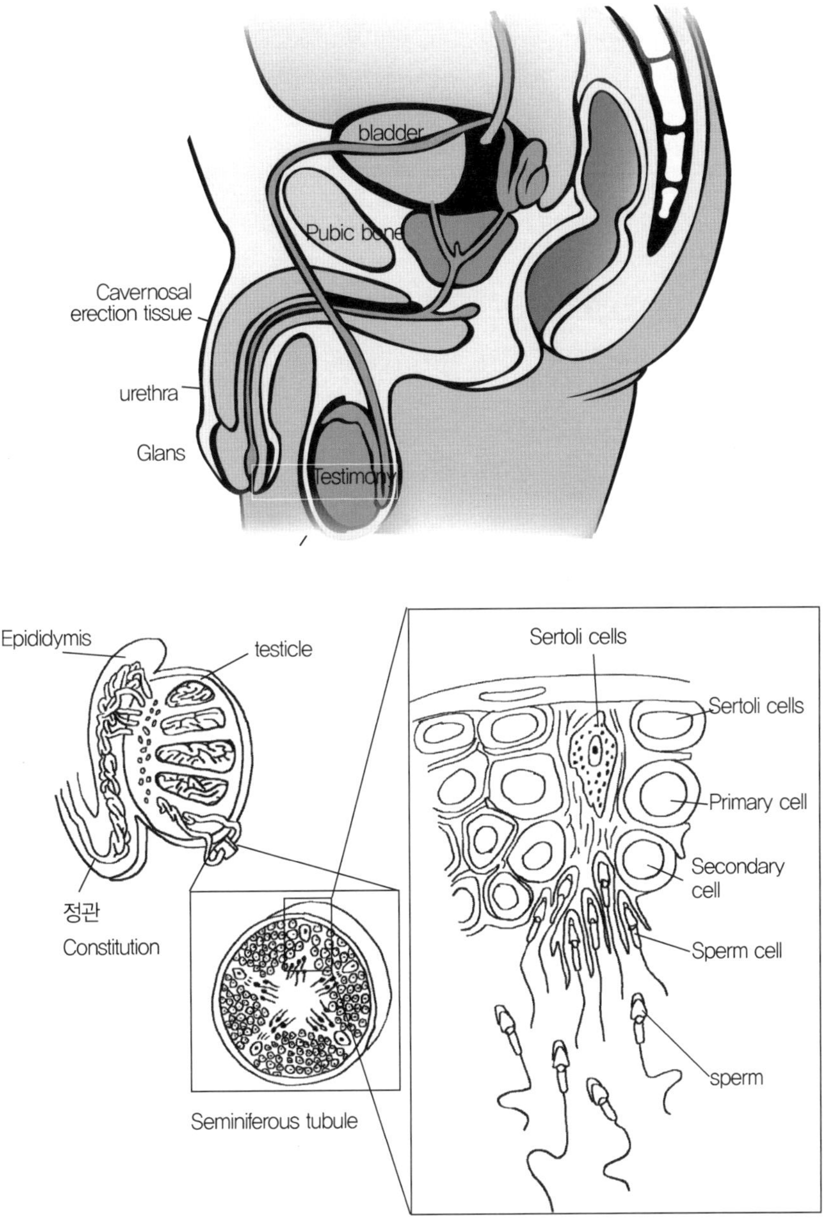

Figure 7-1. Development of male reproductive system and sperm

lumen and become the round heads and the long–tailed sperms. Among the germ cells, there are the Sertoli cells, which surround the germ cells and supply and protect the nutrients.

There is a radial cell around each tubule, which produces the male hormone. In the spermatids, the mature sperms go to the storage place, the amphibian, to develop the mobility and the amphibian that is connected to the urethra . The urethra passes through the penis and goes out of the body. When puberty releases the gonadotropin–releasing hormone (GnRH) from the hypothalamus, the pituitary gland secretes the luteinizing hormone (LH) and the follicle–stimulating hormone (FSH). The testicular Lady's cells begin to produce the testosterone under the signal of the luteinizing hormone. As the concentration of the testosterone increases, the body exhibits a secondary character and exhibits the dramatic changes in the puberty. The voice becomes thicker, the muscles become stronger, the body becomes hairy, and the testicles become mature. After the puberty, the increased testosterone is maintained and then decreased with the aging

7.3. The female reproductive system

The female reproductive system should produce a newborn by producing the sex hormones, maturing the germ cells, supporting and nourishing the developing embryos, and raising the embryos.

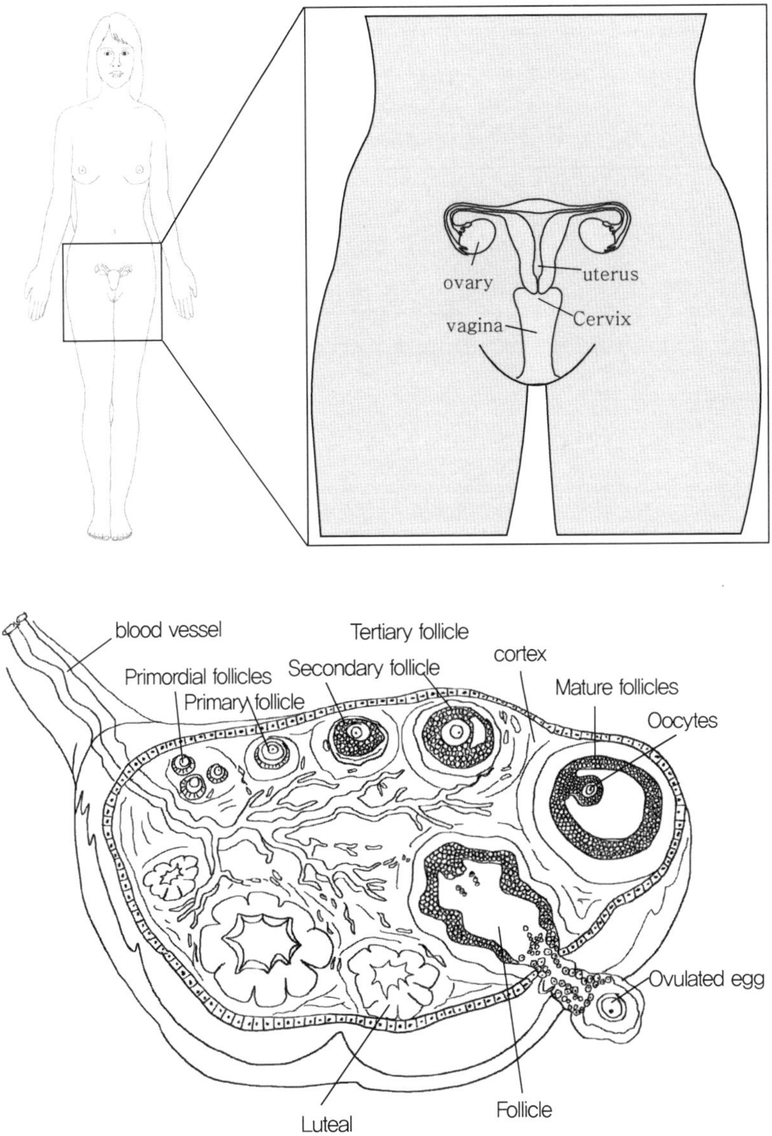

Figure 7-2. Developmental process of female reproductive system and oocyte

The important organs in the female reproductive system are the ovaries, the uterine tubes, the uterus, the vagina, and the external genitalia (Fig. 7–2). The ovary is a small, flat, almond–shaped organ with a length of 5 cm, a width of 2.5 cm, a thickness of 8 mm, and a weight of 6g–8g near the lateral wall of the pelvic cavity. The ovaries produce the immature, female germ cells, secrete the female hormones, such as the estrogen and the progesterone, and secrete the inulin, which regulates the feedback of the pituitary gland's follicle–stimulating hormone.

The ovaries are fertilized in the oviducts and move to the uterus to form the placenta after the implantation. Through the placenta, the fetus receives the oxygen and the nutrients from the mother. The lower part of the uterus is called the "neck", and the lower part is connected to the vagina

7.4. The ovarian cycle and the uterine cycle

At the time of the first birth, there are 1 million ovarian germ cells in the ovaries of the women. When the secondary growth begins, the first oocyte matures and gives birth to another oocyte, approximately every 28 days. The first oocyte in the ovary is surrounded by a layer of the follicular cells, which is called a "follicle" (Fig. 7–3).

Six to twelve follicles are matured each month, and, after one

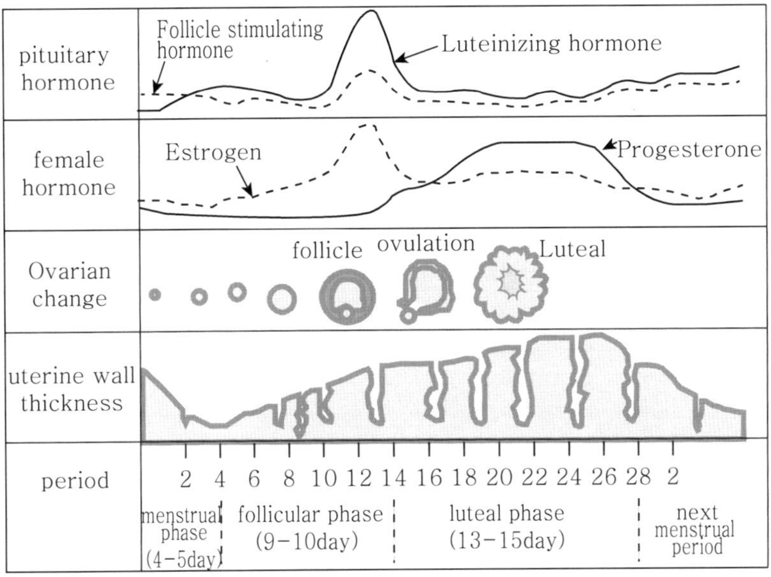

Figure 7-3. Changes in female hormones and changes in the uterine wall

week, the development stops most of the time, with one follicle feeding the nutrients so that only the one continues to grow. Two weeks later, the mature follicles burst and release the eggs. The follicles release, and the remaining follicles turn yellow to produce the estrogen and the progesterone for 2 weeks. When the egg is fertilized, these hormones continue to be produced, and the egg is degraded if it is not fertilized. This is called the "ovarian cycle".

The female, uterine cycle hasthe two stages– the endometrium–growing and the falling–off. After 5 days of the ovarian cycle, the endometrium begins to grow, which is when the fertilization is ready. If the embryo does not reach the uterus while preparing for 14 days after the ovulation, the endometrium will go away. This is called "menstruation". In the natural state, most mammals reabsorb it into the body without making the endometrium fall off, except for the humans.

7.5. The ovarian cycle, the uterine cycle, and the hormones

The ovarian cycle and the uterine cycle are regulated by the hormones. In puberty, a long–named hormone called the "gonadotropin releasing hormone" (GnRH) is released from the hypothalamus, which causes a signal to the anterior pituitary gland to secrete the follicle–stimulating hormone (FSH) and the luteinizing hormone (LH). The hormones released from the pituitary

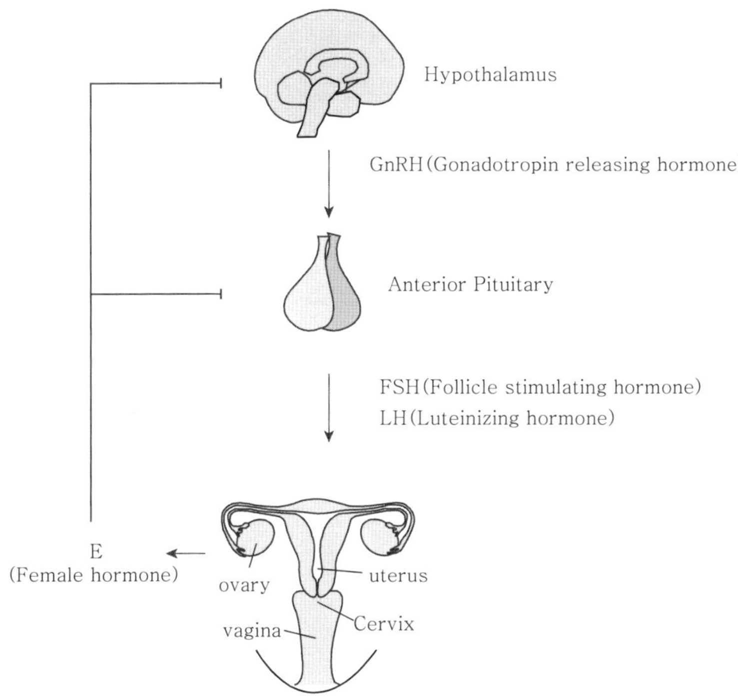

Figure 7–4. Hypothalamus – pituitary–female Female hormone axis (HPG axis) and negative feedback process

When GnRH is released from the hypothalamus, GnRH stimulates the anterior pituitary gland to release FSH (follicle stimulating hormone or follicle stimulating hormone) from the anterior pituitary. FSH stimulates the ovaries and promotes the maturation of the follicles in the ovaries. The mature follicles temporarily turn into endocrine organs and release female hormones. The female hormone released at a high concentration causes the release of LH (luteinizing hormone) from the anterior pituitary gland, and LH weakens the follicle wall of the oocyte, making a hole in the follicle wall to allow the secondary oocyte to exit. This is called ovulation. The follicles after ovulation turn into corpus luteum (yellow lutein).The luteal secretes progesterone (progesterone), and the lutea decays after 12–16 days when LH is not secreted. If pregnant, placental human chorionic gonadotropin (hCG) is released and stimulates the progesterone to continue to release from the corpus luteum. After 5 weeks of gestation, the placenta produces progesterone. In the 10–12 weeks of pregnancy, a lot of estrogen (female hormone) is released from the fetus. Female hormone binds to the female hormone receptor in the hypothalamus and pituitary cells again, thus acting as a negative feedback suppressing the activity of these hormone organs. This stops the new menstrual cycle.

gland stimulate the ovaries to produce the estrogen, and the estrogen causes the secondary manifestations that are characteristic of the adolescence throughout the body.

When the FSH and LH secretions increase in the anterior, pituitary gland, several follicles mature in the ovary and the follicles increase the estrogen production. The increased estrogen allows the endometrium to grow, and, at the same time, it regulates the negative feedback tothe anterior pituitary gland in the first 12 days of the ovarian cycle, thereby, causing the LH to increase and the FSH to decrease, and, again, thereby releasing the oocyte from the follicles

7.6. The modification of the sperm and the egg

Men produce sperm and the male hormones in a pair of the gonads called the "testes", which regulate the male reproductive

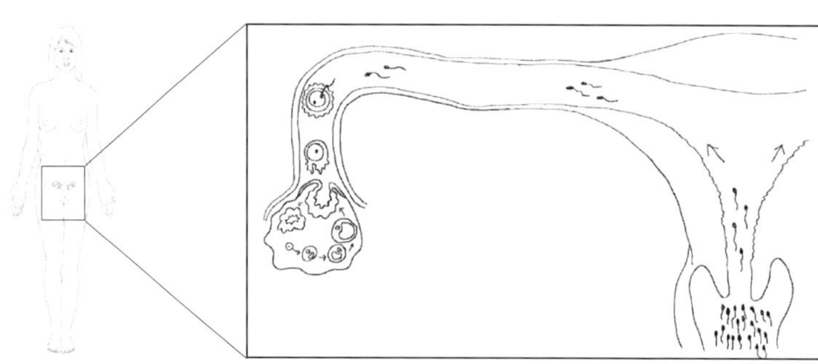

Figure 7–5. The process of fertilization of the sperm and egg

ability. Women secrete the eggs and the sex hormones from the first reproductive organs, the ovaries. A pair of the fallopian tubes arethe conduits that lead the oocyte (immature oocyte) from the ovary to the uterus, where the normal fertilization occurs. The average ejaculation volume is about 3 ml. It contains about 300 million sperms. The sperm life is 1.5 days ~ 3 days after the discharge, and the life time of the eggs is 24 hours after the discharge.

A sperm must pass through three gates until it meets an egg and the egg is fertilized. First, the unhealthy sperms are removed from the mucous membrane of the uterine cervix, which is the first portal, and are eaten by the white blood cells of the uterus in the second portal, the uterus. 300 million sperms start, and 60,000 of them reach the fallopian tube. The small fur cilia in the fallopian tube are directed downward to the opposite direction of the sperm's motion and serve as the third gate. Eventually, more than 100 sperms come to the oocyte and only a single sperm passes through the membrane of the oocyte and combines with the modification. When fertilized, the sperm DNA of the father and the egg DNA of the mother combine to resemble the parents' characteristics.

7.7. Vegetarianism, menstrual cycle, and diminished dysmenorrhea

If we understand the ovarian cycle and the uterine cycle, we can see that ovulation is possible without menstruation. Menstruation is not an integral part of fertility (ovulation). Menstruation occurs in the mammals, including the humans, the ovulation is done, but the endometrial tissue is not removed and is reabsorbed. However, the animal breeding zoos are known to show the menstrual blood.

During the month, 70% of the endometrial tissues usually fall apart, where the blood, the mucus, and the toxins are released together, and the bleeding usually lasts for from 3 days to 7 days. Many women suffer from severe abdominal pain, back pain, depression and nausea, and are exposed to the risk of anemia due to the monthly bleeding. In addition, there are more menstrual blood, hormones, and iron than the other blood, which are lost more as their aging advances. Therefore, if women can reduce the loss of the body nutrition due to menstruation, they will be able to lead a healthier life. If menstruation is caused by a large amount of the body waste, would it not be possible to reduce the blood loss when the amount of the body tissue waste is small? Like other animals, could the endometrium be resorbed into the body and eliminated? There are the studies related to this question.

Soy has the phytoestrogens that play a role that is similar to estrogen in the human body. Phyto means "plant." Phytoestrogens

Table 7-1. Isoflavones intake and menstrual cycle

Menstruation order	Isoflavone group	Milk protein group
1 time	26.27day	27.82day
2 time	27.81day	27.12day
3 time	29.81day	27.55day
3 time-1 time	3.52day increase	0.06day decrease
free estradiol	1.28 pg/ml	1.59 pg/ml

Cancer (2002) 94:1166–74. Free estradiol: a female hormone that is free of transfer proteins

are absorbed by the body and, sometimes, they have a weak estrogenic effect, sometimes binding to the estrogen receptors instead of the estrogen. When the estrogen is excessive, it promotes the proliferation of the breast tissue, and the generation of the breast cancer is increased, so that the weakly acting phytoestrogen prevents the breast cancer. In fact, the traditional Chinese or Japanese women who had consumed less beef and had consumed more beans than the Western women had the fewer breast cancers.

In 2002, Kumar and colleagues at the University of Florida designed an experiment to determine if phytoestrogens affect the menstrual cycle and, thus, prevent breast cancer. The premise of the logic is that the female menstrual cycle includes the follicles and the luteal phase, during which the breast cells proliferate from two to three times faster than the follicles. If the phytoestrogen increases the menstrual cycle, the prolongation of the luteal phase gets longer than that of the luteal phase, and, thus, the proliferation of the breast cells is suppressed and the possibility of breast cancer is lowered.

Usually, the menstrual cycle is 0.77 days in the menstrual cycle and 0.23 days in the luteal cycle. The researchers selected 66 women aged between 25 and 55, and one group received 40 mg of the isoflavone (genistein), a kind of phytoestrogen, while the other group had consumed the same calories of the milk protein as a fake drug [1,2]. The average intake of the isoflavones of the Asian people is from 40 mg per day to 80 mg per day.

The blood samples that had been collected during the three menstrual cycles showed that the estradiol, a kind of estrogen, had been reduced from 1.37 to 1.28 in the isoflavone group, while, regarding the milk protein group, ithad increased slightly from 1.54 to 1.59. In the human body, the sex hormone binds to the sex hormone–binding protein (SHBG), and its action is restricted. A free state that is not associated with the SHBG cannot control its action, but works in the body randomly with the sex hormone function. Thus, a reduction in the liberated estradiol would reduce the proliferation of the breast cells.

In the group taking the isoflavones, the menstrual cycle was 26.27 days at the beginning, but it was 29.81 days at the second time, and it was 3.52 days at the third time, while the menstrual cycle of the milk protein intake group had been decreased from 27.82 days at first to 27.55 days second and to 0.06 days third.

That is to say, as initially predicted, the isoflavones have been shown to increase the menstrual cycle, which may reduce the breast cancer incidence.

The increase in the menstrual cycle of the isoflavone group was 1.46 days, and that of the milk protein group was 0.14 days. The concentrations of the luteinizing hormone (LH) and the follicle-stimulating hormone (FSH) were lower in the isoflavone group. These results suggest that the isoflavones have a long-term effect on the pituitary gland, thereby, resulting in the anti-estrogenic effects [3].

7.8. Changes in vegetarianism and the menstrual period

In addition to the benefits of the isoflavones that vegetarians enjoy, there is, also, the problem of the increased menstrual effects of the animal foods. A problem of the fat in the intake of the animal foods would be that it is consumed too much. Reichman and colleagues had examined whether the menstrual cycle changes according to the amount of the fat that is ingested.

The experiment had consisted of 31 healthy women between the ages of 20 and 40 who had been initially fed a 40% fat diet over four menstrual cycles and 20% fat for the next four weeks. The period of the cycle was measured. In the experiment, 7 of the 31

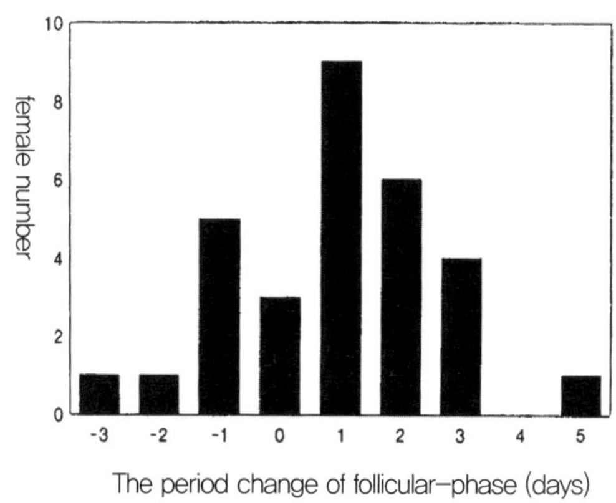

Figure 7–6. The intake of calories was reduced from 40% of fat to 20%

Reducing fat intake, on the average, increases the cell cycle of the ovaries, which lowers the likelihood of developing hormone-stimulated cancers.

healthy women had shown a decrease of the follicle size and 20 healthy women had shown an increase of the follicle size. The average change in the total of the 31 healthy women was 0.9 days (Fig. 7–5). And the average increased period of 20 healthy women had increased to 1.9 days [1].

The type of the food consumed affects the menstrual cycle as well as the menstrual pain. A study had been conducted at a university in Naples, Italy. The researchers had examined the symptoms of menstruation and the types of the foods that had been consumed by 356 female students who were aged from 14 years old to 21 years old. The menstrual cycle had been assessed according to the degree

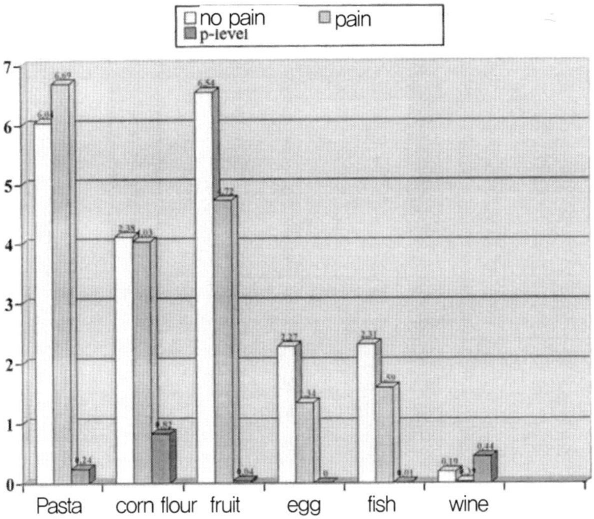

Figure 7–7. Types of Dysmenorrhea and Intakes

of the wetting of the pads, and a questionnaire had been used to determine the degree of the menstrual pain, the pain location, the pain time, the pain duration, the postmenstrual pain, the pain during each cycle, the uterine volume, and the ovarian volume. And the ovarian forms were scanned by ultrasound. According to this survey, 85% of the subjects had dysmenorrhea, 54% had no pain, and, the earlier the menarche started, the greater the menstrual pain and the longer the pain period [4].

The researchers had compared the types of the foods that had been consumed by the women with or without menstrual pain. The women without pain during the menstruation had consumed

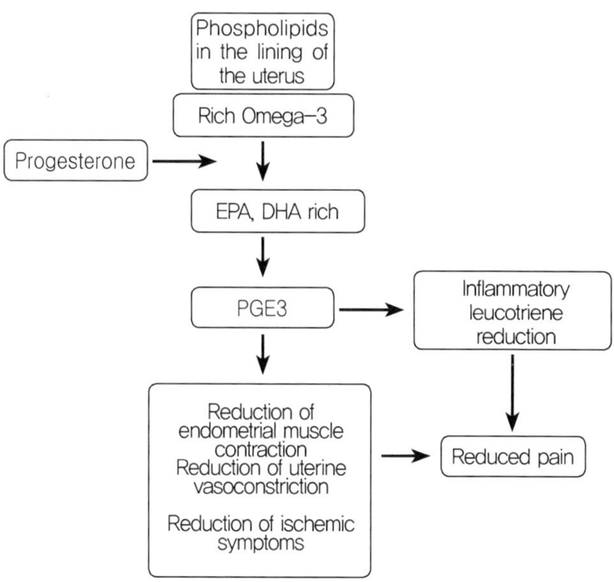

Figure 7-8. Mechanisms of Omega-3 Reduction of Dysmenorrhe

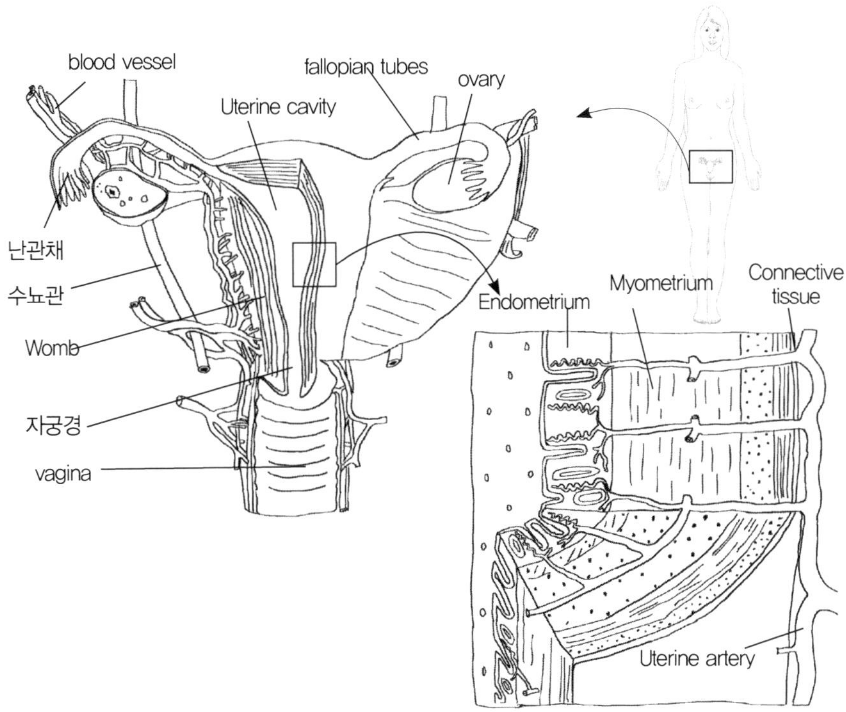

Figure 7-9. The structure of the uterus

more fruits, eggs, and fish, while those with severe pain were those who had consumed pasta (wheat flour), corn powder, and wine (Fig. 7-6). Fruits are known to be rich in antioxidants and various vitamins. Eggs are thought to be calcium and fish omega-3 abundant, and they may have the beneficial effect of pain relief. The omega-6 fatty acids, known as the inflammatory fatty acids, are abundant in corn, while the omega-6 during menstruation produces the prostaglandins and the rucotrienes in the endometrium, thereby, promoting the inflammation. Omega-3, on the other hand, produces the other classes of the prostaglandins and reduces the vasoconstriction and the contraction of the endometrium (Fig. 7−7). These effects inhibit the uterine and the smooth muscle cell proliferation, thus, reducing the menstrual pain and reducing the duration of the menstrual bleeding and the amount of the bleeding, as the researchers estimate. However, the omega−3 fatty acids are not only found in fish, but are more abundant in the perilla, and, next, they are safe, cheap, and easy to ingest through the walnuts and the beans.

A series of studies had explored why the vegetarian women have a long menstrual cycle, the fewer menstrual cramps, the fewer menstrual cycles, and the shorter menstrual periods. And because of the few hormones, the vitamins, the minerals, and the nutrients that are wasted by the menstrual blood, the vegetarian diet makes the body healthier and more vigorous

7.9. Healthy sperm and the environmental hormones.

Healthy sperm are a necessary condition for producing healthy offspring. However, the external environment can interfere with the production of the healthy sperm. Environmental hormones, heavy metals, such as mercury, and the free radicals attack and destroy the germ cells, damage the genes, and destroy their proteins. When the sperm is damaged and the damaged sperm is fertilized, it causes the defects in the newborn baby and the many problems, such as cancer, cardiovascular disease, and infertility. In this chapter, we examine the merits of the vegetarian diet in terms of three elements: The environmental hormones, the heavy metals, and the free radicals, which pose a threat to the healthy sperm.

Evidence is growing that environmental hormones can damage the male reproductive system. These environmental hormones are related to the estrogenic effects that are possessed by the organic, chlorine insecticides, the polychlorinated biphenyls (PCBs), the phenolic compounds, the phthalate compounds (PEs), and the like. The sources of these compounds are mainly the industrial wastes, the soils contaminated with wastes, the agricultural wastes, and the municipal wastes.

PCBs is a halogenated, lipophilic, and aromatic carbon compound with over 200 species that are reported. They are widely used as the insulating materials for the electrical appliances, such as the

PVC, the copying paper, the solvents for recycling the newspapers, and the waterproofing materials. They are found in all ecosystems, including the air, the water, the soil, the fish, the wildlife, the milk, the sperm, and the human fat cells. The PCBs are associated with the problems such as the development, the reproduction, the skin, the hepatotoxicity, the endocrine side effects, the carcinogenic effects, and the metabolic enzymes. A fetus in the uterus that had been exposed to the trace amounts of the PCBs has the very small genitalia.

Polyether sulfone (PEs) is the most widely-used chemical that is used in many plastic products. This chemical weakens male sperm motility and is known to have the mutagenic effects. The mechanism by which these organochlorines affect the fertility is associated with the estrogenic effects. In other words, these environmental hormones play the role of an estrogen, which

Table 7-2. Environmental hormones and standard indicators of infertile male and normal male

Characteristic	Infertile male	healthy fertile male
PCBs Concentration (μg/ml)	7.63	0
PEs Concentration (μg/ml)	2.03	0.06
Number of sperm ($\times 10^6$/ml)	17.04	72.75
One-time sperm volume (ml)	2.5	3.5
Normal form of sperm (%)	38.67	63.46
Single chain of DNA (damaged state)	15.92	4.3

Environ Health Perspect (2004) 112:69-78

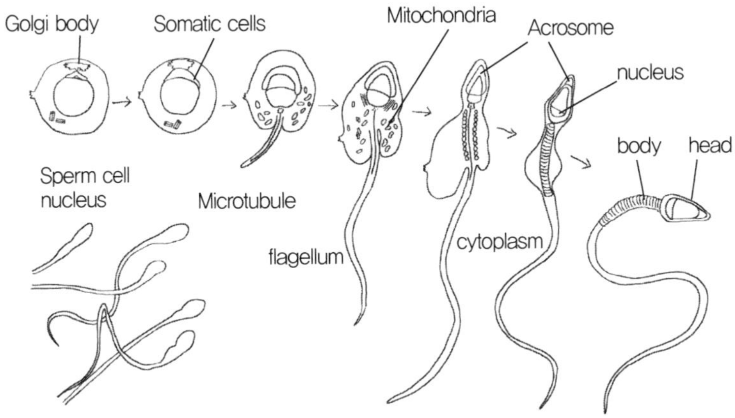

Figure 7-10. Sperm Development Process

inhibits the development process of the Sertoli cells of the fetal testes, and the damaged Sertoli cells, again, have a negative effect on the Leydig cells, which also confuses the production of the male hormones.

The results of a survey of 557 infertile couples in India clearly showed the benefits of vegetarianism regarding the sperm health. The researchers in India had measured the levels of the environmental hormones in the infertile men and the healthy women who had been pregnant, assuming that the environmental hormones will affect the sperm health. As a result of the test, the environmental hormones were detected in the semen of the infertile males but not the males at the reproductive ages. In other words, the PCBs were 7.63 μg / ml for the infertile men, but not

Table 7-3. Environmental hormone concentration and semen quality of infertile male

	Mean PCBs concentration (μg/ml)	Mean PEs concentration (μg/ml)	Mean motility sperm count ($\times 10^6$/ml)
City fish consume	10.49	3.13	0.51
Rural fish consume	5.26	0.77	0.92
City residence vegetarian	4.92	0.57	1.24
Rural resident vegetarian	1.28	0.37	7.5

Environ Health Perspect (2004) 112:69-78

for the men who were fertile, and the PEs were 2.03 μg / ml for the infertile men and 0.06 μg / ml for the fertile men (Table 7-2) [5]. The researchers further divided the infertile men into four groups based on whether or not they eat fish, assuming that the city has the more chances for coming into contact with the environmental hormones than the countryside and assuming that the environmental hormones are usually dissolved in water and accumulated in the aquatic organisms. They, also, had examined the levels of the environmental hormones and the health of the semen in the males in each group.

The highest levels of the environmental hormones were found in the urban areas, with the males eating fish at an average PCBs concentration of 10.49 μg / ml, while the group with the lowest levels of the environmental hormones was the group at 1.28 Ug / ml (Table 7-3). And the residence had been in the country.It was lower in the urban areas when eating fish than when not eating fish [5].

Environmental hormones act like the hormones in the human

body, so they can bind the sex hormone-binding globulin (SHBG) and the male hormone-binding proteins or bind the hormone receptors that are present in the cells to prevent the human hormones from acting. Or, to further enhance the hormonal action of the human body, the endocrine system is disturbed. Because of these problems, the environmental hormones act on the testes and the epididymis, which can affect the normal sperm production and the male hormone secretion. If the normal hormone secretion is impaired in the testes, the hormones associated with these hormones, such as those from the thyroid gland, the pineal gland, and the adrenal glands, will, also, have the side-effects. They,also, act on the white blood cells to release the peroxide anion in an uncontrolled state, which can lead to a damage and a reduction of the sperm

7.10. Heavy metal, sperm, and vegetarians

One of the world's best-known examples of heavy metal contaminations was a mercury contamination in Japan. Mercury from a factory in Minamitaman in the 1950s started to pollute the coastal waters. Since 1955, the offshore people have been consuming an average of 30mg per person per kilogram of body weight every year. Mercury toxicity is known to be from 3 mg to 7 mg per kg of body weight. By 1965, after more than a decade, the mercury had continued to accumulate in the bodies of the

Table 7-4. Fertility and infertility male, vegetarian hair mercury levels (mg/kg)

Group	Age	fertility male	infertility male
non-vegetarian	17-29year	2.445	3.128
	30-39year	3.462	3.867
	40-49year	2.985	5.313
	50-72year	3.762	7.563
vegetarian	0.38		

people, and, soon after reaching the toxic levels, the people with the symptom of mercury poisoning began to appear. The visual, auditory, and verbal inabilities, the ataxia, and the limbic seizures had been seen in these patients, and the main target had been the central nervous system.

Even if the intake is low, mercury accumulates in the body, so it can cause the problem of male infertility when it has been about from 20 years to 30 years . As the industrialization has progressed globally, the pollution of the ocean through the heavy metals has become more serious, especially in the coastal cities where the fish consumption is easy and routine.

The Hong Kong people usually eat fish or shellfish more than four times a week. In 1997, there was a report on the status of the heavy metals contamination and the infertility among the Hong Kong people. The researchers divided the infertile men and the healthy boys, by age, and, also,the vegetarians as a group to investigate the mercury concentration in the hair [6].

As expected, the fertile male had a lower mercury concentration than the infertile male. At the age of the 30s, the male was 3.462 mg/kg forthe fertile male, while the male was 3.867 mg/kg for the infertile male. The mercury concentration of the vegetarians was 0.38 mg/kg, which is very low, at about one tenth of the non-vegetarians (Table 7-4). As the age increases, the accumulated mercury concentration increases, and the difference between the infertile male and the infertile female is, also, increased.

The proportions of the mercury accumulationsin the fish consumptions in this study were 219 in a Bangladesh study in 1996, 149 in a Brazilian study in 2001, and 143 in a Swedish survey in 2004.

In Sweden, the hair mercury concentration in the men who had ingested fish at least once a month was 0.5 g / kg, while at least eight times a month was 3.6 g / kg. As a result of analyzing 37 pairs of the subjects, it was found that the fish intake range of the 35 pairs of the males and the females who had ingested fish was proportional to the hair mercury concentrations [7].

7.11. Oxidizer, sperm, and the vegetarians

The functionally-impaired sperm will be an important cause of male infertility. As described above, the sperm function impairment

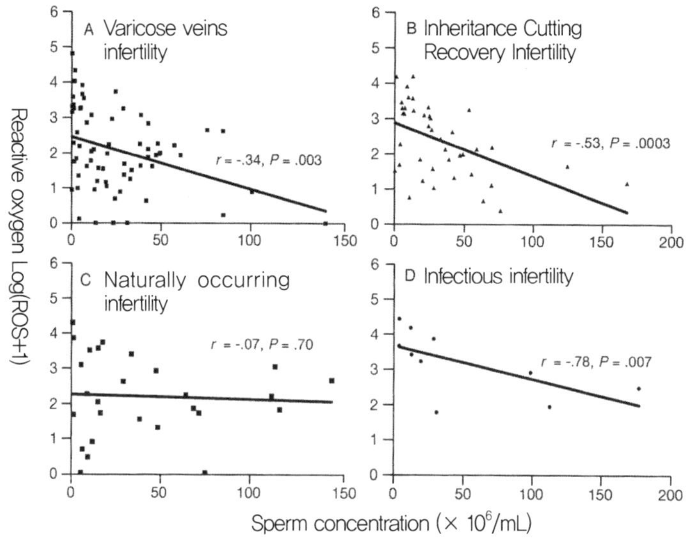

Figure 7–11. Active oxygen and sperm concentration

is caused by the environmental hormones and the mercury, but a functional damage caused by active oxygen is considered to be an important part. Clinically, one of the most important indicators of infertility is the high oxygen stress in the semen.

Active oxygen is produced by burning fuel by using the oxygen in the intracellular organelle called "mitochondria" to produce energy in the cells in the body. One of about 250 oxygens is presumed to be an active oxygen. To prevent the risk regarding the naturally occurring active oxygen, the body makes the antioxidant enzymes and consumes the antioxidants in the form of food. However, if the active oxygen and the antioxidants are not in equilibrium, and, if

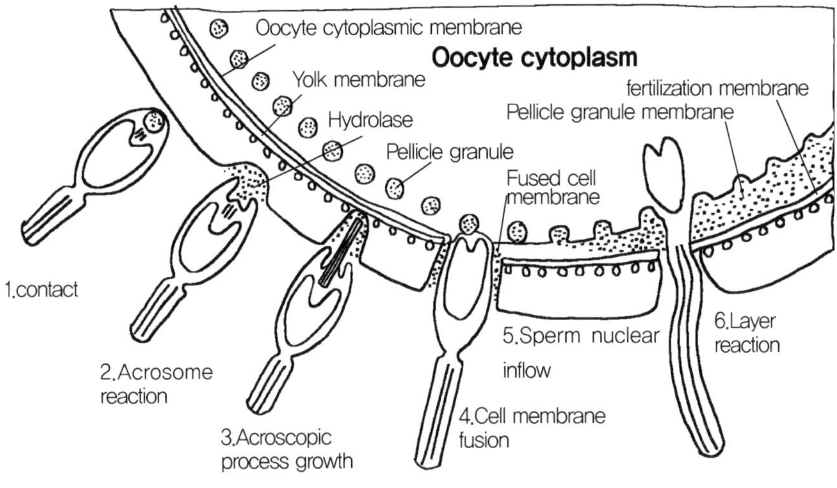

Figure 7–12. Fertilization process of sperm and egg

Table 7–5. Relationship between sperm state and active oxygen

Clinical diagnosis	Sperm concentration ($\times 10^6$/ml)	Sperm motility (%)	Log(Active oxygen+1) (cpm)
Normal	69.42	55.45	1.3
Varicose veins infertility	25.89	38.40	2.2
Inheritance Cutting Recovery Infertility	34.18	28.97	2.4
Naturally occurring infertility	37.53	37.93	2.3
Infection infertility	48.24	48.17	3.2

Fertility and Sterility (2000) 73(3): 459–464

they do not cope adequately with the active oxygen that has been produced, the human cells will be damaged. Of course, this includes the sperm. The testicles, in which the sperm are produced, are particularly rich in the unsaturated fatty acids, which are the good targets for the active oxygen.

Thus, if the sperm is attacked by active oxygen and its normal function is impaired, it cannot pass through the gates, such as the low pH and the leukocyte that is caught in the uterus until it meets the ovum in the oviduct, and the acrosome can be damaged. Even if it is passed, it will be difficult to correct it when the gene is damaged, and it will stop the development process. In other words, the free radicals can lead to fertility by destroying the function of the spermatozoa at the various stages of the process, which is necessary until the fertilization. One study found that, after the infertile males were randomly selected, they had the high levels of the free radicals in the semen, which were 40%–88% of the infertile males (Fig. 7–8, Table 7–5).

From 1997 to 1998, a team of men in Ohio had studied 167 infertile men and had examined the relationship between oxygen

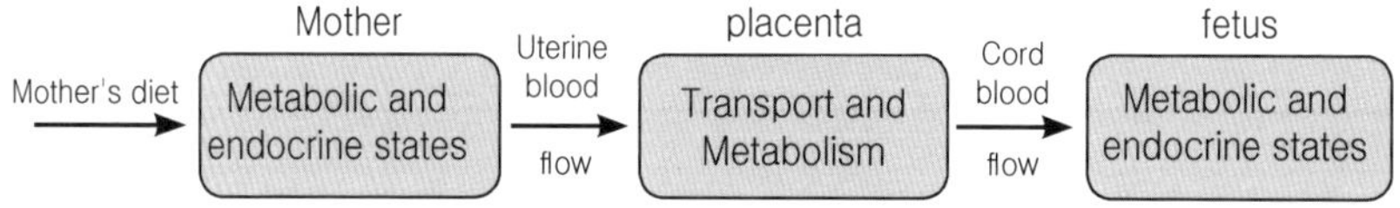

Figure 7–13. Nutrient supply from mother's diet to fetus

and sperm concentration. They were divided into four groups according to the causes of the infertility: The varicosis, the vasectomy, the reconstructive infertility, the spontaneous infertility, and the infertility associated with infection. The results showed that the amount of the reactive oxygen species was higher in all four groups compared to the normal group, especially in the cases of the infections [8].

7.12. Fetal health and the fetal programming hypothesis.

Gradual change from fertilization to maturation is called a "development". The developmental process is surprising because only one cell grows into a highly-organized system of the tissues, the organs, and the organ systems of the several tens of cells. During the development, certain genes are turned on and the others are turned off to allow for the differentiation. To do this, the fetus needs the nutrients. The fetus absorbs the nutrients made by the mother through the placenta and sends the metabolism waste to the mother (Fig. 7-9). Thus, the placenta is the life support device of the fetus. The placenta is divided into the maternal placenta and the fetal placenta, which are not connected to the blood vessels but have the respective, independent regions.

So, how do the mother's nutrients reach the fetus? The placenta is spaced out with the short intervals as if the fingers of the mother

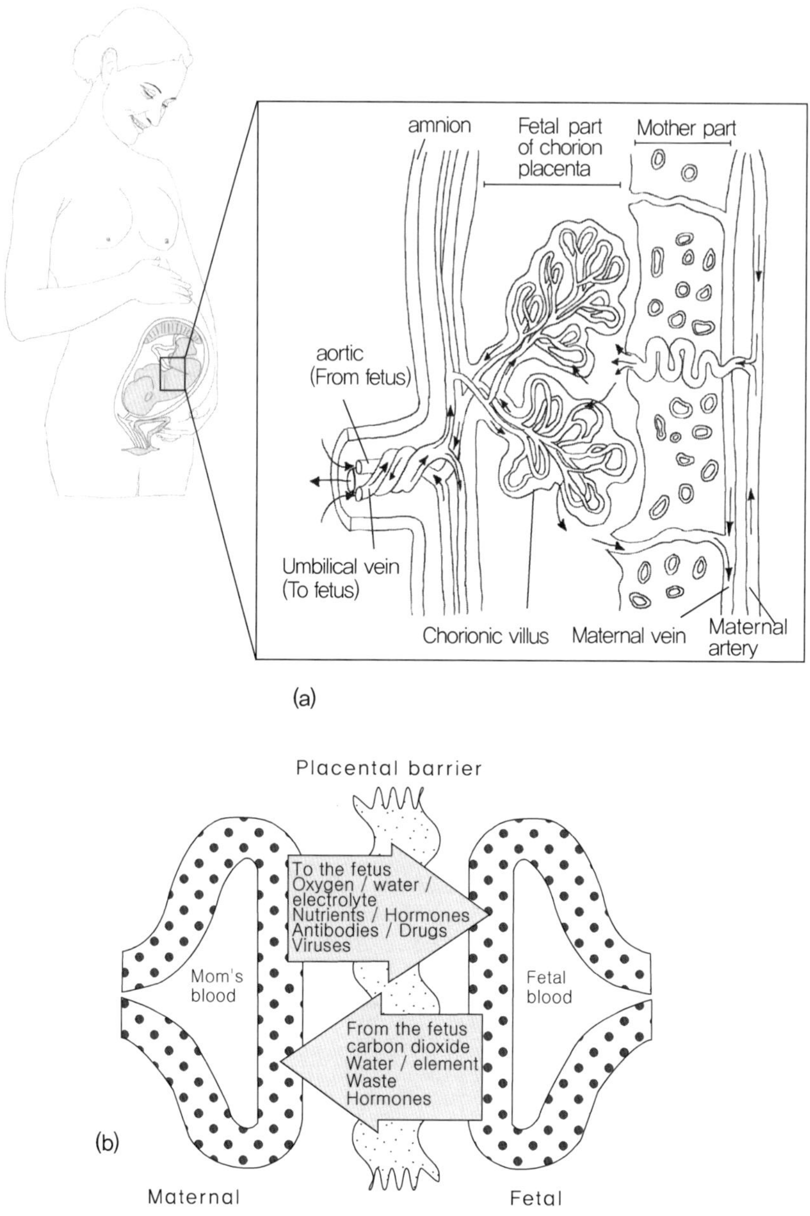

Figure 7–14. Placenta structure (a) and nutrient transfer (b)

placenta are staggered, so that the substances spread between the two villi, and, sometimes, there is an active movement using the energy.

The red blood cells, which are important for the oxygen transfer, are too large to pass between the villi, but the oxygen-binding capacity of the fetal placenta hemoglobin is larger, so that the red blood cells of the maternal placenta remain intact and only the oxygen is delivered toward the fetal placenta. It is because of this placenta that the blood types of the mother and the fetus are different from each other. As such, the placenta should be as clean as possible, just like a home where the fetus is nourished

7.13. The role of the placenta in the fetal programming

The 'fetal origin hypothesis' is the theory that the adult cardiovascular and metabolic diseases are largely influenced by the malnutrition during the fetal period. In other words, if the maternal placenta fails to respond to the fetal nutritional needs, the fetus adapts to its deficient nutritional status so that its body development process can survive. In other words, when the nutrients become insufficient, the fetus changes the flow of the blood for the development of the brain, which is the most important part of the body, to send the nutrients to the brain and, instead, to reduce the blood flow to the heart, the pancreas and the like.This enables

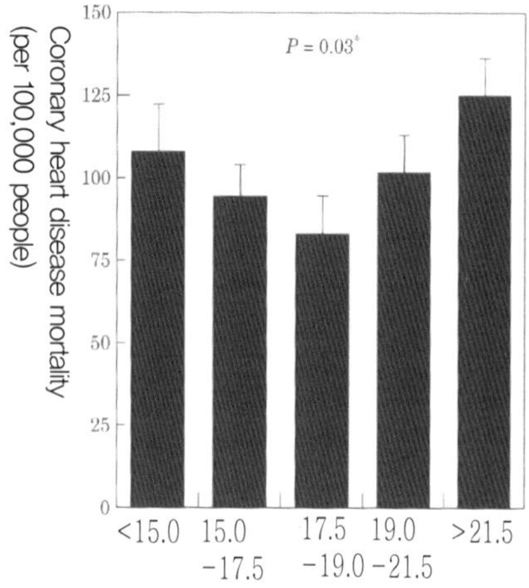

Figure 7–15. Heart disease mortality and placental weight ratio [10]

Table 7–6. Green vegetables, meat, fish intake and diastolic blood pressure (mmHg)

Green vegetable (Times / week)	Meat, fish (times / week)			
	Less than 11 times	12~15	16~21	More than 21 times
Less than 7 times	120	120	123	124
More than 7 times	118	120	120	121
Average	119	120	121	122

the survival. This allows for the immediate survival, but it can be manifested as a pulmonary disease, a cardiovascular disease, and the metabolic syndrome when overloaded after the birth.

This hypothesis was first proposed in the early 1990s and has been supported by numerous epidemiological studies and experimental data to date. In other words, the maternal nutrition can continue to affect the life span after the birth by programming the fetal body.

This programming is made possible by directly altering the nutrients available for the fetus and by indirectly influencing the function and structure of the placenta. In other words, the changes in the placental growth and the vascular resistance change the placental nutrition and the hormone metabolism and cause the changes in the nutrients delivery and the distribution between the maternal, the placenta, and the fetus, all of which are important for the fetal adaptation. This is the central idea of programming [9].

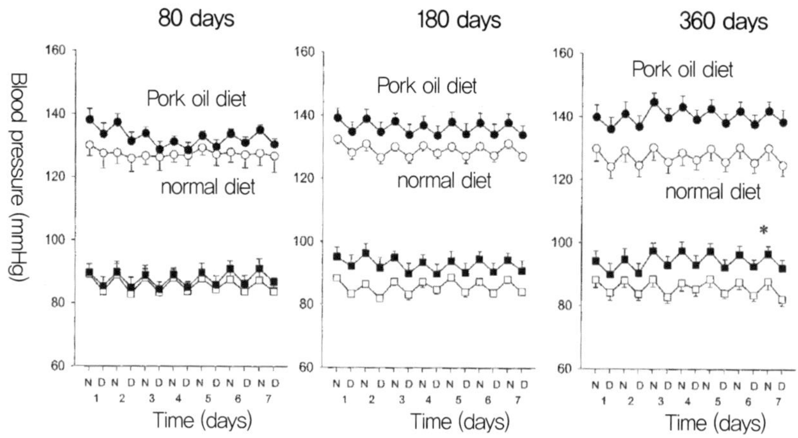

Figure 7–16. Difference in blood pressure according to dietary fat

7.14. The dietary pattern of the mother and the fetal mother's cardiovascular diseases.

The nutrients in the blood of the mother affect the nutrients in the blood of the placenta, which, in turn, determine the nutritional status of the fetus (Fig. 7-10). Depending on the weight of the placenta, the mortality rate of the coronary heart disease varies from mother to mother (Fig. 7-11).

There had been a study of 626 men and women in the Motherwell Province of Scotland. The mothers were admitted to a hospital from 1967 to 1968, and the ages were from 27 years old to 30 years old. The researchers went to the hospital in Motherwell and had obtained the data on the mothers' pregnancies and, later,on the dietary intake, and, then,they analyzed the food items: Meat, fish, eggs, cheese, green vegetables, potatoes, bread, cakes, biscuits, milk, etc. The average daily intake of the animal protein was about 58g. After obtaining the data on the birth weights of the newborn babies born from the mothers, the blood pressure of the subjects who had grown up as the adults had been investigated [11].

According to the research results, the diastolic blood pressure of the offspring was lower if the mother had consumed more green vegetables, and the blood pressure was higher if the meat had been consumed more. As shown in Table 7-6, the offspring of the mothers who had eaten the green vegetables seven times a week and had eatenthe meat less than 11 times per week had a

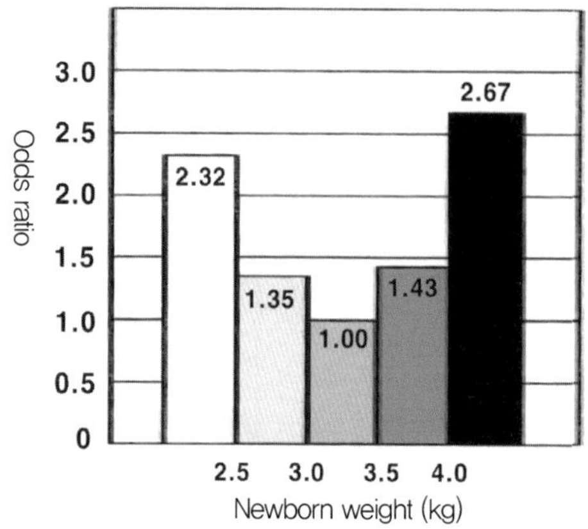

Figure 7-17. Relative Risk of Neonatal Weight and Type 2 Diabetes in School Age

diastolic blood pressure of 118. On the other hand, the offspring of the mothers who had eaten more than 21 meals,including the fish while eating the green vegetables, less than 7 times per week had a diastolic blood pressure of 124 and a difference of 6 mmHg. It is generally known that a 10 mm Hg reduction of the blood pressure reduces the mortality by 30%.

So, why is high maternal protein diet a problem? The essential amino acids are absorbed by the human body and are synthesized or oxidized to be used as an energy source. To be oxidized, vitamin B6 and the folic acid are needed. Thus, the excessive amounts of the essential amino acids are needed to provide the mother with the

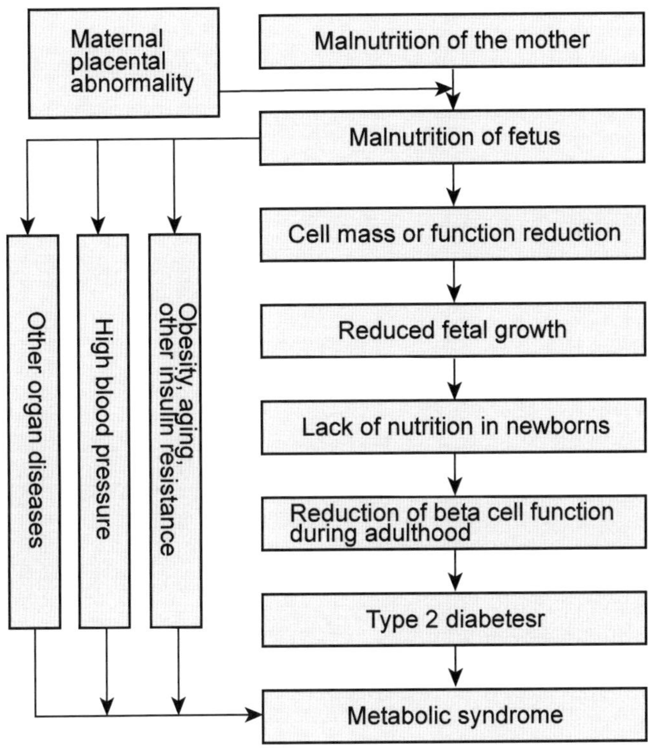

Figure 7-18. Fetal programming hypothesis of metabolic syndrome

metabolic stress, resulting in the changes of the hormones, such as the cortisol in the mother's body (Fig. 7-10). The researchers interpreted that this had been a bad influence on the fetus and that it had affected the developmental process of the fetus and had, ultimately, increased the incidence of the cardiovascular disease. In particular, the offsprings of the mothers who had consumed the fish in the late pregnancy had developed the diastolic blood pressures [11]

7.15. Fatty acid and maternal health

This study examines the changes in the blood pressure according to the type of the lipids consumed by the mother and shows the risk of the animal foods to the fetus during the pregnancy. In 2003, Khan and colleagues reported that, during pregnancy and lactation, 10 days before the pregnancy of the mother rats, one group had been fed a normal diet,with 5.3% of corn oil, and the other group had been fed with 25.7% animal fat, while the protein and the carbohydrates had increased the fat mass. After the offsprings of the two groups of the mothers had weaned, they had been fed the same diet, which had been free to eat, and their blood pressures were measured on the 80th day, 180th day, and on the 360th day. At 180 days, the weight of the dietary fat group was 458.27g, while that of the normal dietary group was 399g. The systolic blood pressure was from 142.1mmHg to 129.7mmHg, and the dietary group was 12.4mmHg lower (Fig.) The researchers estimated that the animal fat resulted in an abnormal function of the vascular, endothelial cells and that this was due to the elevated blood pressure. They, also, mentioned that the DHA is important for the prevention of the cardiovascular disease

7.16. Gestational diabetes and the metabolic syndrome

When the nutrients supplied by the mother are deficient, the fetus will save the blood for the growth of the brain and the other essential organs, which are rich in the nutrients and oxygen, which is called the "brain-saving adaptation". Animal studies have shown that, when hypoxemia occurs, the fetus blocks the umbilical cord's arterial blood and damages the liver and pancreas tissues. The blood thus saved is used for the circulation in the central nervous system.

A survey of the diabetic children who were the school-aged children who were aged from 6 years old to 18 years old from 1992 to 1997 is an example of the fetal programming hypothesis. The researchers randomly selected 1,780 diabetics and 1,966 normal subjects for a fasting glucose test. And the birth weights of the subjects were obtained from the birth registers.

The diabetes risk was found to be 2.32 for the 2,500 g diabetics, 1.35 for the group between 2,500 g and 2,999, and 1.43 for the group between 3,500 gand 3,999 g.Their birth weights were between 3,000 g and 3,499 g. The group with the birth weights of 4,000 g or more had the diabetes incidence of 2.67 (Fig. 7–13) [13]. That is, the healthiest group would be between 3,000 g and 3,499 g if diabetes was not considered, regardless of age, sex, BMI, and genetic or socioeconomic status, and the trend of the diabetes was U–shaped.

If there is the mother's lack of the nutrient supply during the pregnancy, the fetus concentrates the blood flow to the brain and the heart, which are essential for the survival, and supplies the nutrients and the oxygen, which reduces the number of the beta cells in the pancreas and weakens the susceptibility to insulin (Fig. 7–14). However, the weakened beta cells and the low–insulin–sensitive human cells of the underweight–born offsprings fail to overcome the burden of the over–nutrition during the growing season. Eventually, the human body is exposed to the urine and the excessive burden [14].

The nutritional deficiency of the fetus is exposed to the risk of a kidney damage and hypertension in addition to the postnatal diabetes through the changes of the fetal growth, the metabolism, and the vascular system. This is a kind of the metabolic syndrome

7.17. Are the vegetarians, the placenta, and the fetus benefited?

Women lose iron in their menstrual period every month, so their iron storages are less than those of men. Usually, it is 3.2g for males and 2.8g for females. During the pregnancy period, the fetus requires the iron from the mother in order to grow. In the early stages of pregnancy, from 1 mg to 2.5 mg of the iron is increased to 6.5 mg of the iron in the last 3 months of the pregnancy. Can vegetarians meet most of their iron needs from the plant foods and meet the fetal demand with the nonheme iron, which has a lower rate of absorption than the animal meat?

Scientists say that the results are met. The mothers in the Third World, most of whom are the vegetarians, take an average of from 10 mg to 14 mg of the nonheme iron. However, not all of the ingested iron is absorbed. The iron absorption during the pregnancy varies dramatically, with only 7% of the intake being absorbed at 12 weeks of the gestation, but 36% at week 24 and 66% at week 36. In other words, even without the mother's anemia, vegetarians can feed the amount needed by the fetus at each period, which is 9.4 times the ability of the vegetable foods to change the rate of the absorption of the nonheme iron. As already mentioned above, the hemolysis of the animal foods absorbs at up to twice the absorption rate, which is almost constant regardless of the intake.

The reason why hemolysis can be a problem is that the mother's blood must be diluted for the fetus to grow. When a woman becomes pregnant, the heat from the fetal placenta increases the body temperature of the mother. At this time, the mother enlarges the blood vessels of the peripheral part, thereby dissipating the heat. At the same time, the volume of the blood increases and the blood concentration becomes thin.

The blood hemoglobin concentration in pregnant women is 133 g/L on the average, which falls sharply from the 20th week of the gestation to 110 g/L in the 36th gestational week. However, the blood–thinning results in a beneficial effect on the growth of the fetus. As the concentration decreases, the viscosity of the blood, also, decreases because the blood flow between the maternal placenta villi and the fetal placenta villi is accelerated and the fetus is supplied with the sufficient nutrients.

The placenta is separated from the fetal placenta and the maternal placenta, as if the fingers of the two hands are in contact with each other, as if they are staggered, so that the supply of the nutrients and the oxygen is made by widening the gap between them.

However, as the maternal blood volume increases, the total hemoglobin mass and the total erythrocyte mass increase during the pregnancy.

A large–scale survey of 150,000 pregnant women in London from 1988 to 1991 found that the average weight of the newborn babies was high at 85~95 g/L, with the low, maternal hemoglobin concentration at from 95 g/L to 105 g/L.

However, if the plasma volume is not increased enough, the flow of the blood is not fast enough to supply the nutrients to the fetal villi, thus, limiting the fetal growth. In other words, the maternal blood is supplied to the villi spaces by the twisted arteries of the placenta. If the blood pressure rises, the placenta is separated from the uterine wall and impacted, resulting in the bleeding and the lumps of the blood in the placenta. This situation, eventually, leads to the spatial closures between the maternal villi and the fetal villi, for the supply to the fetus, making it difficult to provide the nutrition, while the size of the placenta becomes large. In a poor nutritional environment, the fetus runs the survival programs to survive from the reduction of the blood to the heart, the lungs, the kidneys, and the pancreas and to increase the blood flow to the brain and the central nervous system. This causes many diseases after the birth.

One of the representative examples is a damage to the fetal, cardiac, circulatory system due to the elevation of the fetal hematocrit and the blood viscosity. According to a preliminary study of 38,000 newborns in the United States, the fetal, hematocrit values were higher when the placenta's weight was lower than expected for the newborn's body weight. The physiological changes that occur in an oxygen transfer cause an adaptation process called "the change of the fetal hematocrit", which may lead to a change in the size of the placenta and a change of the oxygen delivery, which may have important consequences for the fetal lung development.

The placental weight (placental weight / newborn body weight) of the newborn's weight, also, implies the placenta's role in the fetal programming. According to Martyn, Barker, and Osmond's 1996 study on the ratio between the U-shape and the heart disease, if the placental weight is too low or too high compared to the weight of the newborn, there is a high risk of death from coronary heart disease after the baby grows up [15].

Preeclampsia, which affects the several species and causes a headache, the proteinuria, the elevated blood pressure, and affects the many organs, increases three-fold when the plasma volume expansion is impaired. The iron deficiency, of course, causes the anemia in the fetus, but, in the industrialized countries, it is more likely that the iron deficiency will cause a blood volume expansion failure. As already mentioned above, the non-hemp iron of the vegetable foods actively changes the absorption rate according to the situation of the human body and fulfills the goal of expanding the volume of the blood of the mother and completes the mission of supplying the necessary iron

7.18. Conclusion

A case of a fully vegetarian mother is known. She had been vegan for several years before she was pregnant, and she had been so clean that her baby did not have to be washed, so many people who were watching the scene were very surprised. The direct voice of the mother was as follows:

"My sister-in-law is vegetarian, and when I went to the hospital with my sister-in-law, the doctor said she had a very positive amniotic fluid that was more positive than those of the other mothers. There is no exact scientific basis, but I think it is not a vegetarian influence. It's the same with my baby."

She did not eat any raw food, like the carp that many pregnant women eat. Instead, she replied in the morning with the organic fruits that had been grown directly, and she ate a lot of the mulberry leaf powder. Mulberry leaves contain six times as much calcium as milk and six times as much iron as spinach.

The fact that a newborn baby was clean enough not to be washed means that the placenta was, also, clean, which means that the oxygen and the nutrients had been well-supplied without any obstruction. There has been no specific investigation into the human body, but, as we have seen above, there had been the case of the intake of the animal fat, the consumption of the vegetables and the carbohydrates, and the low blood pressure of the offsprings of the mothers who had consumed less animal protein, and others of the like. In addition, it can be estimated that it will be very beneficial in the fetal programming, as well.

References

1. Reichman ME, Judd JT, Taylor PR, Nair PP, Jones DY, Campbell WS: Effect of dietary fat on length of the follicular phase of the menstrual cycle in a controlled diet setting. J Clin Endocrinol Metab 1992, 74:1171–1175.

2. McIntosh JE, Matthews CD, Crocker JM, Broom TJ, Cox LW: Predicting the luteinizing hormone surge: relationship between the duration of the follicular and luteal phases and the length of the human menstrual cycle. Fertil Steril 1980, 34:125–130.

3. Kumar NB, Cantor A, Allen K, Riccardi D, Cox CE: The specific role of isoflavones on estrogen metabolism in premenopausal women. Cancer 2002, 94:1166–1174.

4. Balbi C, Musone R, Menditto A, Di Prisco L, Cassese E, D'Ajello M, Ambrosio D, Cardone A: Influence of menstrual factors and dietary habits on menstrual pain in adolescence age. Eur J Obstet Gynecol Reprod Biol 2000, 91:143–148.

5. Chapin RE, Robbins WA, Schieve LA, Sweeney AM, Tabacova SA, Tomashek KM: Off to a good start: the influence of pre- and periconceptional exposures, parental fertility, and nutrition on children's health. Environ Health Perspect 2004, 112:69–78.

6. Dickman MD, Leung KM: Mercury and organochlorine exposure from fish consumption in Hong Kong. Chemosphere 1998, 37:991–1015.

7. Johnsson C, Sallsten G, Schutz A, Sjors A, Barregard L: Hair mercury levels versus freshwater fish consumption in household members of Swedish angling societies. Environ Res 2004, 96:257–263.

8. Pasqualotto FF, Sharma RK, Nelson DR, Thomas AJ, Agarwal A: Relationship between oxidative stress, semen characteristics, and clinical diagnosis in men undergoing infertility investigation. Fertil Steril 2000, 73:459–464.

9. Harding JE: The nutritional basis of the fetal origins of adult disease. Int J Epidemiol 2001, 30:15–23.

10. Forsen T, Eriksson JG, Tuomilehto J, Teramo K, Osmond C, Barker DJ: Mother's weight in pregnancy and coronary heart disease in a cohort of Finnish men: follow up study. BMJ 1997, 315:837–840.

11. Shiell AW, Campbell-Brown M, Haselden S, Robinson S, Godfrey KM, Barker DJ: High-meat, low-carbohydrate diet in pregnancy: relation to adult blood pressure in the offspring. Hypertension 2001, 38:1282–1288.

12. Khan IY, Taylor PD, Dekou V, Seed PT, Lakasing L, Graham D, Dominiczak AF, Hanson MA, Poston L: Gender-linked hypertension in offspring of lard-fed pregnant rats. Hypertension 2003, 41:168–175.

13. Wei JN, Sung FC, Li CY, Chang CH, Lin RS, Lin CC, Chiang CC, Chuang LM: Low birth weight and high birth weight infants are both at an increased risk to have type 2 diabetes among schoolchildren in taiwan. Diabetes Care 2003, 26:343–348.

14. Hales CN, Barker DJ: The thrifty phenotype hypothesis. Br Med Bull 2001, 60:5–20.

15. Martyn CN, Barker DJ, Osmond C: Mothers' pelvic size, fetal growth, and death from stroke and coronary heart disease in men in the UK. Lancet 1996, 348:1264–1268.

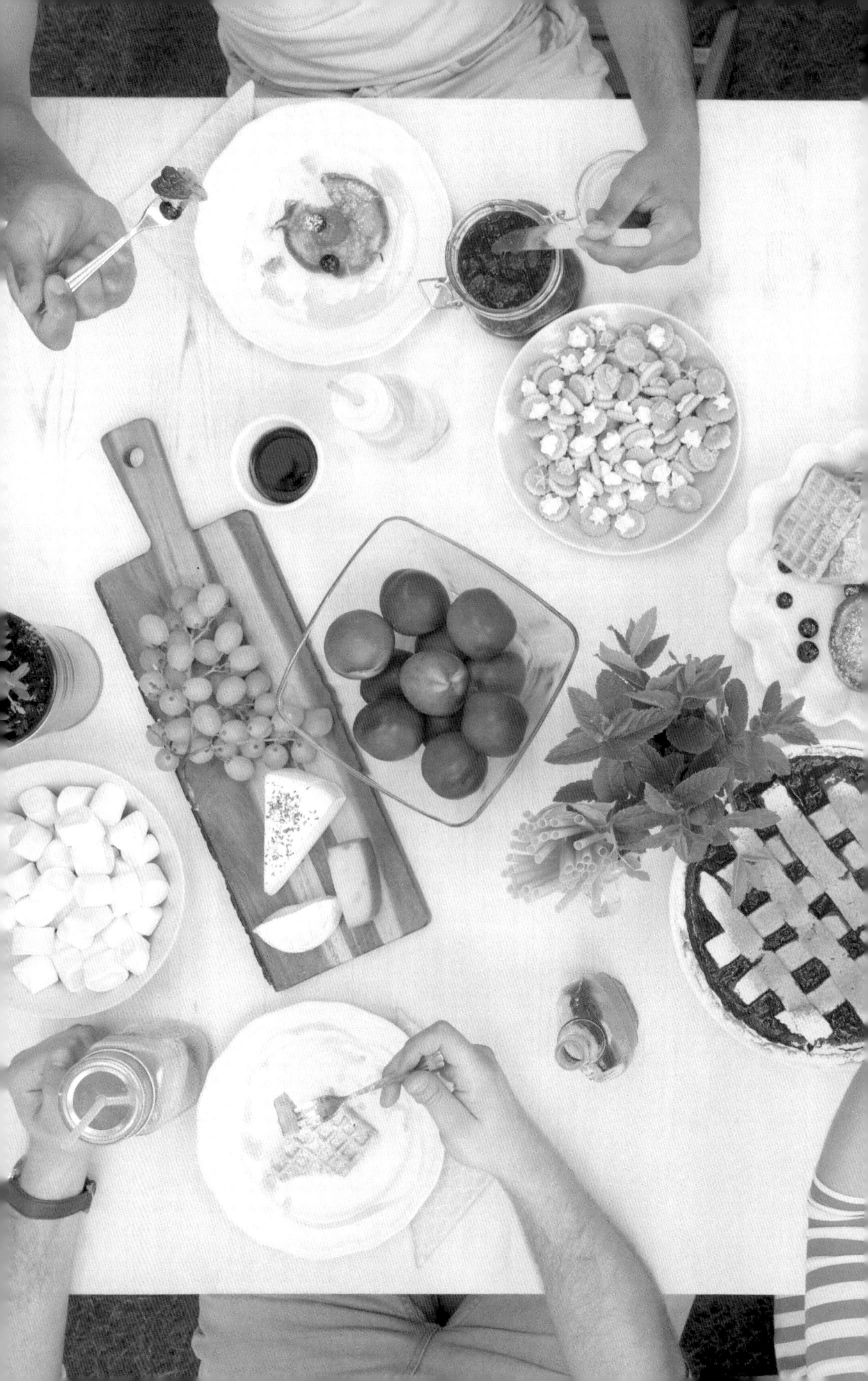

Chapter 8. Immune System and Vegetarian Diet

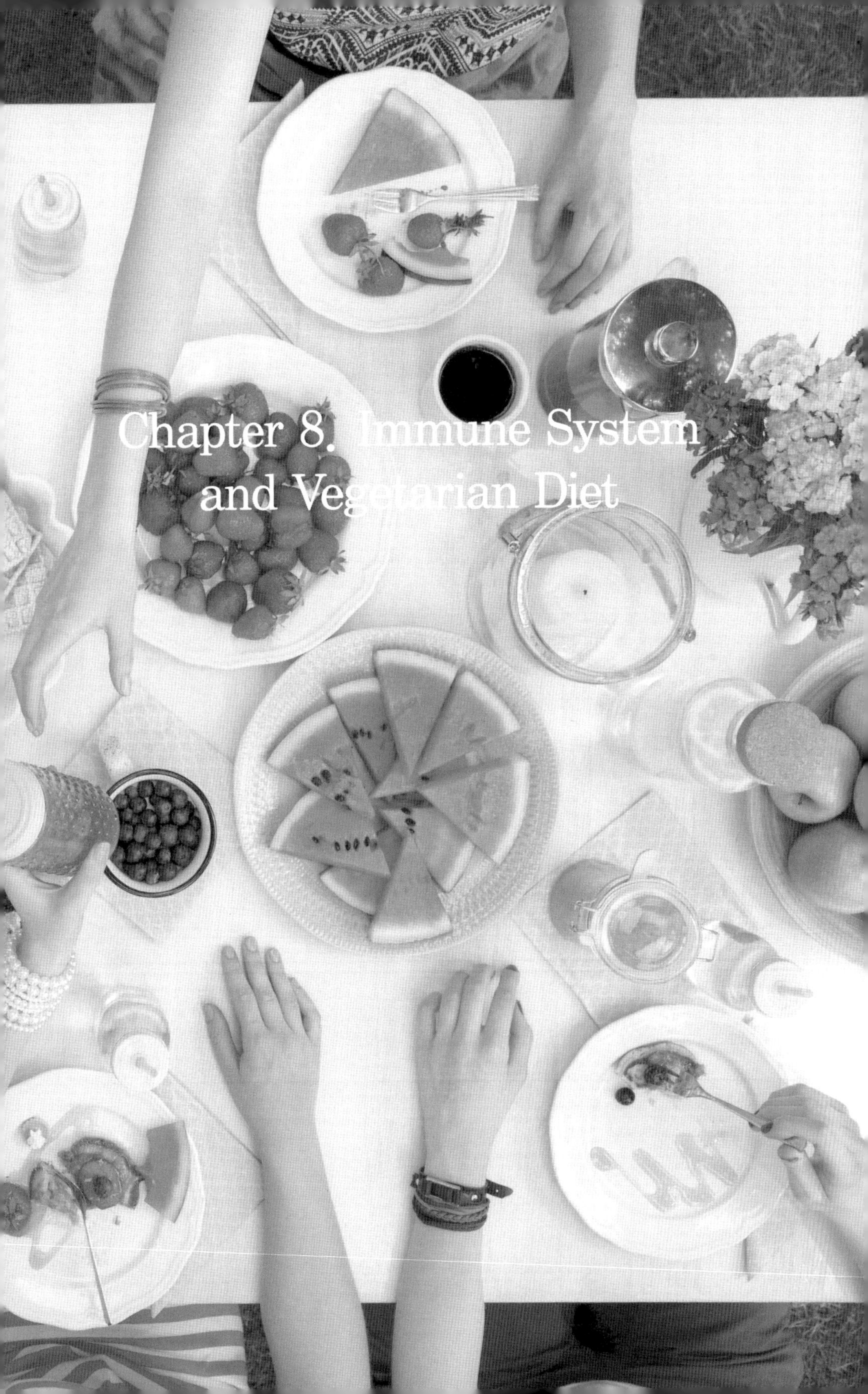

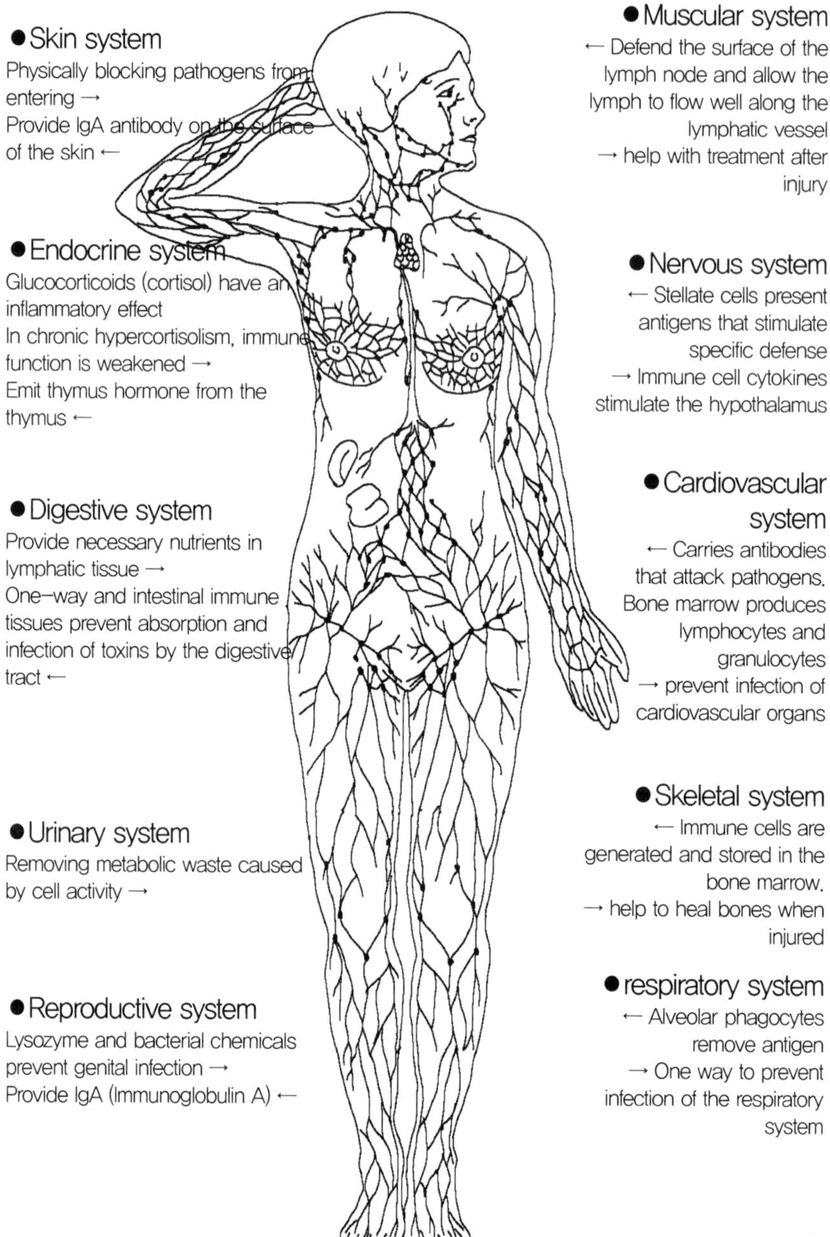

● Skin system
Physically blocking pathogens from entering →
Provide IgA antibody on the surface of the skin ←
● Endocrine system
Glucocorticoids (cortisol) have an inflammatory effect
In chronic hypercortisolism, immune function is weakened →
Emit thymus hormone from the thymus ←
● Digestive system
Provide necessary nutrients in lymphatic tissue →
One–way and intestinal immune tissues prevent absorption and infection of toxins by the digestive tract ←
● Urinary system
Removing metabolic waste caused by cell activity →
● Reproductive system
Lysozyme and bacterial chemicals prevent genital infection →
Provide IgA (Immunoglobulin A) ←
● Muscular system
← Defend the surface of the lymph node and allow the lymph to flow well along the lymphatic vessel
→ help with treatment after injury
● Nervous system
← Stellate cells present antigens that stimulate specific defense
→ Immune cell cytokines stimulate the hypothalamus
● Cardiovascular system
← Carries antibodies that attack pathogens. Bone marrow produces lymphocytes and granulocytes
→ prevent infection of cardiovascular organs
● Skeletal system
← Immune cells are generated and stored in the bone marrow.
→ help to heal bones when injured
● respiratory system
← Alveolar phagocytes remove antigen
→ One way to prevent infection of the respiratory system

Chapter 8. The immune system and the vegetarian diet

8.1. The definition of the immune system

Immunity is a struggle between me and myself. This struggle is seen to have existed from the beginning of life. The way in which the microorganisms break down the viruses to protect their genes makes this inference possible. Through the process of evolution, the struggle between me and the non–existent has continued to interact and evolve together. The traces can still be confirmed vividly in our body. A typical example is that we have the two systems, the innate immunity and the adoptive immunity. In other words, the system which is called the "immune immunity" or the "innate immunity" includes the immune recognition patterns that the human beings have from their births. The immune system recognizes the cell walls and the genes of about 13 kinds of the microorganisms from the time of the birth. The representative immune cells are the dendritic cells, the macrophages, the granulocytes, and the natural killer cells (Fig. 8–1, Table 8–1).

However, the microbes are constantly mutating and transforming to deceive the immune system, so it is impossible to remember all those patterns. So, it is the adaptive immunity or the acquired immunity that creates the awareness of the microbe and does not invade after the birth. The typical, acquired immune cells are the T (thymus) cells and the B (bone marrow) cells. The innate, immune system and the acquired immune system interact with each other to protect the human being. It is the digestive tract and the respiratory tract that are important. So, evolutionarily, the immune system starts from the digestive organs. Even now, the largest and wider area of our human body is the superficial immune system and the organ immune system.

When we eat food, the activity of the immune system in the body increases rapidly. The human body has developed a tolerance system because it has to be accepted for the survival of the individual, though it is not. It is not me, but I am tolerated to make it mine. The immune cells interact with the nervous system and the endocrine system. As a result, the physical health can affect the psychology, while the psychological state can affect the immune system.

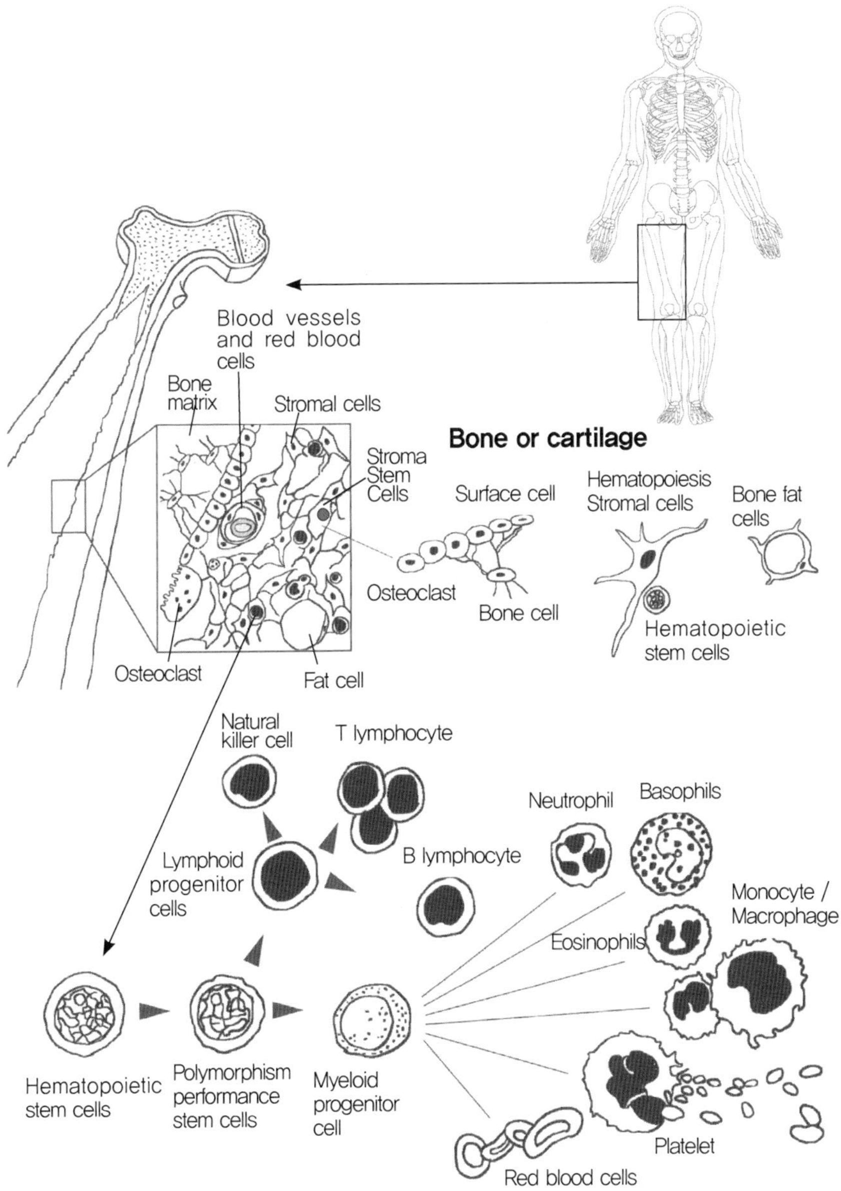

Figure 8–1. Cellular composition and differentiation of endogenous (innate immunity) and adaptive (specific) immunity

8.2. Structure and function of the immune system

The lymphatic organ.

Not only are the many microorganisms alive in our world, they are trying to live in our bodies. The disease-causing microorganisms are called the "pathogens", which are classified into the viruses, the bacteria, the fungi, and the parasites. The immune system finds the pathogenic bacteria and the harmful substances that invade the outside of the body so that all the cells, tissues, and organs of the body can function, and it recognizes and removes the abnormally deformed cells. The pathogens have the different ways of life, attacking the body in a special way and others of the like, and the immune system has developed the various ways to fight them.

The immune system consists of the four main parts: The lymphatic fluid, the lymphatic duct, the lymphocyte, and the lymphatic organs. The lymphatic system, starts from the peripheral tissues and ends up connecting the veins, constantly circulating and helping to remove the strange intruders from the lymphatic organs. The lymphatic organs connect the lymphatic vessels and contain a large number of the lymphocytes. The lymph is a plasma-like liquid, but the concentration of the suspended protein is much lower.

The lymphatic organs are divided into the primary lymphoid organs and the secondary lymphoid organs. The primary lymphoid

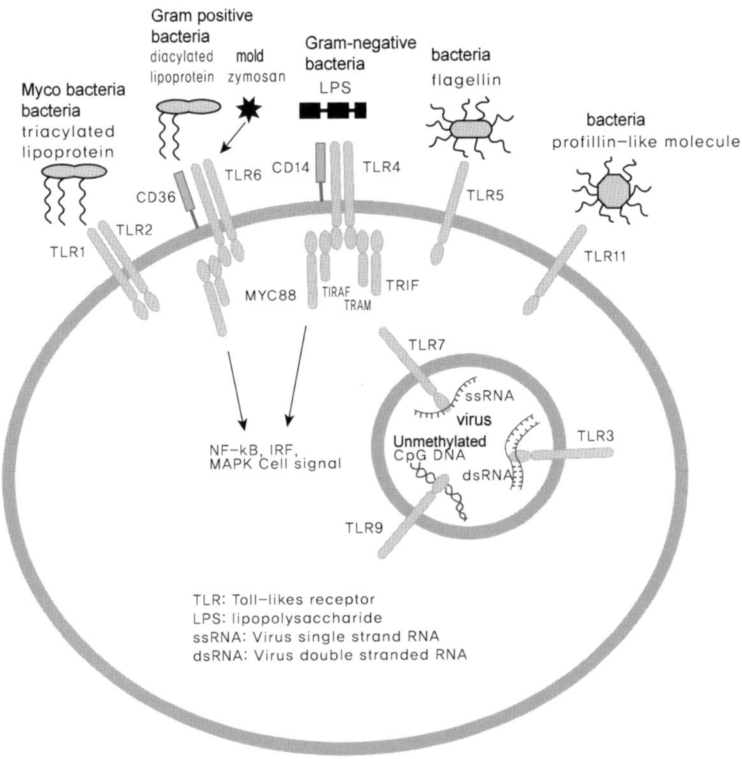

Figure 8-1. Toll-like receptors responsible for the innate immunity (innate immunity) system

Toll-like receptors (TLRs) store pattern information for some basic constituents of bacteria or viruses in the human gene so that the immune system can function from birth. Thirteen different TLRs have been found.

Table 8-1. Comparison of intrinsic and adaptive immunity

division	Innate immunity	Adaptive immunity
Reaction time	Minute, reaction in time	Day unit response
Specificity	Non-specific	Very specific
Diversity	little	Very much
Accuracy	perfect	Sometimes mistakes
Memory function	none	have
Major involved cells	Macrophage natural killer cell, Dendritic cell	B cells, T cells

organs, also called the "central, lymphatic organs", consist of the bone marrow, the thymus, the B lymphocytes in the bone marrow, and the T lymphocytes in the thymus.

The secondary lymphatic organs, also called the "peripheral lymphoid organs", consist of the lymph nodes, the spleen, the intestinal lymphoid tissue, the organ–related lymphoid tissue, and the mucosal–associated lymphoid tissue.

Nonspecific immunity and specific immunity

The number of the red blood cells in a single ml of blood is 5 billion, and the number of the white blood cells in a single ml of blood is 7 million. All the cells in the blood are differentiated into the cells as the omnipotent, hematopoietic cells in the bone marrow and the others. The various types of the white blood cells can be divided into the two types– ie, the phagocytes and the lymphocytes. The phagocytes are responsible for the innate immunity or the nonspecific immunity, and the lymphocytes are responsible for the specific immunity.

Congenital immunity is the recognition of the unchanged parts of the microbial evolution. In the phagocytes, the macrophages and the neutrophils recognize the common, pathogen–related molecules throughthe cell surface receptors and capture and digest

Table 8-2. The difference between necrosis and apoptosis

	necrosis	apoptosis
stimulus	Hypoxia, toxin, ATP depletion, damage	Genetically regulated physiological signal
ATP demand	none	none
Cell change	Expansion, intracellular organelle destruction, Death of organization	Chromatin condensation, membrane saturation, Single cell death
DNA damage	Random fragments	2Cut to 200bp size
Plasma membrane	rupture	Bubble shape
The fate of dead cells	Feeding by phagocytes	Absorbed by surrounding cells
Reaction in tissue	Inflammation	No inflammation

the pathogens. The eosinophils, the mast cells, and the natural killer cells release the soluble, antimicrobial factors and attack the pathogens.

On the other hand, the specific immunity is carried out by the T cells and the B cells. The specialized cells responding to the various antigens can recognize only one antigen. Thus, there are the various types of the T cells and the B cells that can recognize the millions of the antigens.

In an infected area of the blood, the tissue, the epithelium, or others of the like, the antigen that is caught in the phagocyte is transferred to the naive lymphocytes. The lymphocyte receiving the antigen information is comprised of the effector cells and the memory cells.

The immune function of the T cells

The average lifespan of a body cell is from 10 months to 1 year. The lifespan of each cellis different, but it is about one week in the digestive tract, and it almost lives the whole life in the heart or the brain. Therefore, the treatment of the cells that have reached the end of their lives in the human body, which must maintain the certain body, is an important task. To this end, the human body has developed the three programmed cell death mechanisms: Necrosis, apoptosis, and autophagy.

Necrosis is the destruction of the cells through a physical or chemical damage, where the dead tissues release the inflammatory signaling molecules around them to produce the inflammation, or they are destroyed by the phagocytosis, thereby, clearing the site. The other is the programmed cell death, or apoptosis, which is divided into the five to twelve as the cells are degraded by themselves. The most important feature is that the DNA of the nucleus is cut off and is divided into the 200 bp's. At this time, the cell fragments generated are neatly reused in the surrounding cells. And the autophagy is that, when the energy supply is cut off from the outside, it eats itself and starves to death (Table 8-2).

Initially, the T cell development occurs in the bone marrow, but the maturation occurs in the thymus just above the heart. 98% of the T cells that reach the thymus die for the cell immunity defense (self-tolerance) and only 2% are released. That is, among the T

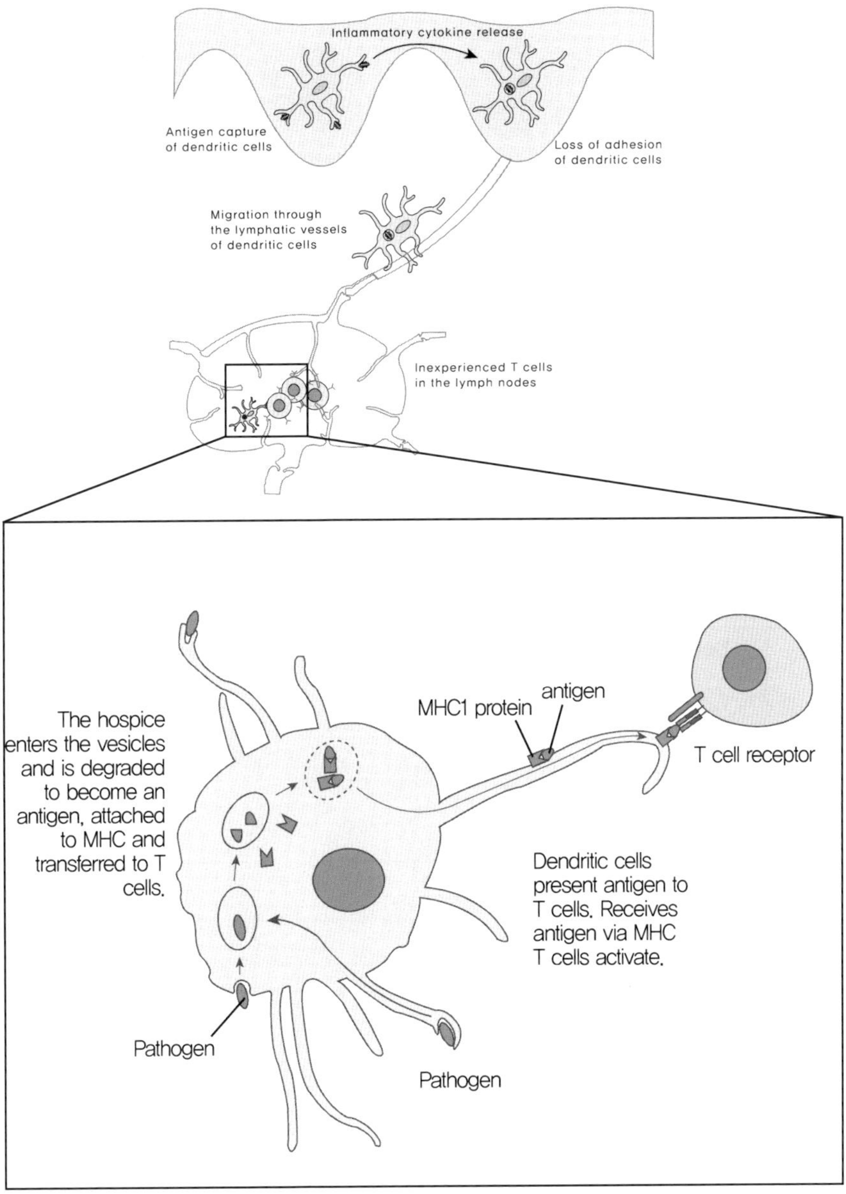

Figure 8-3. Adaptive Immunity and MHC

cells that are randomly generated, the T cells that attack themselves are removed, and the T cells that do not recognize their own cell markers are, also, removed. This is called the "positive selection" in that only the T cells capable of recognizing the 'negative selection' and their major histocompatibility complex (MHC) antigen are differentiated. The main histocompatibility complex (MHC) is a protein that is presented together around the antigen when an infected cell presents an antigen to the surface. If the MHC is called "kimbap", the antigen will be about the size of the kimbap. The MHC is recognized by the T cells, so that the antigen presented

Table 8-3. Chronic inflammatory disease associated with cancer development

cancer	Inflammatory disease	etiology
Bladder cancer	cystitis	Chigger, urinary catheter
Colon cancer	Inflammatory bowel disease, Crohn's disease, colitis	
Lung cancer	bronchitis	Silica, asbestos, smoking
gut-associated lymphoid cancer	Sjogren's syndrome, Hashimoto's thyroiditis	
Melanoma	Skin inflammation	UV-rays
Mesothelioma, lung cancer	Asbestosis, cushioning (a type of pulmonary manifestation)	Asbestos fibers, silica particles
Esophagus cancer	Esophagitis, barrette esophagitis	Stomach acid
구강인세포암	Gingivitis, psittacosis	
Pancreatic cancer	Chronic pancreatitis, hereditary pancreatitis	Alcoholism, trypsin enzyme mutation
Salivary gland cancer	Salivary gland inflammation	
Genital adenocarcinoma	Dry sclerosis	

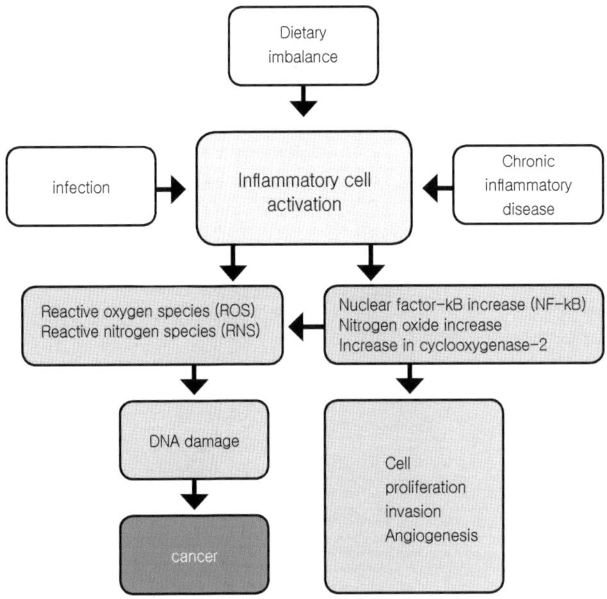

Figure 8-4. The process of inflammation leading to cancer

by the infected cells can be recognized. As for the MHC type 1, it is present in almost all cells, which are recognized by the cytotoxic T cells (Fig. 8-2). The MHC type 2 is only in the macrophages or the B cells, and these cells are called "the antigen-presenting cells" (APCs). The antigen presented by the antigen-presenting cell with the MHC2 is activated by the immune response while the T-cell recognizes it.

The T lymphocyte, starting from the thymus, passes well through the two choices of the voice selection and the positive

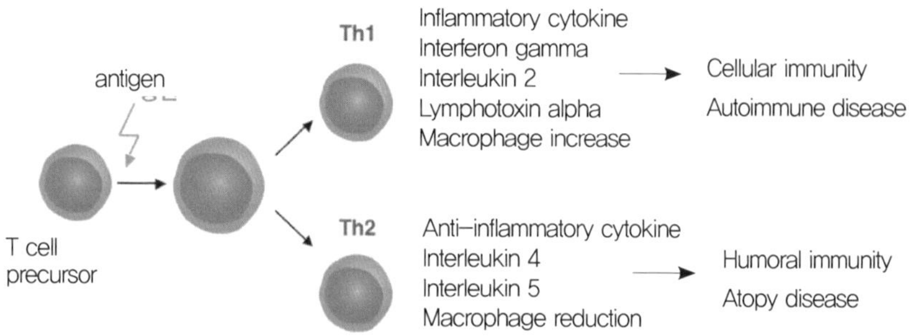

Figure 8-5. Differentiation of T cells into secondary T1 (Th1) or secondary T2 (Th2) effector cells

selection, and receives a piece of antigen presented by a specialized, cell-presenting cell, such as the dendritic cell, in a secondary immune system such as the lymph nodes. Depending on the type of the antigenic fragment, the T cells are specialized, or differentiated, into the cytotoxic T cells.

The activated, cytotoxic T cells detect the abnormal cells that are infected by the cancer viruses and signal them to do the cell death. The proteins produced by the bacteria, the parasites, and the viruses that grow in the cells move to the cell surface. The cytotoxic cells recognize the antigen presented by the main histocompatibility complex (MHC) on the surface of the infected cells, which is the apoptosis (self-death).

The helper T cells (Th cells) help the activity of the other cells, such as the B cells or the macrophages. The Th1 cells stimulate the macrophages to kill the infected cells by causing the vesicles containing the microbial enzymes and the antimicrobials to fuse with the parasites of the bacterial parasites. The Th2 cells activate the B cells to destroy the extracellular pathogens. The natural killer cells (NK cells) are classified into an internal immune system by eliminating the foreign substances without the antigen–specific receptors.

8.3. Chronic inflammation and cancer formation

Many chronic, inflammatory diseases are an important cause of the cancer development and progression. For example, the inflammatory bowel diseases (IBDs), such as ultrathin colitis (UC) and the Crohn's disease (IBD), increase with the Westernization of the diet, which increases the risk of colon cancer and the like through the chronic inflammation. Barrett's esophagitis, also, increases the likelihood of developing the esophageal adenocarcinoma and colon cancer, and the hereditary pancreatitis is prone to the cancer through the chronic inflammation.

The results of the chronic pancreatitis and the chronic hepatitis infection all go through the inflammatory pathway to cancer. It is estimated that 15% of the tumors worldwide are due to infection. It is presumed that the chronic, inflammatory disease through infection is closely related to cancer development (Table 8–3).

In fact, inflammation is the mechanism by which the body prevents infection. The primary barrier of the body is the skin. If the skin, the respiratory organ walls, or the digestive organ walls are damaged by any cause, the underlying mast cells are damaged and release the histamine. The histamine expands the capillaries to increase the permeability, which facilitates the migration of the phagocytes and eliminates the invading bacteria and the others of the like.

The cells from the injured or infected tissues also emit the cytokines that signal the neutrophils, followed by the monocytes. When the monocytes are excited, they immediately turn into the macrophages, like an angry Hulk, and differentiate into the swallowing, external bacteria or the invading substances. Instead of becoming enormous and exciting, the cells then secrete the various cytokines to attract the other white blood cells, which is the beginning of a specific immune response. The common pus in the inflammation is the dead neutrophils, the dead human cells, the body fluids, etc. In the normal cases, the macrophages digest them, and they disappear gradually.

In other words, the cytokine is a small, soluble protein that is secreted by the immune cells and many other cells. It is a signaling substance of the immune cells that changes the properties and actions of themselves or the other cells. Thus, the release of the cytokines that signal the other cells to protect the body from a trauma or an infection is an essential part of the hosting for the self–protection, but the uncontrolled, overexpressed cytokine is a potential source of the many diseases, including cancer. . Thus, the inflammation usually produces the anti–inflammatory cytokines (Th2 cytokines, IL–1, IL–10, IL–13, etc.) almost immediately after the production of the inflammatory cytokines(Th1 cytokines). These cytokines then act as the signals to the hypothalamus, thereby releasing the cortisol from the adrenal cortex through the hormone axis of the hypothalamus–pituitary–adrenal gland, where the cortisol enters into the immune cells and inhibits the immune response. This is called the "cytokine–HPA feedback" and is widely known as a typical interaction between the immune system and the nervous system. This is the mechanism of the action of the steroid drugs prescribed for the various inflammatory diseases. However, if any problems occur, such as the maintenance of the cytokine initiation factors or the failure of the lysis, the inflammation may worsen and a chronic inflammation may progress.

One of the ways to defend the immune cells against the invading microorganisms is to produce and destroy the active oxygen and the nitrogen species, which can damage the DNAs and overproduce the lipids. In other words, the mutation is caused by a DNA damage, and the action of the immune cells due to the chronic inflammation paradoxically becomes an important possibility of a cancer cell progression. Breast cancer, colorectal cancer, pancreatic cancer, thyroid cancer, bladder cancer, skin cancer, etc., are associated with inflammation. Here, we find that an important regulatory action of

Table 8-4. Nutrients that affect asthma [5]

nutrient	Potential Mechanism of Effect	Source
vitamin A,C,E	antioxidant; Prevent endogenous, exogenous oxidative inflammation	
vitamin C	Prostaglandin inhibition	Sour fruits, tomatoes, potatoes, Broccoli, strawberry, cabbage, spinach
vitamin E	Membrane stabilization, suppression of IgE production	brown rice, whole wheat, nuts, fruits, vegetables
Flavone, Flavonoid	antioxidant; Mast cell stabilization	
magnesium	Smooth muscle relaxation, mast cell stabilization	Nuts, legumes, brown rice, whole wheat
Selenium	Antioxidant cofactor of glutathione peroxidase	Algae, nuts, seeds, Brown rice, whole wheat
cupper, zinc	Antioxidant cofactor of SOD	Algae, nuts, brown rice, whole wheat
Omega-3 fatty acids	leucotriene substitute stabilizes cell membrane inflammation	Perilla, Beans, Walnuts
Omega-6 fatty acids	Increase eicosanoid production, causing inflammation	Corn oil, edible oil
Salt	Increases smooth muscle contraction, inflammation occurs	Processed foods, etc.

Am J Respir Crit Med (2004) 170:725-729

the excessive inflammatory response is being an antioxidant. The various fruits and vegetables are the antioxidants and act as the ligands for the ligand-dependent gene regulators called the "nuclear receptors". The ligands are the small molecules that control the behavior of the larger polymers, such as the hormones, which are a kind of the ligand. For example, when your body becomes irritated and depressed, you can see that the inflammation sinks within a few hours after mixing with the blueberries, the strawberries, the carrots, a little bit of the nuts, a little bit of the sun salt, and a little bit of water. Of course, the various fruits and vegetables have

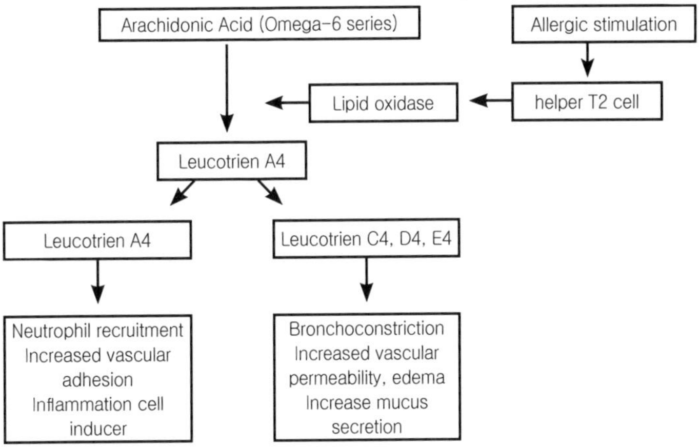

Figure 8-6. Physiological effects of Omega-6 fatty acids in airway

the anti–inflammatory properties, so you can choose a variety of the foods to suit your taste.

Inflammation is not only the beginning of cancer, but, also, plays an important role in the cancer proliferation such as the cancer cell differentiation and the blood vessel formation around the cancer cells. In the absence of the inflammatory cytokines, the limited inflammation occurs, thereby limiting the angiogenesis and the tumor growth. However, the abundance of the inflammatory cytokines promotes the new blood vessel formation around the cancer and the rapid growth of the cancer. Under certain conditions, the balance of the inflammatory cytokines and the anti–inflammatory cytokines changes, which translates into the excessive inflammation and the antiangiogenic and tumor regressions [1].

The activation of the inflammatory cells involves the balance of the ancillary Th1 cells and the secondary Th2 cells with the infection and the dietary factors. An important part of the inflammation–related dietary factors are the plant–rich omega–3 fatty acids and the antioxidants

8.4. Asthma and the omega–3 fatty acids

The infection–free immune diseases include the allergies and the autoimmune diseases. The autoimmune diseases include the asthma, the atopy, and the rheumatoid arthritis, which are

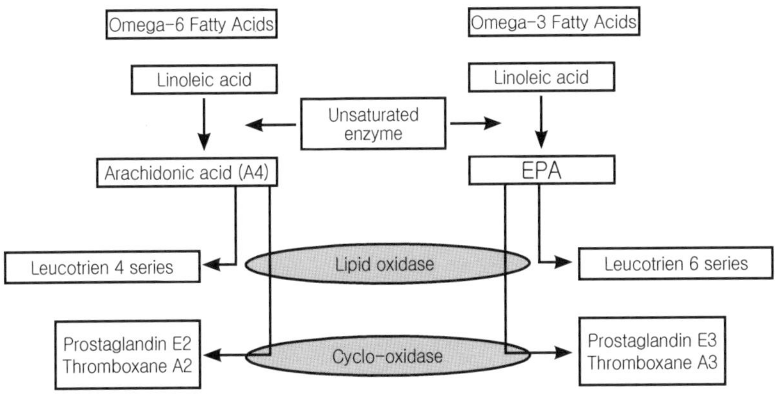

Figure 8-7. Enzyme competition of omega-3 fatty acids and omega-6 fatty acids

associated with the abnormal, inflammatory responses. As a typical example, asthma is a chronic, inflammatory disease of the respiratory tract that manifests as the seizure dyspnea, in which the respiration accelerates and shortens. Initially, it starts with a cough, but, over time, the lumps of the mucus and the mucus come out. In acute conditions, the difficulty in breathing, the severe vomiting, the body temperature rise, and the shocks come.

Asthma is especially important in the balance of the supplements Th1 and Th2. The process by which the inexperienced T cells that do not meet the antigens are differentiated into the complementary cells of the Th1 or the Th2, which is regulated by a sophisticated mechanism through a wide variety of the factors, is not yet clear. However, it is known that the various factors, such as the cytokines and the peptides that occur during the infection, affect the differentiation.

One hypothesis is as follows:The dendritic cells, the macrophages, and the NK cells release the interleukin 2 (IL–2) and the interferon gamma (IFN–γ) cytokines while attacking the viruses or the specific, intracellular bacteria, Th1, and, at the same time,the production of the auxiliary cells, Th2, is inhibited. On the other hand, when the IL–4 and the IL–5 are present, they are differentiated into the secondary cell Th2, and the change to the secondary cell Th1 is suppressed.

Studies on the T helper cells in the blood and the bronchoalveolar lavage have shown that the blood of the atopic asthmatics is biased toward the production of the supp cell Th2, an inflammatory T cell. In this case, the omega–6 lipids are involved in the activation of the Th2, secondary cells. That is, when the Th2 auxotrophs are exposed to any stimulus, the Th2 auxotroph activates alipid–oxidizing enzyme to convert the arachidonic acid, an omega–6 fatty acid, into a substance called the "leukotriene A4". The leukotriene A4 is again differentiated into the leukotriene B4, C4, D4, and E4. The leukotriene B4 is a kind of the eicosanoid that strongly attracts the leukocytes and aggregates the neutrophils and the inflammatory cells (Figure 8–5). And the leukotriene C4, D4, and E4, which bind to the specific receptors in the lung cells to constrict the bronchi, secrete the mucus into the respiratory organs and the mast cells, and, also, increase the vascular permeability. [2].

Table 8-5. Epidemiological studies on atopy, asthma and dietary antioxidant effects [7]

Target (age)	effect
adult (30)	Ingestion of vitamin C prevents rough breathing and bronchitis
child (8–13)	Some selenium intake has a preventive effect
adult female (34–68)	A large amount of vitamin E intake is effective in preventing asthma
adult (18–70)	The intake of large amounts of vitamins C and E is beneficial for lung function
child (8–11)	Fresh fruit intake is beneficial to lung function
child (6–7)	Vitamin C-rich fruits are beneficial for rough breathing even when consuming small amounts

Medical Hypotheses (2004) 63, 280–290

8.5. The principles of the asthma treatment through the intake of the omega-3 fatty acids

Patients with asthma produce a considerable amount of the leukotriene-4 family compared to the normal people, and, thus, the regulation of the production of the leukotrienes is an important part of the treatment of asthma. This is the principle of the action of commercially making available the anti-asthmatics. However, the omega-3 fatty acids, which can be regulated through dietary intake, can reduce the production of the leukotriene-4 family, like the antihistamines.

The omega-3 fatty acids have a protective effect on the inflammatory diseases, such as asthma, because they have a competitive and inhibitory effect on the biosynthetic pathway of the omega-6 fatty acids. The reason for this effect is that the omega-3 and omega-6 families share the same unsaturated enzyme and the same lipid oxidase. That is, when the linolenic acid becomes the EPA and the linoleic acid changes to the arachidonic acid, they use the same enzyme (Figure 8-6). Therefore, if the amount of the linolenic acid is changed to the linolenic acid EPA, the use of the unsaturated enzymes, as much as that, and the amount of the linoleic acid are changed so that the arachidonic acid is relatively less. In addition, the numerically increased EPA produces the leukotriene-5 family using the lipid oxidase, which reduces the formation of the leukotriene-4 family of the arachidonic acid, thereby inhibiting the abnormal concentration of the neutrophils and the inflammatory cells help reduce the inflammation.

In addition, the arachidonic acid is made from the prostaglandin E2 and the thromboxane A2 using the cyclo-oxidase, which stimulates the T lymphocytes to produce the immunoglobulin E (IgE). Thus, when the EPA is converted to the prostaglandin E3 and the thromboxane A3 using the cyclooxygenase, the metabolic pathway of the arachidonic acid is reduced and, thus, the production of the IgE is, also, reduced. The patients with asthma have a higher level of the IgE, which is known as the beginning of an allergic reaction to an antigen. The EPA can reduce the incidence and symptoms of asthma by inhibiting the production of the IgE and by reducing the allergic response through the cyclooxygenase pathway

8.6. Asthma-healing diet

Will the lipid composition in the body cells change depending on the type of the food actually consumed, and will the production of the leukotriene, the prostaglandin, and the thromboxane be different?

According to the results of a study, the daily supplementation of 200 mg of the EPA and the DHA for two months resulted in a significant decrease in the daytime asthma, a decrease in the concentration of the hydrogen peroxide in the exhalation, and a maximum increase in the excretion [3].

Whether the polyunsaturated fats released from the cell membranes are omega-3 or omega-6 depends on the dietary pattern. According to another study, the omega-3 had maintained in the cell membrane well when it had been supplemented continuously for 2 weeks. The omega-6 had accumulated in the cell membrane when it had been supplemented for 6 weeks.

In other words, the dietary fat intake changes the lipid composition of the cell membrane and changes the type of the eosinogen production, which, in turn, affects the cellular inflammatory response. Further studies have shown that when 3 g of the EPA had been fed into the diet per day, the synthesis of the arachidonic acid had been inhibited by the inhibitory effect of the unsaturated enzyme pathway [4].

As the lipid-oxidizing enzyme triggers the omega-6 arginine

acid, it can be expected that the dietary antioxidant system will prevent the occurrence of asthma. Studies have shown that vitamin C, vitamin E, beta-carotene, and fruits prevent the oxidative inflammation by the antioxidant effects, that vitamin C inhibits the production of the prostaglandins, and that vitamin E stabilizes the membrane, resulting in the inhibition of the IgE production. −5). Selenium, copper, and zinc are, also, important as the cofactors for the antioxidant enzymes.

Illness caused by inflammation is not limited to asthma. There are the numerous cardiovascular and diabetic diseases, including rheumatoid arthritis, atopic dermatitis, and the chronic, inflammatory diseases that progress to cancer. Inflammation is a necessary action to prevent infection, but the overeating of omega-6 due to meat, cooking oil, and the diets lacking the antioxidants increases the likelihood of producing an unnecessary inflammation in the human health

8.7. Vegetarian diet to relieve atopic dermatitis.

Is this diet really effective for atopic dermatitis? If so, what is the immunological mechanism? A study of thishad been carried out in Japan. The subjects were 14 males (mean age 25 years) and 6 males and 15 females aged between 15 years old and 36 years old. Five had had asthma, and one was asthmatic at the time of the experiment.

Ten patients had had, or had been suffering from, rhinitis. 65% of the patients had the family history of an allergy. All participants stopped the steroid or the antihistamine drug two months before the admission.

All patients had received the same meals, and, in the mornings, they received 250 grams of the fresh vegetable juice (vegetable juice consisted of several vegetables, such as spinach and cabbage). At lunch, they ate 5 grams of the seaweed on the brown rice porridge that was equivalent to 10 grams of the sesame seeds, 200 grams of tofu, and 80 grams of brown rice. Dinner was the same as lunch, but 2.5 grams of the sun saliva had been consumed daily.

The energy intake was 1,085kcal, which was 55% of the recommended dietary allowance, protein was 75%, calcium was 180%, iron was 130%, vitamin C was 250% and vitamin E was 110%. An interesting point was that the persimmon tea had been drunk instead of water. This diet had been performed in a private hospital for 2 months. The skin conditions had been measured weekly by two doctors using the European Task Force on Atopic Dermatitis (1993) method, which had been used to diagnose atopic dermatitis.

The results were as follows:The diagnostic indices were significantly lower and the eosinophil counts had been lowered before the experiment and 2 months after the experiment [6]. The eosinophils are the inflammatory cells that play a role in dermatitis formation. And the number of the natural killer cells (NK cells) had, also, been lowered.

The authors say that the low–calorie–based, vegetarian diets significantly reduce the skin inflammation. In the experiment, the number of the eosinophils and the number of the neutrophils, which are the inflammatory cells, had decreased compared to before the dermatitis had improved (Fig. 8–7 (b)). In general, a low calorie or fasting reduces the neutrophil counts in the peripheral blood vessels.

The lactate dehydrogenase (LDH), the peripheral neutrophil count, and the serum IgE levels are known to be the indicators of the severity of the atopic disease. After the vegetarian diet, the activity of the NK had decreased, while the synthesis of the interleukin–4 / interferon–γ in the peripheral blood T cells had been slightly lower [6]. The prostaglandin E2 (PGE2) produced by the activation of the B cells induces the synthesis of the immunoglobulin E (IgE) and the conversion of the inexperienced T cells into the Th2 cells. And these molecules are a key factor in the immunological abnormality of the atopic patients. The two months of the vegetarian diet had improved the IgE levels and the Th1 / Th2 balance by reducing the amount of the PGE2 that had been produced by the peripheral, mononuclear cells, leading to the symptoms of the atopic disease. The researchers conclude that the vegetarian diets are very useful as the alternative therapies for the atopic diseases

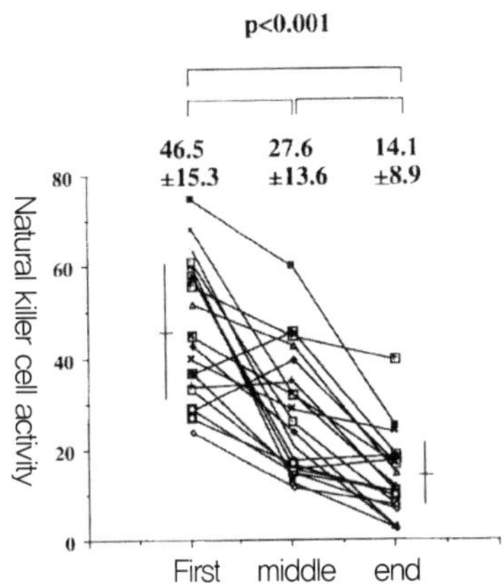

(a) Decrease natural killer cell activity after vegetarian diet

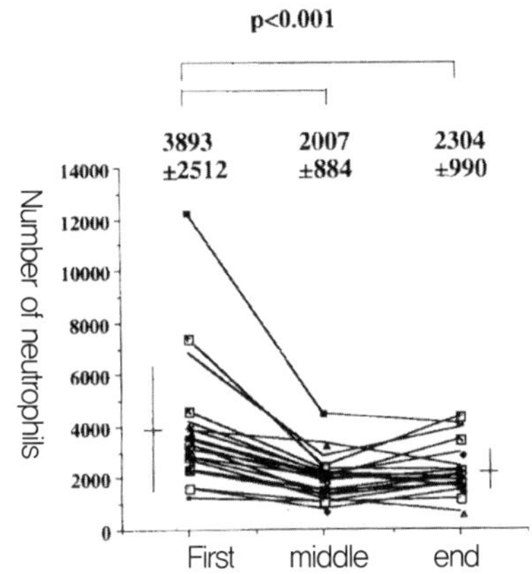

(b) Decrease in neutrophil count after vegetarian diet

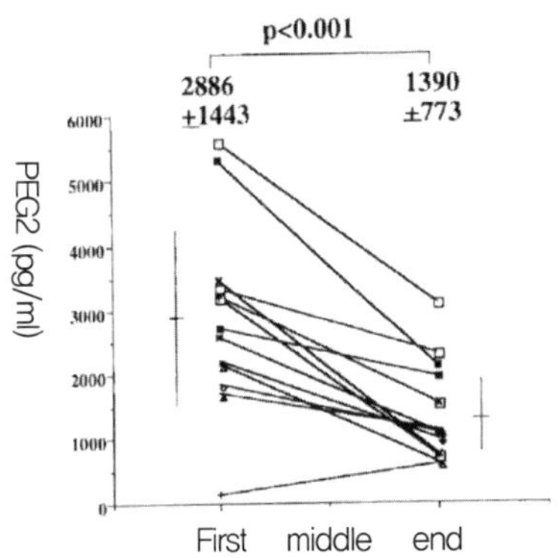

(c) Decrease in PGE2 after vegetarian diet

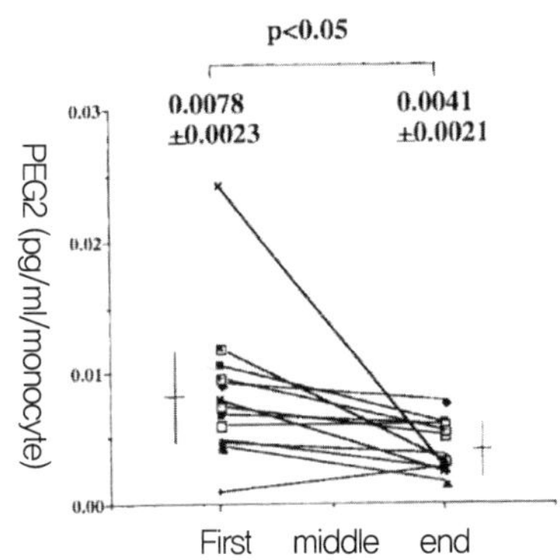

(d) Decrease in PEG2 / mononuclear cells after vegetarian diet

Figure 8-8. Physiological improvement after vegetarian diet for atopic dermatitis patients [6]

8.8. Vegetarianism to improve rheumatoid arthritis.

This experiment had beencarried out at a university hospital in Oslo. The volunteers were randomly divided into two groups, one group receiving the vegetarian diet and the other receiving the non–vegetarian diet for 13 months, the results of which had been observed. The vegetarian diet group was 27 persons and the non – vegetarian diet group was 26 persons.

The vegetarian diet group started a four–week program by fasting at a health farm. Then, after receiving the vegetarian diet, they returned home and the vegetarian diet had been continued for

Table 8–6. Food items conducted after fasting

	vegan (3.5 months)	lacto–ovo vegetarian (12 months)
vegetable	All vegetables except tomatoes and cucumbers	All vegetables
Root vegetables	Potatoes, carrots, beets, turnips	Same as vegan
fruit	All kinds of dried fruits, Fresh pear, peach, banana, melon	All kinds
grain	Sorghum, buckwheat, rice, corn starch (Except gluten)	All kinds
Seedling	Sunflower seeds, flaxseed, sesame seeds, pumpkin seeds	Same as vegan
Oil	All kinds	Same as vegan
Legumes	All kinds	Same as vegan
dairy product	Do not ingest	All kinds
beverage	Herbal tea, vegetable soup, vegetable soup	Same as vegan + Fruit juice, Alcoholic beverages, except wine
Sugar	Honey, a little brown sugar	Same as vegan

12 months (Table 8–6). The non–vegetarian group had spent four weeks in a nursing home and had continued the usual daily meals for 12 months. Prior to entering the health farm and the nursing home, respectively, and at 1 month, 4 months, 7 months, 10 months, and 13 months, the physicians underwent a clinical testing and a blood collection.

Dietitians surveyed the diet at 2.5 months, 5.5 months, 8.5 months, and 11.5 months, and the two groups of the vegetarians and the non–vegetarians, if possible, had the same conditions except for the meals. The vegan diet group had a strict vegetarian diet for three and a half months after fasting, after which time the gluten–containing meals,the milk, and the dairy products had been, also, allowed.

One month after the experiment, there was a sudden change in almost all the items. The vegetarian diet showed the beneficial results, but the responses to the diet was divided into the two groups of the superior and the inferior. That is, in the vegetarian group, 12 persons out of the 27 persons had been significantly improved, while, in the non–vegetarian group, 2 persons out of the 26 persons had improved.

First, we can see that the vegetarian group was much better than the non–vegetarian group. The painful time of the vegetarian group was reduced to less than 3 hours in one month after the vegetarian diet and in the 5th hour before the vegetarian diet, while it returned to less than 4 hours in the non–vegetarian group. (Fig.

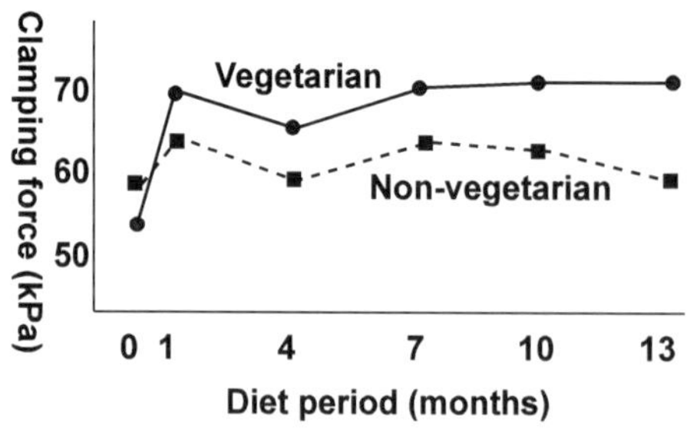

(a) Vegetarian diet and tightening power

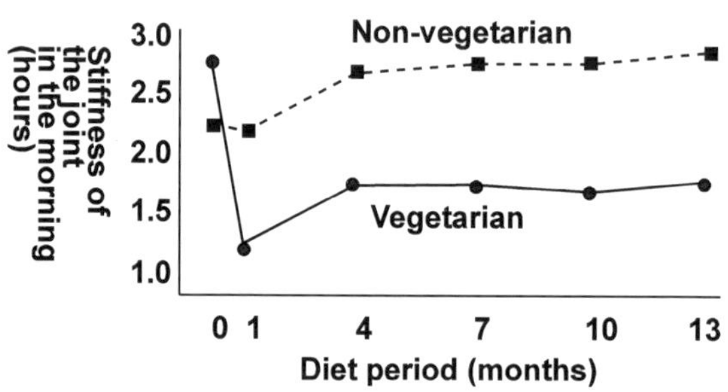

(b) Reduces vegetarian diet and pain time

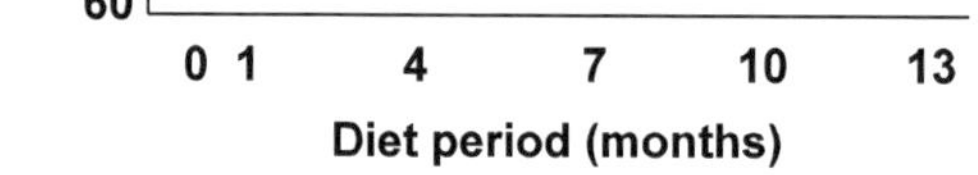

(b) Reduces vegetarian diet and pain time

Figure 8–9. The sins of vegetarian and non–vegetarian groups of patients with rheumatoid arthritis are the ratio of clamping force(a), stiffness of joint(b), weight (c)

8–8(b)). The feeling of the joint stiffness in the morning that the rheumatic patients commonly feel had been reduced to 2.7 hours for the non–vegetarian group after 13 months, but had been reduced to 1.7 hours for the vegetarian group (Fig. 8–9(a)). Especially, at the time of one month after the vegetarian diet, which had been a whole vegan diet, it had decreased to 1.2 hours. This seems to be consistent with the other finding that vegetarian diet is more effective regarding rheumatoid arthritis.

In a survey of the hand grip strengths, there was a difference between the vegetarian and non–vegetarian groups. The vegetarian group showed a stronger grip strength, increasing from 55kPa before the vegetarian diet to 70kPa after 13 months of the vegetarian diet, while the non–vegetarian group had been staying at 60kPa (Figure 8–8 (a)) [8].

In the case of the body weight, the first time the vegan diet was administered, it had decreased rapidly from 70 kg to 64 kg after 1 month, but it had recovered over time, and there was no statistically significant difference in the body weight from the non–vegetarians after 13 months.

The number of the leukocyte counts showed little change in the non–vegetarian group, while, for the vegetarian group, it had decreased rapidly after the first month of the diet, and it had gradually recovered in the 13th month, but it was still less than that of the non–vegetarian group (Fig. 8–9) [8]. The reduction of the number of the white blood cells in a vegetarian group is a common.

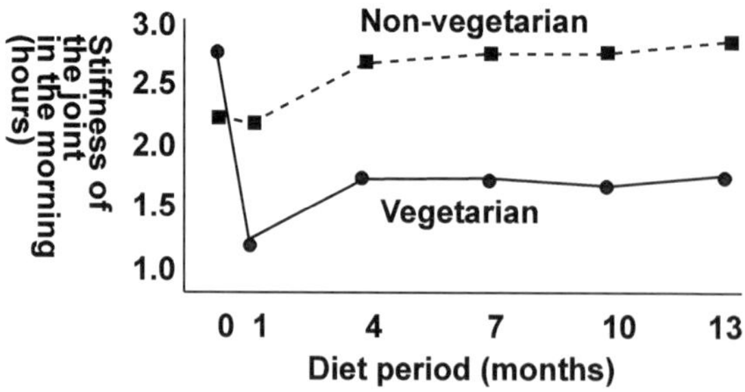

(a) Reduces vegetarian dietary and joint stiffness time

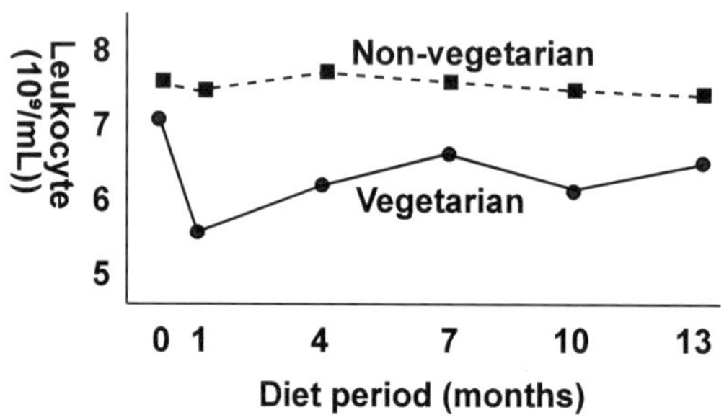

(b) Reduce vegetarian diet and white blood cell count

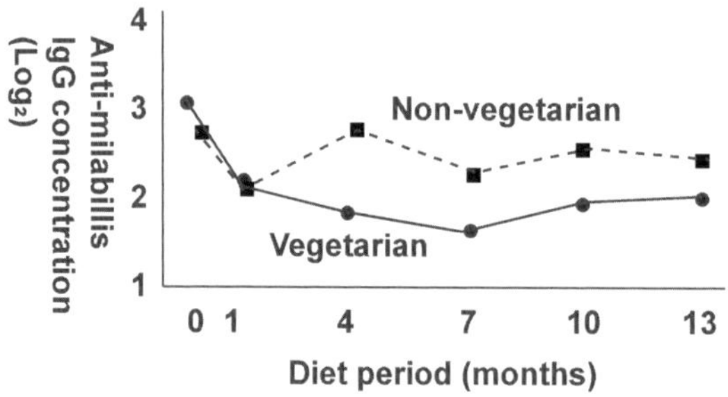

(c) vegetarian diet and reduced anti-milabillis IgG concentration

Figure 8-10. Comparison of arthroplasty time (a), leukocyte count (b) and anti-milabilis IgG concentration in vegetarian and non-vegetarian groups of patients with rheumatoid arthritis

8.9. Autoimmune diseases and vegetarianism

Ulcerative colitis and the Crohn's disease are the typical, inflammatory bowel diseases and the autoimmune diseases. They mainly affect the Westerners, and they are known to be the rare diseases among the Asia-Pacific peoples. Recently, however, the incidence of these diseases has increased at an unprecedented rate not only in Japan, China, but, also, in Korea.

According to a survey conducted by the NHS, ulcerative colitis and the Crohn's disease have tripled over the past decade since the early 1990s. This tendency is not an exception in Korea, and the number of the persons per 100,000 persons from 1986 until 1988 had increased by 6.1 times to 1.23 persons from 1995 until 1997 [9] (Fig. 8-10).

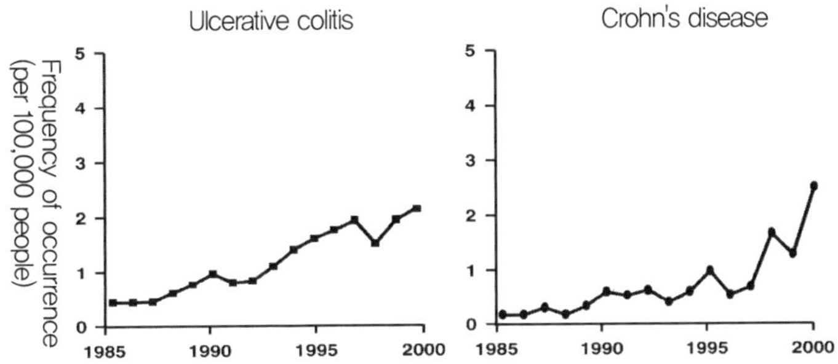

Figure 8-11. Ulcerative colitis and Crohn's disease prevalence in Songpa area, Seoul for 15 years [9]

Table 8-7. Autoimmune disease and autoantigen [10]

Organ-specific disease	Known antigen
Edison's disease	21-Hydroxylase
Celiac disease	Tissue glutamine converting enzyme
Type 1 diabetes	insulin
Graves hyperthyroidism	Thyroid stimulating hormone receptor
Hashimoto thyroiditis	Thyroid peroxidase, thyroid globulin
Myasthenia gravis	Acetylcholine receptor
Goodpasture syndrome	Type 4 collagen
pemphigus	Mesmoglene 3
Malignant anemia	Intrinsic factor
Gallbladder	E2 PDC
백반	Tyrosine enzyme
Multiple sclerosis	Myelin protein, Glycolipid
Somatic disease	**Known antigen**
systemic rupus	splysome snRNP
Erythema	Erythema, DNA
Sjogren's syndrome	Ribonuclease particles
Polymyositis	Muscarinic receptor
Dermatomyositis	Cyclin peptide
Generalized sclerosis	Isomerization enzyme
Focal somatic sclerosis	Centromere protein

Lancet (2004) 363:1544-46

In the 1960s, Buckets reported that the autoimmune diseases were very rare among the African Ugandans who had the vegetarian diet with the abundant fiber and that the symptoms were not severe even when they appeared. On the other hand, in

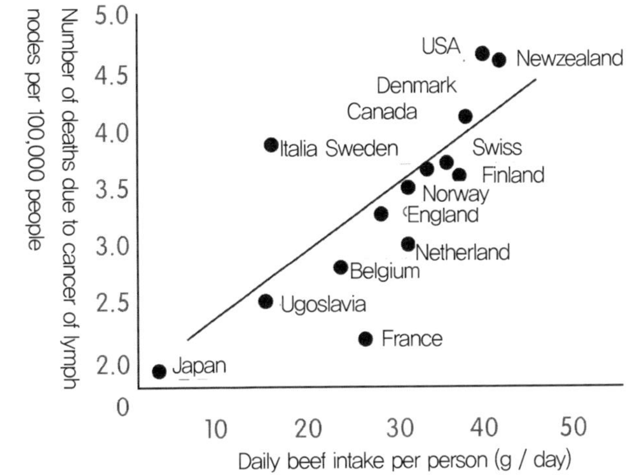

Figure 8–12. Proportion of beef intake and lymph node cancer mortality rate (1963–65)

the meat-centered Western societies, the autoimmune diseases are severe and their symptoms are extremely painful. In Korea, recently, the meat consumption has increased to be as much as that of the West.And is this not a diet that is related to the occurrence of such autoimmune diseases? What causes the autoimmune diseases? And why?

Are the eating patterns related? To understand this, it is necessary to understand the process of generating the immune cells called the "double selection". In other words, the immune cells should not attack me, but should attack me. Only the cells that meet these two conditions can move out of the bone marrow and the thymus and travel through the body

phenomenon in the other studies, and it can be an advantage for the autoimmune diseases. The restrictions of the total intake of the calories, the protein, the antioxidant vitamins, and the minerals that are important in the role of suppressing the immune responsesare known to suppress the immune responses to the autoimmune diseases as a kind of the immune suppression that is effective. In other words, the vegetarian diet can provide the effective, nutritional support and the antioxidants to the human body, while lowering the total calorie intake safely.

Proteus mirabilis is an intestinal microorganism that produces the hemorrhagic toxic peptides on the surface membrane. It acts as an antigen and causes an inflammation through a stimulation to the natural killer cells and through the activation of a complement. In the measurement of the immunoglobulin G (IgG) concentration for this antigen, the vegetarian response group showed a much lower value than the non-vegetarian group.

8.10. The dual selection process of the immune cells

The bone marrow–derived T cells migrate to the thymus, where it takes about a week to differentiate into the mature T cells. In the adult mice (rats), 50 million T cells are produced daily from the thymus, and only about 10,000 are matured. The remaining 98%, or 49 million T cells, die from the thymus. So, why is this wasteful work going on? This is because the newly–generated T cells must undergo a negative selection of the self–tolerance and a positive selection of the restriction of the major histocompatibility complex (MHC). The positive selection here is to live only with the MHC–recognizing T cells presenting the antigen when the cell is infected. In other words, the T cells that are able to attack the invading outsiders, but not the T cells that cannot attack, are not needed, and they die without having to go outside the thymus. (Fig. 8–11 (c)).

On the other hand, the voice selection is a task in which, when the normal cells are recognized as an antigen, an autoimmune disease occurs and the cells are killed before they are released from the thymus. (Fig. 8–11 (d)).

The bone marrow–derived T cells reach the thymus, and they will take about a week to differentiate. In the adult mice, 50 million T cells are produced daily in the thymus, but only about 10,000 are matured. The remaining 98%, or 49 million T cells, die at the thymus.

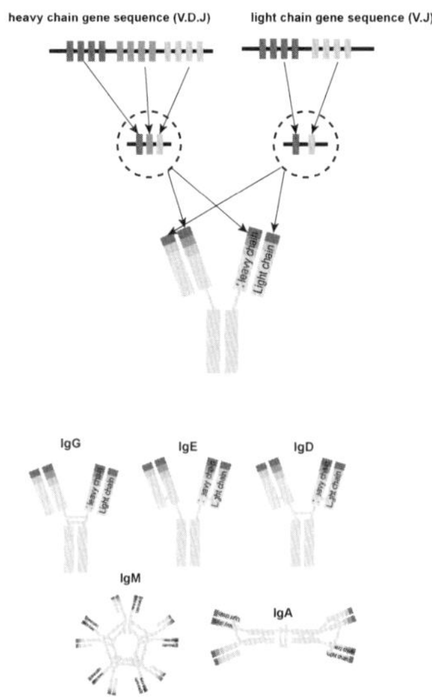

Figure 8–13. Random VDJ recombination process of T cell receptor (TCR) and B cell antibody

So, why is this wasteful work going on? This is because the newly–generated T cells must undergo a negative selection of the MHC restriction, a positive selection, and the self–tolerance. The positive selection means that the MHC–unrecognized T cells that present the antigens when the cells are infected cannot cause an immune response, so they only live with the MHC–recognizing T cells. On the other hand, the voice selection is the task of allowing the cell to die before it is released from the thymus, since the autoimmune disease occurs when it recognizes its normal cells as an antigen. Because of these two mechanisms, only 2% of the T cells that are produced are mature and come out of the thymus and become immune to the body.

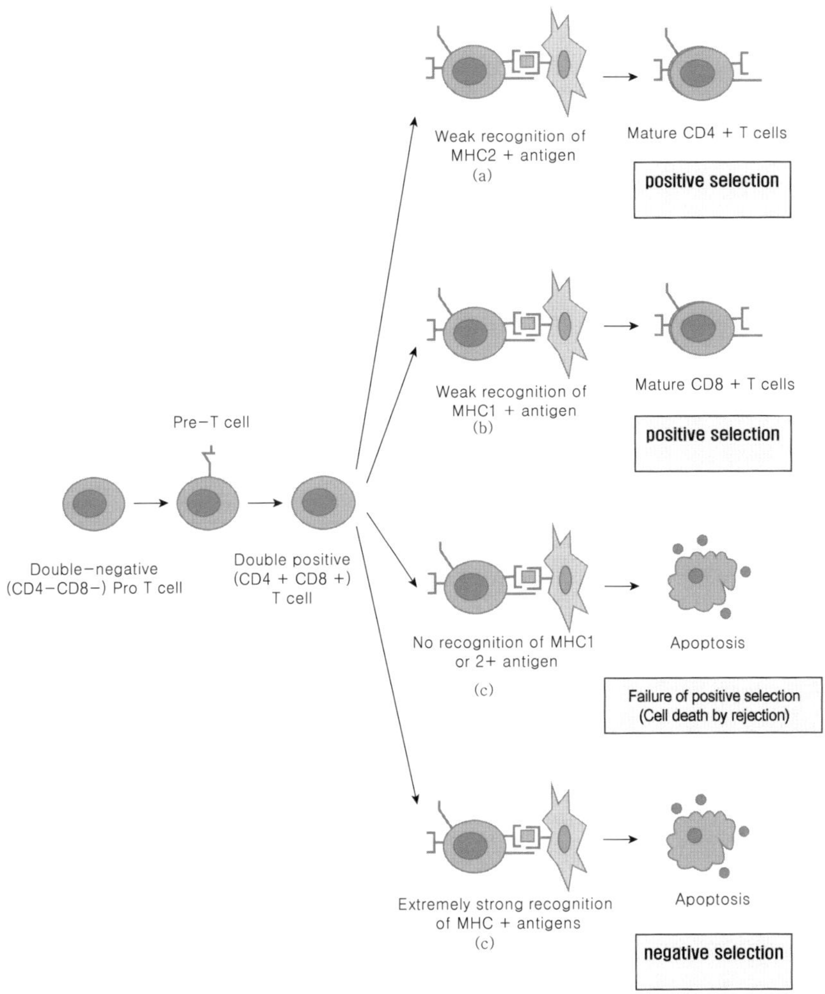

Figure 8-14. Positive selection and negative selection of T cells

8.11. Autoimmune disease

Many diseases of the human body are caused by an attack called "autoimmunity", which has lost the self-tolerance. The autoimmune diseases are divided into the organ-specific, autoimmune diseases and the systemic, autoimmune diseases. The tumor-specific autoimmune diseases include the thyroid disease, the type 1 diabetes, and the anemia, and the autoimmune diseases include the erythema, the polyposis, and the rheumatoid arthritis [10].

Here, it is noteworthy that, when the autoimmune diseases occur, there are many other types of the autoimmune diseases. For example, in the case of the type 2 APS, the major disease is the Edison's disease, with the chronic thyroiditis occurring in 56.1% and the Graves' disease in 21.1%. The co-occurrence of these autoimmune diseases is called the "autoimmune polyglandular

Table 8-8. Autoimmune disease of type 2 APS [11]

Endocrine disease	Prevalence(%)
Edison's disease+Chronic thyroiditis	56.1%
Edison's disease+Graves' disease	21.1%
Edison's disease+Type 1 diabetes	10.9%
Edison's disease+Chronic thyroiditis+Type 1 diabetes	9.6%
Edison's disease+Graves' disease+Type 1 diabetes	2.0%

Clin Exp Immunol (2004) 137:225–233

syndromes" (APS) [11] (Table 8-8).

If something has a common cause and if it includes the food it eats, the vegetarian diet may be involved in the healing of the autoimmune diseases.

McCarty found that the insulin-like growth factor-1 (IGF-1) and the IGF-binding protein (IGFBP) are the most important factors that can lower the risk of the autoimmune diseases-the rolactin, the vitamin D, the omega-3 fatty acids, and the green tea. In contrast to the vegetarians, the non-vegetarians have a high secretion of the IGF-1, which inhibits the controlled cell deaths and releases the immune cells that can attack the autoantigens. One of these actions is to increase the survival of the autoreactive T lymphocytes by interfering with the negative selection in the thymus, and the other is to enhance the function of the monocytes, the neutrophils,the mature T cells, and the mature B cells.

In addition, the non-vegetarians have a low production of the IGF-binding protein, which increases the amount of the unbound IGF-1 and, therefore, increases the intolerant action of the IGF-1, thereby, also, reducing the normal cell deaths, thereby, further increasing the risk of the autoimmune disease.

A second advantage of the vegetarian diet, which benefits from the autoimmunity, is that the mechatia is called the "prolactin", and prolactin is a growth factor for the lymphocytes. The T lymphocytes, the thymocytes, the thymic, epithelial cells, the B lymphocytes, and the progesterone receptors in the monolayer promote the maturation of these cells. He points out that women with the high prolactin levels in the blood have an increased autoantibody level, that the autoimmune disease has begun, and that the rats that had been prescribed the prolactin had become more aggressive.

In 1981, Bruce and his colleagues, who had measured the hormones of the 41 vegetarians and 45 non–vegetarians who were aged from 50 years old to 79 years old, found that the vegetarian, plasma prolactin levels had averaged 6.0 μg/L, while the non–vegetarians had averaged 7.1 μg/L. And it was 16% higher for the non–vegetarians [12].

Prolactin, also, stimulates the production of the lymphocytes that attack the self–antibodies, but it can, also, increase the deformation of the lymphocytes themselves. According to a study published in 'Lancet' in 1976, there was an almost proportional relationship between the small intestinal protein intakes from 1963 to 1965 and the lymph node cancer deaths [13].

The omega–3 intake is, also, important for the autoimmune disease. Omega–3 is involved in the gene regulation as well as the anti–inflammatory effects, thereby promoting the apoptosis in the negative selection process of the thymus and thereby reducing the response to the autoantigens. I infer that, in addition to this, there may be an overproduction of the steroid hormones by eating meat. This is because, in the double selection process, the steroid hormones can affect the gene regulations of the immature, immune cells, which, in turn, can lead to the incomplete immune cells, resulting in an increase of the autoimmune diseases in the body. Further research is needed.

8.12. Comparison of the immune status between the vegetarians and the non-vegetarians.

There had been the vegetarian diets that had been effective against the various diseases, and there was also a survey on the specific immunity index of the vegetarians and the non-vegetarians. A study had been conducted by a research team from the University of California, Linda, USA, who published their

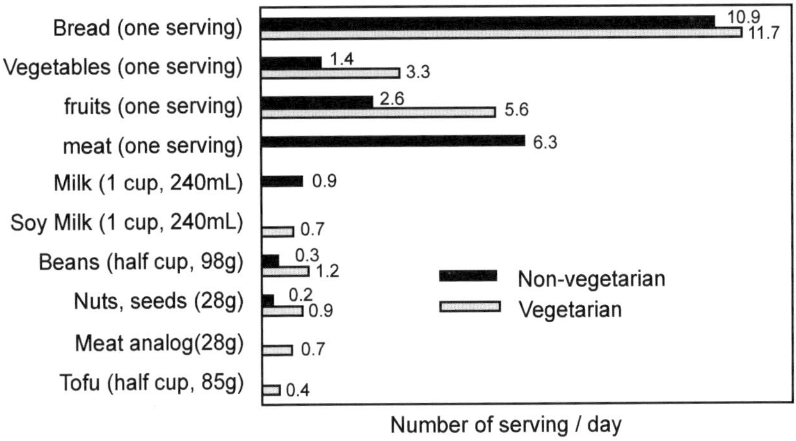

Figure 8-15. Comparison of vegetarian and non-vegetarian eating patterns

paper in the American Journal of Clinical Nutrition in 1999. The subjects of study were 45 healthy adult volunteers, consisting of the students from the Roma Linda University and the employees of the local health care organizations.

The age was between 20 years old and 60 years old, within 120% of the ideal weight, and the current dietary pattern had been maintained for more than one year. In addition, they had excluded the cases that could affect the nutritional status, such as having the metabolic diseases, taking the drugs, smoking, drinking more than once a day, exercising more than 7 hours a week, and the others of the like.

There were 25 vegans, 10 males, and 15 females, and the vegan period ranged from 1 year to 25 years, with an average duration of 4.2 years. Before the vegan diet, with the average of 12.1 years, the Uranus vegetarian diet had ranged from 1 year to 37 years. A total of 20 non-vegetarians (10 men and 10 women each) had been taking the usual, multivitamin tablets. Among the vegans, 4 had been the multivitamin supplements, while 9 of the 25 supplements had been the vitamin B12 supplements. The participants had learned how to accurately record the items and the quantities of the food they had ingested from the skilled researchers. The results are shown in Figure 8-12.

Compared to the non-vegetarians, the vegetarians had consumed the vegetables, the fruits, the nuts, the soy milk, and the plant analogues, while they did not eat meat and milk. The clinical, biochemical measurements of the blood had been performed in a standard manner by the Clinical Laboratory of the Roma Linda Medical School.

The plasma levels of the leukocytes, the lymphocytes, the platelets, and the complement factors were lower in the vegans than in non-vegetarians, while the levels of the serum albumin were very high and the blood urea nitrogen levels were low among the vegans (Table 8-9) [14]. The researchers found that, even though the serum albumin is not a sensitive indicator of the protein intake, a high level of the protein in a vegan diet is sufficient for the enough protein intake. The NK cell activity of the vegans was higher than that of the non-vegetarians, and the dissolution rate of the vegans was higher than that of the non-vegetarians. The researchers had reserved a clear interpretation of these differences

Table 8-9. Correlation between Immune Index and Diet

variable	Beta value (β)	Explanatory power (R^2)	P value
	Lymphocyte count		
Diet	0.34	0.12	0.02
BMI	0.09	0.12	-
	Complement factor 3		
Diet	0.51	0.26	0.000
BMI	0.23	0.29	-

Table 8-10. Immune status of non-vegetarian and vegan people

	non-vegetarian (n=20)	vegan (n=25)	based on non-vegetarian	
			Difference	Rate of change (%)
		Leukocyte count ($\times 10^9$/L)		
white blood cell	5.83	4.96	0.87↓	14.9↓
Lymphocyte	1.90	1.56	0.34↓	17.9↓
Neutrophil	3.47	3.04	0.43↓	12.4↓
Monocyte	0.24	0.19	0.05↓	20.8↓
Eosinophils	0.17	0.14	0.03↓	17.6↓
Basophils	0.05	0.04	0.01↓	20.0↓
Platelet	270	235	35↓	13.0↓
Albumin	46.9	49.3	2.4↑	5.1↑
Blood urea nitrogen				
		Immunoglobulin (g/L)		
IgG	13.5	13.6	0.1↑	0.7↑
IgA	29.0	23.0	6.0↓	20.7↓
IgM	18.5	20.0	1.5↑	8.1↑
Complement Factor 3 (g / L)	0.75	0.63	0.12↓	16.0↓
		NK cell cytotoxic activity		
Effector ratio to target (% dissolution)	31.6	33.6	2.0↑	6%↑

Am J Clin Nutr 1999;70(suppl):586S-93S

8.13. The enzyme nutrition.

As shown above, the number of the immune cells, such as the leukocytes, the lymphocytes, the neutrophils, the protein spheres, the eosinophils, and the basophils,had been reduced from 20.8% to 12.4%, while the cytotoxic activity of the NK cells was about 6% higher than that of the non–vegetarians. An understanding of this phenomenon can be helped by the enzyme nutrition hypothesis, which had been widely circulated in the 1930s.

In 1934, Howell claimed that the enzyme, itself, in the food helps the digestion process in the body. If you eat fresh fruit or vegetables, the enzyme contained in the food, itself, will work in the digestive system of the body, making it better to absorb, and the body will not need to increase the white blood cells. On the other hand, if you eat too much food, all the beneficial enzymes contained in the natural food are destroyed, and the human body needs to take charge of the digestion of the food that is completely consumed, and the aging of the human body is accelerated. In addition, when the human body has the excessive protein and uric acid, the number of the enzyme–rich, white blood cells increases to help the digestion [15].

The digestive organs of the human body are considered to consist of the largest immune system because the areas of the surface of the stomach and the intestines of the body are between 300m2 and

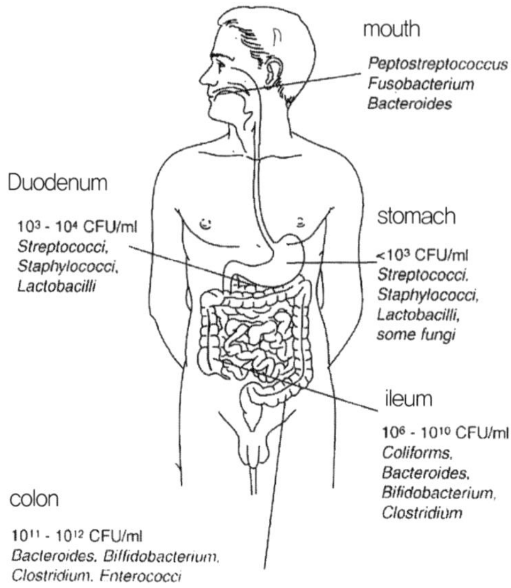

Figure 8–16. Microorganisms of the digestive tract

400m2, which contain more than 10 times more microorganisms than the over 1000 kinds of the human cells (Figure 8–13) [16]. The gut–associated, lymphoid tissue (GALT), present in the lower part of the surface of the digestive tract, is considered to be one of the largest immune tissues in the human body. The GALT is very important in the immuno–nutrition because the surface structure of the digestive tract is exposed to the high concentrations of the dietary factors. Food is essentially 'nothing', and the immune system is initiated by the defensive action against 'what is not', so the initial immune system starts from the field evolutionarily.

The major, basic structure of the GALT is Peyer's patch, where the M cells and the T cells form the epithelial barriers between the intestinal tissues and the lymphatic tissues. The antigens are selected, and the antigens in the digestive tract are transferred to the peyer's patch (Figure 8–14). The B cells in the facial patches secrete the antibodies to the mucosa that is attached to the intestines, and the T cells defend the pathogens that have penetrated across the mucosal barrier. However, the GALT is exposed to the large amounts of the food antigens, and the antigen–specific inhibitory cells are present to prevent the mucosal, immune responses to the food and the normal, fungal bacteria to prevent the inappropriate, inflammatory responses.

The beneficial fungi, also, protect the body from the immense antigens of the food and the microbes coming from the outside, and these fungi are a kind of the bifidus that grows well and eats the fibrin. However, a flesh–less diet lacking the fiber can weaken the composition of the healthy, intestinal microbes and multiply the pathogens that are harmful to humans. Therefore, the non–veggies will be exposed to more pathogens and toxins which they produce, and more antibodies and white blood cells will be needed than the vegans.

The peripheral, lymphatic organs are structurally located where the lymphocytes are collected, and they act to capture the pathogens that have moved from the site of the infection. In

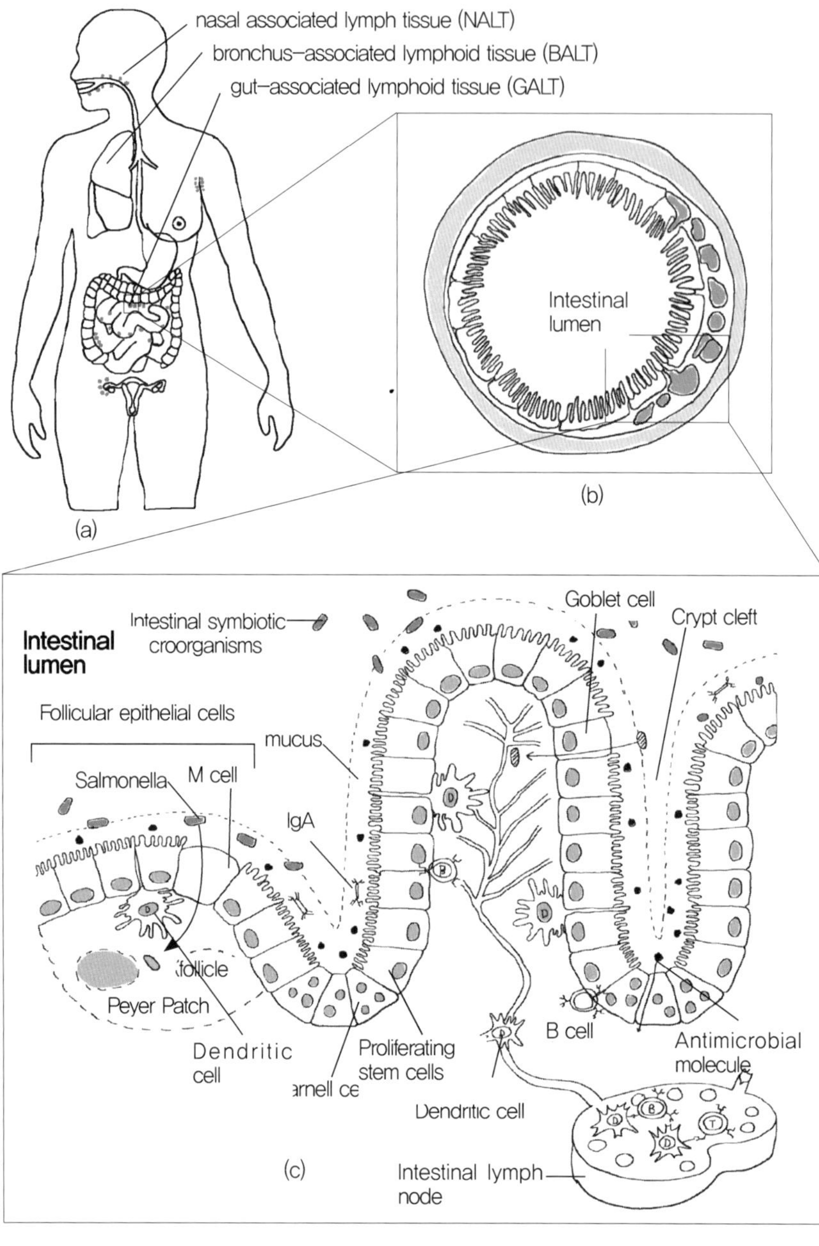

Figure 8-17. Immune system of gastrointestinal tract, gut-associated lymphoid tissue (GALT)

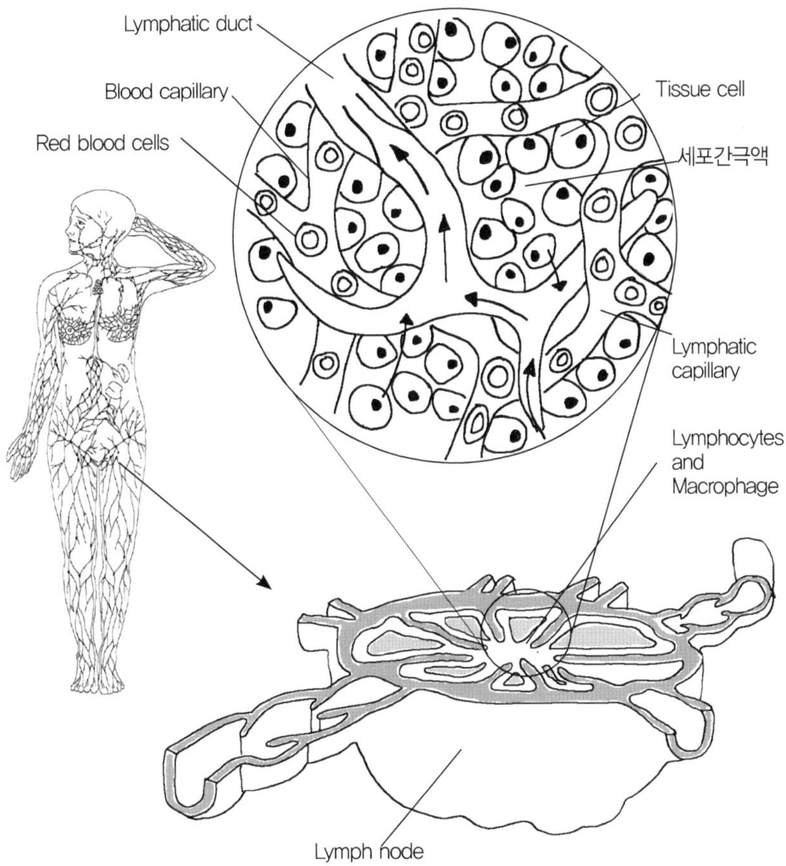

Figure 8–18. Models of lymph nodes

the lymphoid tissues, the lymphocytes stop the circulation and differentiate into the effective B cells or T cells in order to recognize the specific antigens on the surface of the bovine. In comparison to the vegetarian diet, the non–vegetarian diet will be easier to multiply and the human body will need more lymphocytes. And the non–vegetarian blood has the higher cholesterol and lipid content than that of the vegetarian, and the blood sugar concentration and the iron concentration are high, which slows the flow of the blood. Therefore, the leukocyte migration rate and activity will be slowed, and the count of the leukocytes against the antigens will be relatively higher. A vegan diet can make the blood flow more effectively, thereby, increasing the leukocyte activity and the speed of the movement, so that fewer white blood cells are sufficient to perform the same function.

Other hypotheses related to the neuroendocrine system are possible. That is, the steroid hormones are involved in the negative and positive selection processes in the thymus of the T cells. Compared to the vegetarians, the non–vegetarians have a very high level of the cortisol, which affects the selection process of the T cells, which can produce the large amounts of the T cells that are capable of producing the autoimmune diseases and that can be released into the circulatory system. The mechanisms for the dual selection are not yet known in detail, and further studies are needed in the future

8.14. Conclusion

Much is still unknown about the immune system. In particular, the relationship between the nutrition and the immunity is an important area to be studied in the future. The antioxidants that are rich in the various plants are beneficial to almost all of the diseases of the human body, such as cancer, diabetes, dementia, arthritis, and cataracts by alleviating the inflammatory reaction. Meat, by feeding cholesterol, disturbs the hormones of the body, including the five steroid hormones. This again has a detrimental effect on the development of the immune cells and can be one of the causes of the various diseases in the human body. An in-depth study is needed. Some plant components inhibit the formation of the new blood vessels in the development of cancer. Understanding the dietary and immune needs is important because it is important to prevent cancer in advance, rather than treating it after the disease has occurred

References

1. Philpott M, Ferguson LR: Immunonutrition and cancer. Mutat Res 2004, 551:29–42.

2. Wong KW: Clinical efficacy of n–3 fatty acid supplementation in patients with asthma. J Am Diet Assoc 2005, 105:98–105.

3. Emelyanov A, Fedoseev G, Krasnoschekova O, Abulimity A, Trendeleva T, Barnes PJ: Treatment of asthma with lipid extract of New Zealand green–lipped mussel: a randomised clinical trial. Eur Respir J 2002, 20:596–600.

4. Villani F, Comazzi R, De Maria P, Galimberti M: Effect of dietary supplementation with polyunsaturated fatty acids on bronchial hyperreactivity in subjects with seasonal asthma. Respiration 1998, 65:265–269.

5. McKeever TM, Britton J: Diet and asthma. Am J Respir Crit Care Med 2004, 170:725–729.

6. Tanaka T, Kouda K, Kotani M, Takeuchi A, Tabei T, Masamoto Y, Nakamura H, Takigawa M, Suemura M, Takeuchi H, Kouda M: Vegetarian diet ameliorates symptoms of atopic dermatitis through reduction of the number of peripheral eosinophils and of PGE2 synthesis by monocytes. J Physiol Anthropol Appl Human Sci 2001, 20:353–361.

7. Kalantar–Zadeh K, Lee GH, Block G: Relationship between dietary antioxidants and childhood asthma: more epidemiological studies are needed. Medical Hypotheses, 62:280–290.

8. Kjeldsen–Kragh J: Rheumatoid arthritis treated with vegetarian diets. Am J Clin Nutr 1999, 70:594S–600S.

9. Inoue G, Horiike N, Michitaka K, Onji M: Hepatitis C virus clearance is prominent in women in an endemic area. J Gastroenterol Hepatol 2000, 15:1054–1058.

10. Scofield RH: Autoantibodies as predictors of disease. Lancet 2004, 363:1544–1546.

11. Betterle C, Lazzarotto F, Presotto F: Autoimmune polyglandular syndrome Type 2: the tip of an iceberg? Clin Exp Immunol 2004, 137:225–233.

12. Armstrong BK, Brown JB, Clarke HT, Crooke DK, Hahnel R, Masarei JR, Ratajczak T: Diet and reproductive hormones: a study of vegetarian and nonvegetarian postmenopausal women. J Natl Cancer Inst 1981, 67:761–767.

13. Cunningham A: LYMPHOMAS AND ANIMAL–PROTEIN CONSUMPTION. The Lancet 1976, 308:1184–1186.

14. Haddad EH, Berk LS, Kettering JD, Hubbard RW, Peters WR: Dietary intake and biochemical, hematologic, and immune status of vegans compared with nonvegetarians. Am J Clin Nutr

1999, 70:586S–593S.

15. Hawell: Enzyme Nutrition.

16. Young RJ, Huffman S: Probiotic use in children. J Pediatr Health Care 2003, 17:277–283.

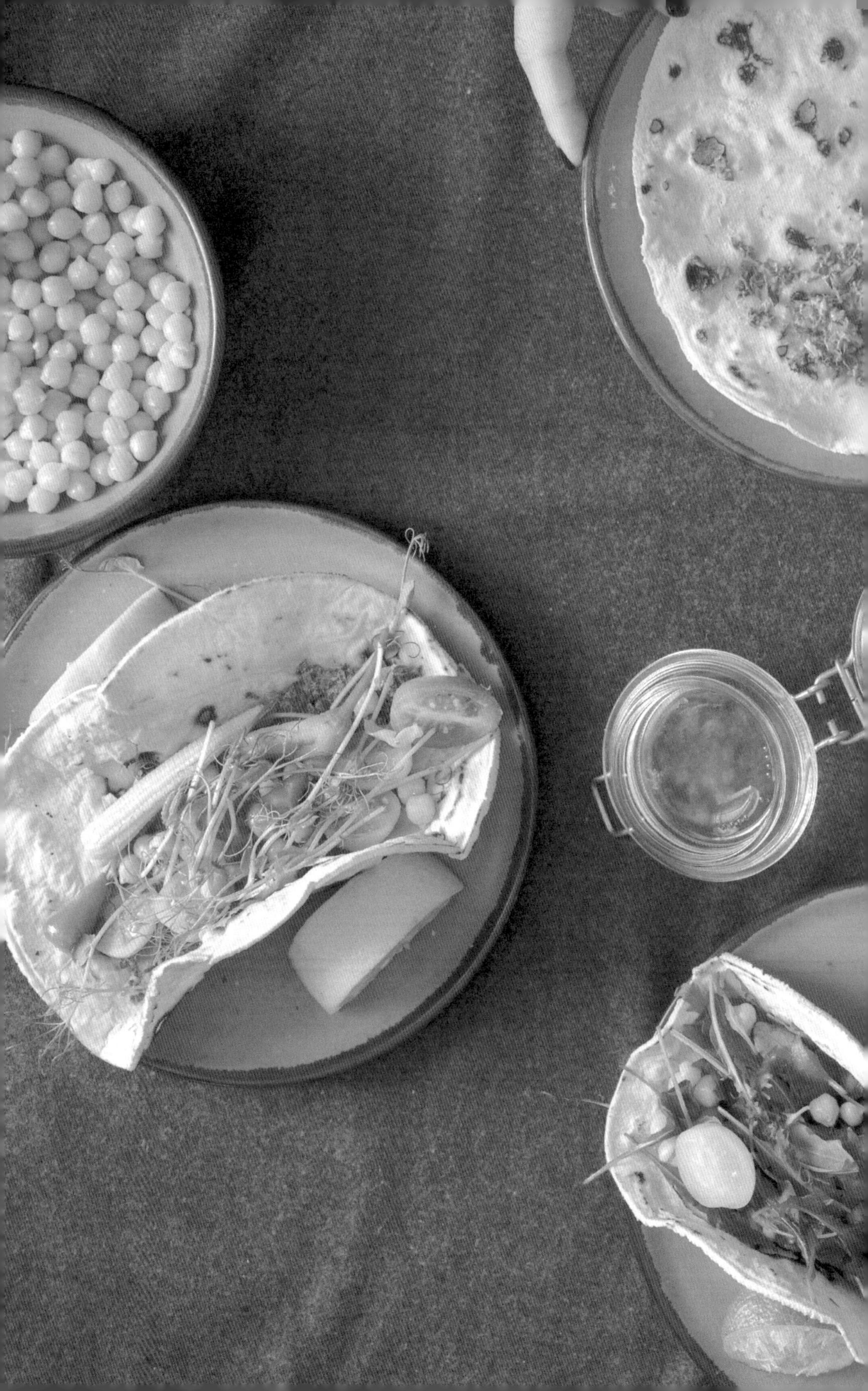

Chapter 9. Endocrine System and Vegetarian Diet

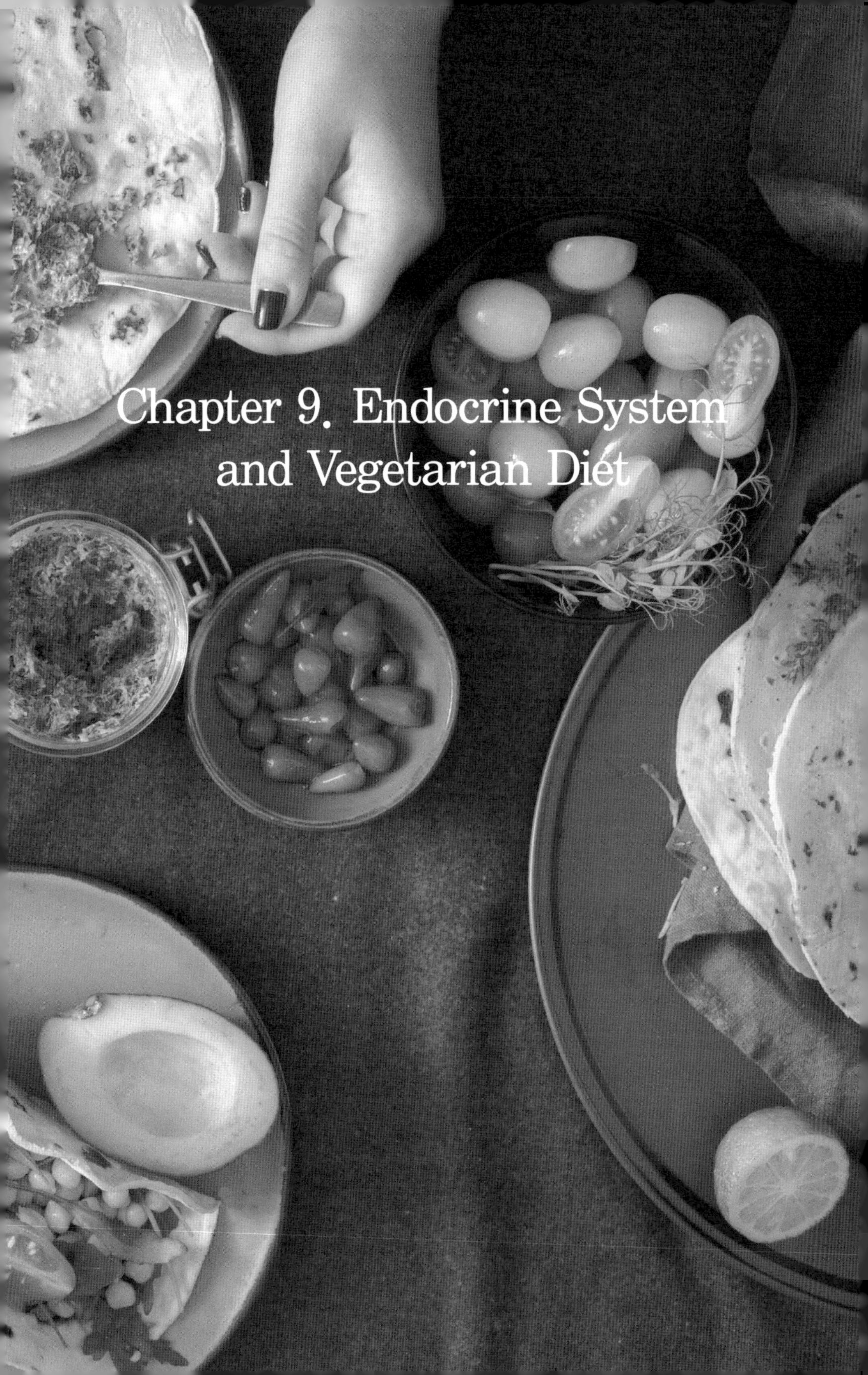

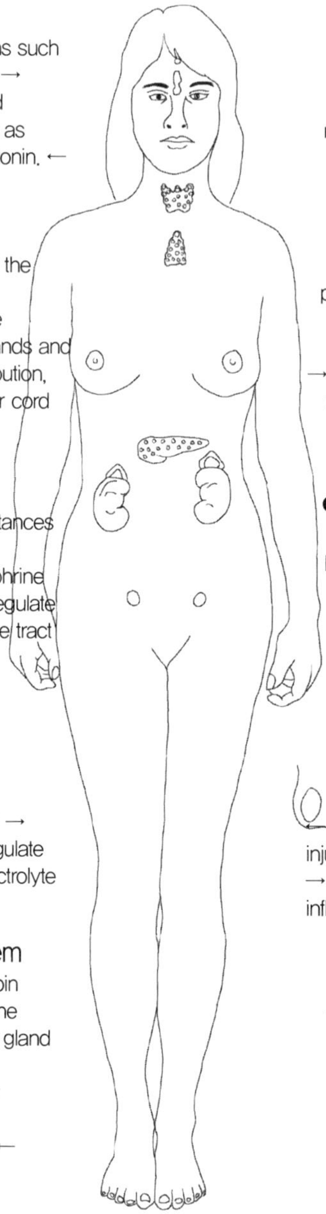

● Skeletal system

Protecting endocrine organs such as brain, chest, and pelvis →
Skeletal growth is regulated by various hormones such as parathyroid hormone, calcitonin. ←

● Skin system

Protect the table surface of the endocrine organ →
Sex hormones promote the activation of sebaceous glands and affect hair growth, fat distribution, and activity of the glandular cord ←

● Digestive system

Provide nutrients and substances for endocrine cells →
Epinephrine and norepinephrine control the sphincter and regulate the pressure in the digestive tract ←

● Urinary system

Kidney cells secrete renin, erythropoietin, and calcitriol →
Aldosterone, ADH, ANP regulate blood flow velocity and electrolyte ←

● Reproductive system

Steroid hormones and inhibin inhibit secretory activity in the hypothalamus and pituitary gland →
Hypothalamus and pituitary hormone control sexual development and function ←

● Muscular system

← Skeletal muscle protects several endocrine organs
→ hormones regulate muscle metabolism, energy production, growth

● Nervous system

←The hypothalamus directly controls the secretion of the pituitary gland and indirectly the secretion of other endocrine organs
→ Some hormones affect neuro–metabolism Hormones regulate fluid, electrolyte balance

● Cardiovascular system

← Circulatory system delivers hormones throughout the body
→ erythropoietin (EPO) regulates the production of red blood cells.

● Immune / lymphatic system

← Lymphocytes infect and repair injuries
→ glucocorticoid shows anti–inflammatory effect

● respiratory system

← Supply oxygen and remove CO_2
→ epinephrine and norepinephrine regulate respiratory activity

Chapter 9. The endocrine system and the vegetarian diet.

9.1. The types and the functions of the endocrine system.

Single cells or small organisms directly receive the necessary substances and energy from the environment and release the waste, after the cell metabolism, directly into the environment. However, a multi−celled organism composed of the many cells cannot directly exchange the environment, matter, and energy. For example, the mean diameter of a human cell is 1 micrometer. Even if the thickness of the breast is 10 cm, it must pass more than 50,000 cells from the outer environment surface to the central cell. Therefore, thestructure like the human body has created an internal environment in which all the cells can function. The extracellular fluid is the primary, internal environment that forces all the cells to become like the locked solutions.

Keeping the temperature, pH, nutrients, and the electrolyte concentration constant as the internal environment is a key factor for the stable and efficient operation of the sanitary napkins, including the energy metabolism, and it is called a "homeostasis".

Stressor is the factor that breaks a homeostasis, and there are the various factors, such as the physically inflammatory reactions and the psychologically dangerous situations. The main purpose of a homeostasis is to generate the energy that life requires. The human body has created the two types of the cell tissues that are dedicated to the internal, environmental, regulation. It senses the changes in the internal and external environments of the human body, sends the signals to the human cells to maintain the homeostasis, is electrically nervous, and is chemically endocrine.

The endocrine contrasts with the exocrine pancreas, which means a method for delivering a signaling substance in a way that diffuses into the flows of the body fluids without any special peculiarities, like the sweat or the saliva. The endocrine cells are a collection of the cells that make the hormones. The hormones are released

Table 9-1. Types and functions of the hypothalamic hormones

	hormone	Function
Releasing hormone	Thyroid stimulating hormone releasing hormone (TRH)	Stimulate thyroid stimulating hormone release
	Gonadotropin releasing hormone (GnRH)	Stimulate the release of FSH and LH
	Growth hormone releasing hormone (GHRH)	Stimulate growth hormone release
	Adrenocorticotropic hormone-releasing hormone (CRH)	Stimulate the release of adrenocorticotropic hormone
	Prolactin (PRL) releasing hormone	Stimulate prolactin release
Inhibitory hormone	Growth Hormone Releasing Hormone	Suppress growth hormone release
	Melanocyte stimulating hormone releasing hormone	Melanocyte stimulating hormone Suppress release
	Prolactin releasing hormone	Suppress prolactin release

Table 9–2. Types and functions of hormones in the pituitary gland

	hormone	Function
Anterior	Thyroid stimulating hormone (TSH)	Thyroxine secretion regulation of the thyroid gland
	Follicle stimulating hormone (FSH)	Follicular maturation, promote estrogen secretion
	Luteinizing hormone (LH)	Ovulation, promotion of progesterone secretion
	Growth hormone (GH)	Promotes bone and muscle growth
	Adrenocorticotropic hormone (ACTH)	Promoting corticoid secretion
	Lactate stimulating hormone (PRL)	Development of breast milk and lactation promotion
Posterior	Vasopressin	Increase blood pressure, promote absorption of water bonsai
	Oxytocin	Uterine muscle contraction during labor

Table 9–3. Types and Functions of Hormones in the Peripheral Hormone Organs

Endocrine		hormone	function
thyroid		Thyroxine	Promote cell metabolism (catabolism)
		Calcitonin	Decrease in plasma calcium
Parathyroid gland		Paratormone	Calcium concentration in plasma increases
pancreas	α cell	Glucagon	Increase in blood sugar (glycogen → glucose)
	β cell	insulin	Decrease in blood sugar (glucose → glycogen)
Adrenal	cortex	Glucocorticoid	Increase in blood sugar (protein, fat → glucose)
		Mineral corticoid	Na^+ reabsorption in kidney, promotion of K^+ secretion
	medulla	Adrenaline (epinephrine)	Increase in blood sugar (glycogen → glucose)
gonad	Testimony	Testosterone	Expression of secondary sex of male
	ovary	Estrogen	Female secondary manifestations, uterine wall development
		Progesterone	Ovulation Suppression, Pregnancy Maintenance

into the extracellular fluid that passes through the endocrine system, which is then spread to the body through the blood of the circulatory system. Receiving the key signal of a specific hormone is the arrest of the target cell. The receptors recognize and bind the hormones. In most cases, the peptide hormone is in the cell membrane, and the receptor of the steroid hormone is in the cytoplasm. The hormones can act in very small amounts, and they can function in about 1 gram of water and, also, in 100 tons of water.

The vertebrate animals have twelve important endocrine glands, including the hypothalamus, the pituitary gland, the pineal gland, the thyroid gland, the parathyroid gland, the thymus, the adrenal gland, the pancreas, the heart, the kidneys, the digestive tract, and the gonads (testes, ovaries).

The central part of the endocrine system is the hypothalamus, called the "femoral gland". The hypothalamus is a chemical substance in the anterior pituitary gland and an electrical signal in the posterior pituitary gland. The posterior pituitary gland receives the electrical signals from the hypothalamus, secretes the antidiuretic hormone and the oxytocin, and the anterior, pituitary gland releases nine hormones.

The nine types of the hormones are classified as the gland-stimulating hormones and the other hormones that stimulate the other endocrine-gland-stimulating hormones released from the endocrine gland. For example, the thyroid-stimulating hormone

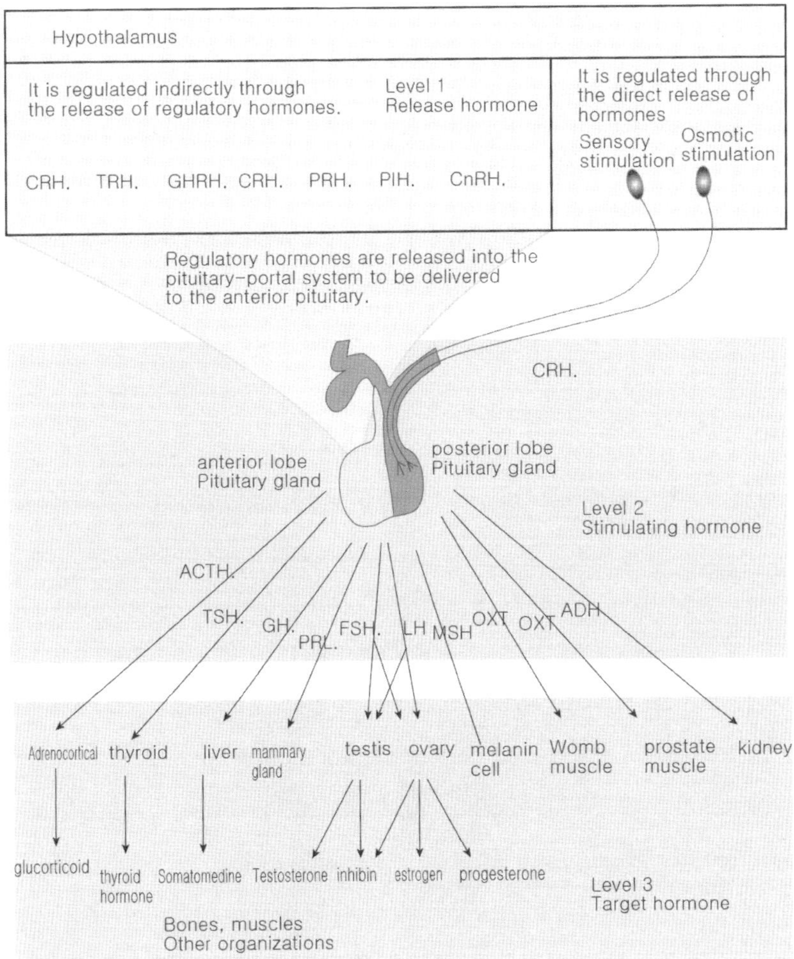

Figure 9-1. Hormone Three Step Process

HPA: Hypothalamus-Pituitary-Adrenal Axis, / HPG: Hypothalamus-Pituitary-Gonad,

HPT: Hypothalamus-Pituitary-Thyroid / HPS: Hypothalamus-Pituitary-Somatotroph,

E2: Estradiol, GC: Glucocorticoid, GH: Growth Hormone

stimulates the thyroid gland to release the thyroid hormones, and the corticosteroids stimulate the cortex to release the cortisol (glucocorticoid) or the aldosterone (mineral corticoid). And the hormone stimulating the reproductive organs to stimulate the formation of the follicles is a follicle-stimulating hormone, and the hormone that stimulates the formation of the lutein is a luteinizing hormone

9.2. The neuroendocrine and hormone three-step signaling.

The endocrine system that releases the action potential and the hormone-releasing hormone is integrated into the neuroendocrine system by sharing the hypothalamus and the pituitary gland. This can be understood through the connection between the anatomical structure of the hypothalamus and the other brain regions. The hypothalamus is as small as 4 grams, accounting for less than 1% of the total brain volume, that is located below the thalamus and at the lower floor of the third ventricle [1].

The hypothalamus is anatomically involved in the diencephalon and is functionally regarded as the limbic system. The hypothalamus receives the somatic and visceral-afferent signals from the periphery via the ventral striatum, the brainstem, and the spinal cord, and receives the afferent signals from the thalamus. The thalamus, the cortex, the limbic system (hippocampus and amygdala), and the nerves are directly interconnected to react to the external and internal environment of the body and to maintain the internal homeostasis [2]. In addition, the hypothalamus indirectly interacts with the basal ganglia that is associated with the limbic system, which can, also, affect the emotions and the psychology.

The signals of the endocrine system are amplified through a three–step process. That is, when the released hormones come out from the hypothalamus, they take a signal from the pituitary gland and release the stimulating hormone. The stimulating hormones stimulate each hormonal organ through the circulatory system, and the hormonal organs emit the target hormones, which affect almost all cells in the body. The purpose of this three–step process is largely understood to be the synthesis of the various signals from the human body and the amplification of the chemical signals that descend from the central to the peripheral (Fig. 9–1).

In other words, the signals inside and outside the human body are synthesized in the nervous system, and, ultimately,they determine the degree of the signaling in the hypothalamus for the human homeostasis. Through each step, the signal is amplified about 1,000 times, and the endocrine organs produce a chemical signal that is 1 million times as much, as it can affect the whole body. The hormones at the distal end of the hypothalamus and the pituitary hormone receptors, again,go through a negative feedback to maintain a value within a certain range.

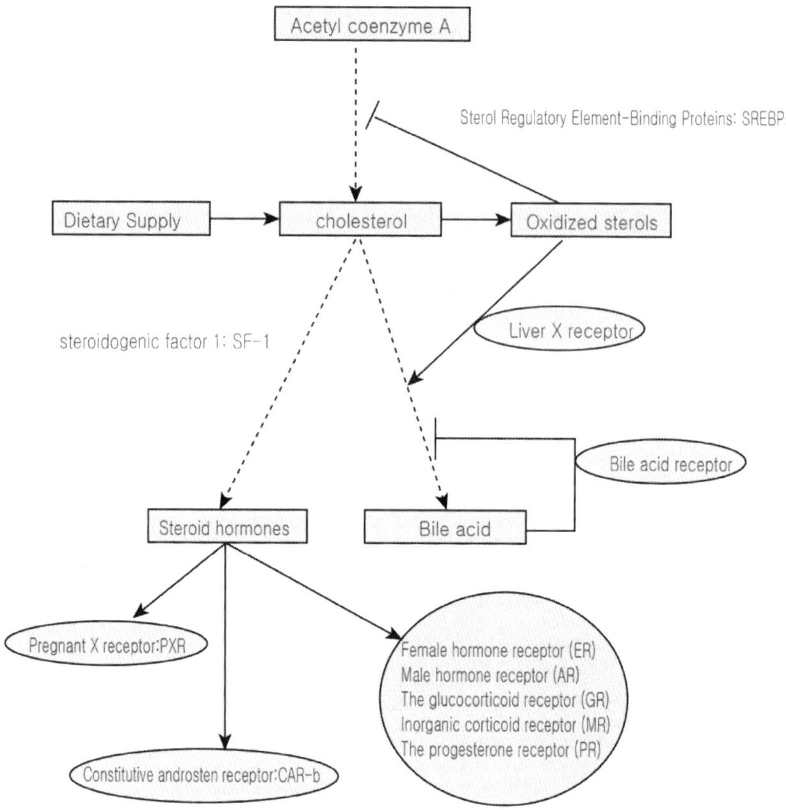

Figure 9–2. Cholesterol metabolism intermediates

The sexual hormones of the genders, cortisol, and aldosterone of the adrenal glands, also, affect the human metabolism, and the various diseases are related to the endocrine system. The importance of this is widely known as the immunosuppression of the cortisol. Chrousos et al. emphasized the importance of the hormonal system in relation to the metabolic syndrome [3, 4].

The endocrine system has long been of interest to the humanity, the sociologists, the public, as well as the biologists in order to influence the psychology and the behaviors of the animals.

The effect of the steroid hormone on the serum through the dietary cholesterol.

The human hormone system has five steroid hormones. The steroid hormones affect almost all cells in the body, including the nerve cells and the immune cells, along with the blood. When they cross the cell membrane and bind to a hormone receptor in the cytoplasm, the hormone receptors move into the nucleus within the cytoplasm and regulate the switches of the hundreds of the genes, thereby creating the long-term changes. The basic skeleton of the steroid hormones is cholesterol, which is actually synthesized from the cholesterol as a raw material. Thus, it can be expected that the nutritional value of the five steroid hormones may be affected by the nutrients that were ingested. Studies have shown that the low-density lipoprotein (LDL) inhibits the 3-hydroxy-3-

methylglutaryl,co-enzyme A reductase, a rate-limiting enzyme in the cholesterol synthesis [5, 6]. Thus, the meat intake affects the entire human body and psychology through the changes in the levels of the various steroid hormones in the body (Fig. 9-2) [7, 8].

9.3. Sex hormones, cancer, and the vegetarian diet

It has been argued that the occurrence of breast cancer is related to the function of ovulation. The results of the epidemiological in vitro experiments and biopsies conducted over the past 50 years show that the steroid hormones, such as the male hormone and the female hormone, regulate the cell proliferation and play an important role in promoting breast cancer. Scientists have found that a variety of the hormones and factors have been linked to the breast cancer outbreaks. The risk of breast cancer was high when the low levels of the sex hormone-binding globulin (SHBG) were found at the high concentrations of the free estradiol, the total estradiol, the total testosterone, and the other estrogens and androgens, which were not associated with protein. In addition, a variety of the epidemiological studies have shown the high risks of breast cancer, prostate cancer, colorectal cancer, and ovarian cancer when the plasma concentrations of the IGF-1 (similar insulin growth factor) hormones were high.

Table 9-4. Comparison of the average of hormonal changes in vegetarian and non-vegetarian [9]

	group (person)	1January	June	change(%)	p-value
SHBG (nmol/l)	vegetarian(50)	36.03	45.10	25.2	0.0001
	non-vegetarian(49)	36.32	37.61	3.6	
Testosterone (ng/ml)	vegetarian(50)	0.41	0.33	-18.3	0.004
	non-vegetarian(49)	0.42	0.39	-6.4	
female hormone (pg/ml)	vegetarian(50)	8.62	7.07	-18.0	0.13
	non-vegetarian(49)	8.30	7.84	-5.7	
Free testosterone (ng/ml)	vegetarian(50)	0.006	0.005	-28.6	0.0001
	non-vegetarian(49)	0.010	0.010	-8.2	
free female hormone (pg/ml)	vegetarian(50)	0.23	0.17	-23.4	0.05
	non-vegetarian(49)	0.22	0.21	-6.8	
Fasting insulin (μIU/ml)	vegetarian(50)	4.82	4.31	-10.4	0.14
	non-vegetarian(49)	4.63	4.87	5.1	
Fasting blood sugar (μg/dl)	vegetarian(50)	91.66	86.47	-5.7	0.026
	non-vegetarian(49)	93.55	92.44	-1.2	
Growth hormone (ng/ml)	vegetarian(50)	1.25	1.92	54.2	0.22
	non-vegetarian(49)	1.10	1.20	9.5	
Growth hormone binding protein(ng/ml)	vegetarian(50)	0.94	1.21	29.1	0.002
	non-vegetarian(49)	0.89	0.65	-26.8	
IGF-1 (ng/ml)	vegetarian(50)	146.65	138.00	-5.9	0.64
	non-vegetarian(49)	135.18	129.29	-4.4	
IGFBP-1 (ng/ml)	vegetarian(50)	40.07	45.73	12.2	0.015
	non-vegetarian(49)	48.07	44.98	-6.4	
IGFBP-2 (ng/ml)	vegetarian(50)	6.15	8.02	30.4	0.0004
	non-vegetarian(49)	6.11	6.52	6.6	

SHBG: Sex hormone binding globulin / IGF-1: Insulin like growth factor-1

* The blood androgen levels in the breast, prostate, colon, and ovarian cancer patients are high.

The free estradiol concentration is high.

The total estradiol concentration is high.

The low levels of the sex hormone–binding protein.

The IGF–1 levels are high.

The IGF–1–binding protein concentration is low

The IGF is a water–insoluble, hydrophobic, peptide hormone that stimulates the cell proliferation and inhibits the programmed cell death (apoptosis). The primary function of the IGF–1 in the body is to promote the body metabolism and growth, as well as the plasma levels of the available steroids (sex hormones). In the experimental studies, the IGF–1 had promoted the growths of both the normal and tumor cells in the breast tissue. In vitro, the IGF–1 and the insulin had inhibited the synthesis of the sex hormone–binding globulin (SHBG) and had stimulated the synthesis of the male hormone and the androgens in the adrenal glands and the ovaries. This effect of the IGF–1 appears equally in both the men and women

9.4. The vegetarian diet patterns and the cancer research experiments

If cancer development is affected by the hormones and the hormone production is affected by the diet, the risk of breast cancer will change with the dietary changes. The related experiments had been conducted in Milan, northern Italy. Berito and colleagues recruited 312 healthy, postmenopausal women between the ages of 50 and 65 from January 1996 to June 1996.

The conditions for the participating women had to be at least 2 years of menopause, at least one ovary, and no hormone-replacement therapy for at least 6 months before the experiment. The women had never been vegetarian before participating in the experiment, they were divided into the two groups of 52 people, one group receiving a Mediterranean vegetarian diet, or a meal of longevity, and the other group receiving no dietary guidance.

The vegetarian group was taught how to get the essential amino acids, the vitamins, and the minerals as a plant starter instead of meat, eggs, and milk, and they were made to not eat these more than once a week. The carbohydrates had been replaced by the complex carbohydrates, such as whole wheat instead of the wheatgrass, and the fruits and the fermented cereals had been recommended, and fat or salt had been rarely added during the cooking. At least once a day, the soybean foods, such as soy milk, miso soup, tofu, and tempeh, were eaten. It was not milk fat, but

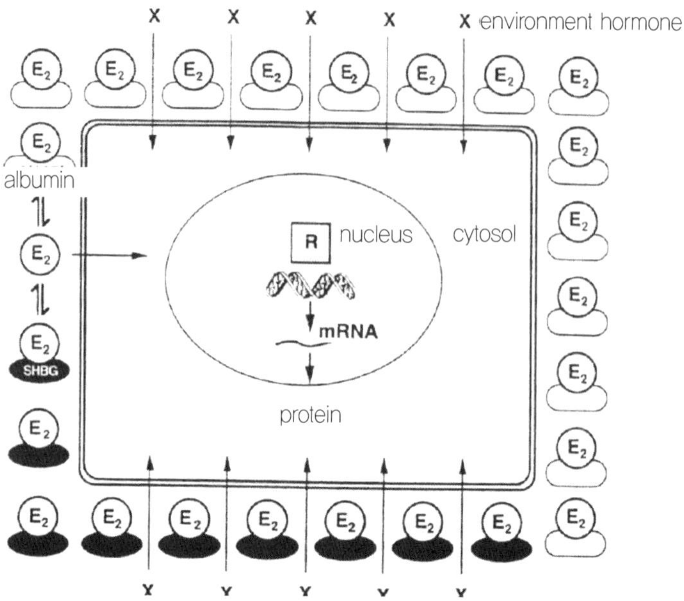

Figure 9-3. Hormone action model in blood [10]

SHBG(Sex hormone-binding globulin), E_2(Female hormone, estradiol), R(Nuclear receptor, Hormone receptor)

the various seeds and the olive oil. The women who had participated in the experiment received 1 kg of bread once a week, which was made by adding 8% of the whole wheat and the flaxseed (rich in omega-3 fatty acids and accounting for a half of the powder). The estimated intake of the isoflavones was 40 mg in the vegetarian group compared to 2 mg in the non-vegetarian group, which is the average intake of the Asian women.

The dietary composition of the vegetarian group lowers the intake of total fat, sugar, and refined carbohydrates and increases the intake of the monounsaturated fats, the omega-3, polyunsaturated, fatty acids, the low glucose, the brown rice, the soybeans, and the vegetables to lower the plasma insulin levels. In addition, the diet had been rich in the endogenous androgen (male hormone) and the phytoestrogens, such as the isoflavones and the lignans, which are the important factors in lowering the estrogen level. The ultimate goal of this experiment was to determine whether a long-term vegetarian diet that reduces the risk of breast cancer is worthwhile.

The results after the 5 months of the vegetarian diet were surprising. The weight loss had been −4.06 kg (vegetarian group) versus −0.56 kg (non-vegetarian group) and the plasma growth hormone level had increased by 54.2% in the vegetarian group only. The growth hormone-binding protein had increased in the vegetarian group, while that of the non-vegetarian group had decreased [9]. And the sex hormone-binding globulin had increased by 25% in the vegetarian group and by 18% in the non-vegetarian group (Table 9-4). The free testosterone (male hormone) and the estradiol (female hormone), which were not associated with the sex hormone-binding globulin, had decreased by 28.6% and 18.0%, respectively, in the vegetarian group. In contrast, the non-vegetarian group had decreased by 8.2% and 5.7%, respectively. Taken together, these results suggest that the vegetarian diets have a beneficial effect on the hormone levels that are associated with the cancer development in the humans.

9.5. The sex hormone–binding protein (SHBG) and the phytoestrogen.

Sex hormones begin to be produced when the fertilized fish are at 7 weeks of age. When the male and female Y chromosomes are signaled to produce the androgen, the reproductive system of the fetus develops into a male, and, when the androgen is not produced, it develops into a female. Until puberty, the gonadotropin–releasing hormone suppression of the hypothalamus due to the gonads does not produce a lot of the sex hormones at the age of 13 and at the age of 14 to suppress the hypothalamus and increase the production of the sex hormones.

The male increases the level of the luteinizing hormone in the testosterone, which is known as the male hormone androgen, which makes the voice thicker, makes the stronger muscles, makes the facial and body hair, and makes the testicles and the penis grow. In the case of the females, the increase of the luteinizing hormone and the follicle–stimulating hormone causes the production of a female hormone in the ovary, the growths of the uterus and the breasts, the increase of the subcutaneous fat, and the start of the menstrual cycle.

The steroids, which are poorly water–soluble in the skeleton, bind with a transport protein called the "sex hormone binding globulin" (SHBG) or the "albumin" when they want to move through the blood. The sex hormones in the body are 99% bound and the

Table 9-5. Production of SHBG according to the concentration of genistein

Genistein dose (unit: micromolar)	Production rate of SHBG per cell (%)
Control	100
5	143
10	153
20	426
30	772
40	343

J Clin Endocrinol Metab (2000) 85:2797-2800

Table 9-6. Isoflavone content in various foods [11]

Food	Total amount of isoflavones*
Soybean	84.0 (13.8-153.4)
soy milk	9.6 (1.26-21.1)
Bean cheese	31.3 (3.33-21.1)
Soy Yoghurt	16.3
Korean Miso	31.5 (3.31-59.4)
tofu	39.0 (22.63-67.49)
Tempe	43.5 (6.88-62.5)
Miso	42.6 (6.88-62.5)
Natto	58.9 (46.4-87.0)

Table 9-7. Changes in serum SHBG levels according to dietary patterns

	non-vegetarian	lacto-ovo vegetarian	vegan	p-value
SHBG	42.6 (226 person)	44.6 (237person)	50.9 (233person)	0.001

remaining 1% are free (free of the binding proteins). This liberated sex hormone is not regulated and enters the cells randomly.

As shown in Figure 9–3, the released hormone, which is not associated with the foreign environmental hormones or proteins, can pass through the cell membrane easily and give a signal to the gene regulator, the nuclear receptor, which can have a very small impact. On the other hand, the sex hormones associated with the SHBG do not function because they do not enter the cell even if they have a large amount of blood. In other words, when the less SHBG is produced, the number of the free sex hormones is increased and the hormone response is more affected by the free hormone level than the total hormone level [10]. The amount of the SHBG is higher in childhood than in adulthood and lower in obesity in childhood than in adulthood. Experimentally, the amount of the SHBG is reduced when the insulin secretion is increased

9.6. Phytoestrogens and the SHBG.

The phytoestrogens are the compounds that act like the hormones in the human body, which are produced by the plants. They are abundant in the plants, such as vegetables, fruits, and grains, and, especially, in the soybean plants and the nuts. The plants that are rich in the phytoestrogens include the isoflavones and the lignans, which are in, and similar to, the endogenous hormone of the estrogen , and, thus, they act as the estrogen receptors, sometimes as the competitors, and sometimes as the complementaries. Thus, the phytoestrogens have the protective effect regarding the cervical cancer, the ovarian cancer, the prostate cancer, the osteoporosis, and the heart disease, and the phytoestrogens inhibit the progression of the menopausal syndrome.

The phytoestrogens, also, affect the synthesis of the sex hormone-binding globulins. In 2000, researchers in Chile had looked at the amounts of the SHBGs that had been produced by the tissue cultures of the human cancer cells and the genistein, a kind of the phytoestrogens. As shown in Table 9-5, the SHBG had increased to 143% when the 5 micromolars (mols) of the genistein were added to 100% of the amount of the SHBG that was produced in a control group to which no genistein was added, and the SHBG had increased to 153% when the 10 micromolars (mols) of the genistein were added to 100% of the amount of the SHBG that was produced in a control group to which no genistein was added, respectively. In other words, the more the phytoestrogens in a plant are taken up to a certain amount, the more the SHBG becomes in the human body, and these proteins bind with the sex hormone and prevent the sexual hormone from acting in a disorderly manner. The SHBG levels, also, increase when fasting. On the other hand, the SHBG production is lower when the high protein is consumed than when the high carbohydrate is consumed [13].

Table 9–6 shows the content of the isoflavones in the various foods. The soybean contains 84 mg of the isoflavones per 100 g, which was the highest value as followed by Natto, Tempe, and Tofu. Table 9–7 shows that the sex hormone–binding globulins (SHBGs) in the blood, according to the dietary pattern, were 44.6 and 44.9, respectively, compared to the 42.6 for the non–vegetarians and the 50.9 for the vegans, which were statistically significant. That is, depending on the dietary pattern, the level of the free state, separated from the protein of the sex hormone, changes, suggesting the possibility of a disturbance in the regulation processes of the various genes in the human body.

9.7. Bertolt's rooster experiment

The first scientific study involving the hormones was Bertolt's rooster experiment [14]. In 1948, Bertolt divided six young roosters into three groups of two each. And, when the first group of the chickens were castrated on both sides of the testicles, they had shown the monotonous tone of their criesas the young roosters, not trying to fight with the other chickens and not showing any mating activity. The roosters' heads and bodies were small, and the color of the crests and the gravy (the roots hanging from the necks of the chickens, etc.) had been faded and had shrunken in size.

Bertolt then experimented with the second group of the chickens.They were reassembled after the testicles were removed. Surprisingly, all of these chickens showed the normal cock behaviors and appearances (Fig. 9–4).

"They tried to fight against each other,they had cried vigorously, and they had shown the normal mating reactions to the hens. Their appearances were, also, distinguished from the appearances of the other young cocks. They were large and heady, crested high, and bright red. "

The third group of the roosters were, also, castrated, and they were transplanted the testicles of the different roosters.They had developed and behaved as the normal roostersjust like the second group [14].

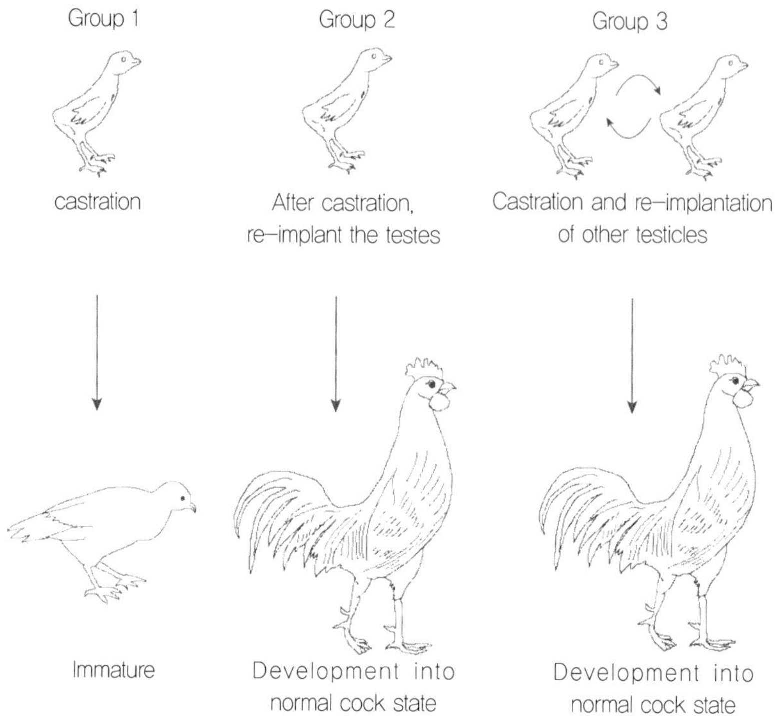

Figure 9–4. Bertolt's experiment with hormones and behavioral changes through rooster castration

9.8. The various functions of the testosterone.

Male hormones are related to the physiological characteristics of the human body and are related to the various symptoms, such as baldness and hair loss. Male hormones not only affect the physiological function, but, also, act on the cranial nerves and can give the various psychological influences. For example, the average testosterone levels of the sex offenders are high, and those of the rebels are particularly high [15].

Aggression is a social behavior that occurs due to a combination of the various social and biological causes. Biologically, aggression is related to the actions of the endocrine system and the nervous system. A few behavioral endocrinology studies have shown that the high levels of the blood testosterone have a positive correlation with the aggressive behavior. The social dominance with the impulsive aggression and the hyperactivity in handling the situations are the same phenomena for both men and women with the high testosterone levels.

As shown in Figure 9–5 and Table 9–8, it can be seen that, as the level of testosterone increases, the visual cognitive ability increases (+) while the auditory cognitive ability decreases (–). And, as the testosterone level increases, the DHT increases, followed by a tendency to baldness, while the hair becomes more hairy. Testosterone affects psychologically to increase the aggressiveness and the self–esteem, while a too low testosterone level can lead

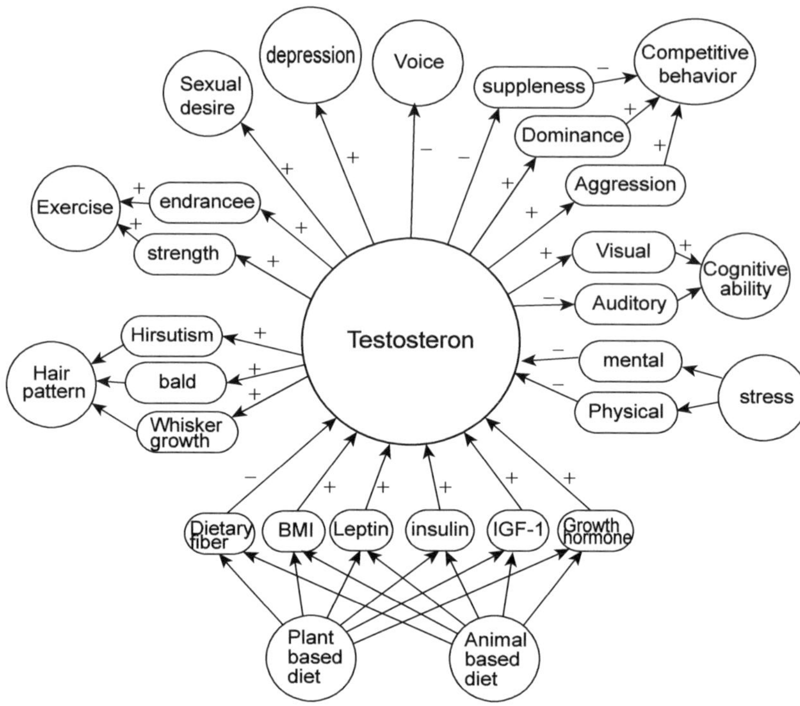

Figure 9–5. Testosterone and feedback mechanisms of behavior, body, and physiology [15]

The + sign affects the positive, and the – sign affects the negative. Testosterone increases sexual desire. Testosterone increases visual cognitive ability, but weakens auditory cognitive ability. As age increases, testosterone levels decrease. Increased testosterone levels also increase aggression. Decreased testosterone levels increase depression. Physical and mental stress lowers testosterone levels. Increased testosterone levels result in increased baldness and increased number of beard.

to depression. These diverse functionsare due to the fact that the receptors acting on the testosterone are present in almost all cells of the body. In other words, the testosterone acts as a kind of the ligand, which acts on the nerve cells, the immune cells, the muscle cells, etc., and causes the various functional changes, such as changing the expression regarding the hundreds of the genes.

Table 9-8. Testosterone levels and physical characteristics [15]

Range of testosterone levels				
type	characteristic	low	middle	high
Hair pattern	bald		●	● ●
	Whisker growth		●	● ●
sexual desire	Non-abuse		●	●
	Criminal aspect			●
Physical ability	reinforce		●	● ●
	endurance	●		
depression		●		
stress		●		
Social behavior	Aggression		●	●
	Physical violence		●	●
	Dominance		●	●
	obey	●		
	Visual perception		●	
Recognition characteristic	Linguistic ability	●		
voice	bass		●	● ●
	Treble	●		
Residential altitude	mountain	●		
	Sleep		●	
Aging		●		
Diet	vegetarian	●		
	Western style		●	

●: related, ● ●: Fairly relevant

European Journal of Endocrinology (2001) 144:183-197

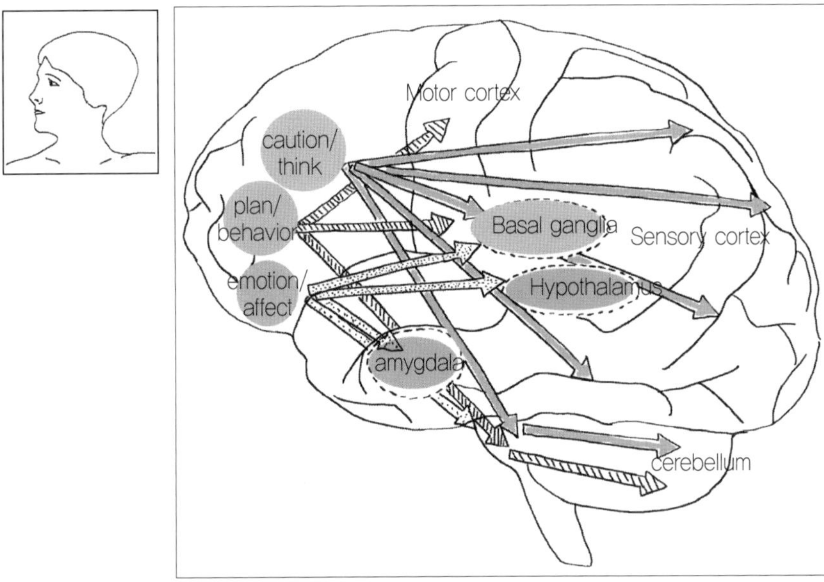

Figure 9–6. Prefrontal, orbital frontal function

9.9. Franzel's aggression experiment and testosterone.

Neurologically, aggression is associated with the orbital, frontal cortex. The orbital, frontal cortex located behind the eyebrows is the brain region involved in the self-regulation and the impulse control. The orbital, frontal lobe is known to be the nerve site where the myelinization lastly occurs.

Studies have shown that, when the activity of the orbital, frontal cortex increases, the level of the reactive aggression decreases, whereas, when the orbital, frontal cortex is removed, the impulsive behavior and the overaggression occur. Based on the trine brain hypothesis of McLean, it can be deduced that the orbital, frontal lobe has the behavioral characteristic when the lower limb system and the reptilian brain are well controlled. Patients with the neurological diseases with the high levels of the reactive aggression had decreased the activity of the orbital, frontal cortex [16].

Franzwell et al. had focused on the characteristics of the endocrine system and the nervous system that are associated with aggression and have hypothesized that, as the level of the testosterone increases, the activity of the orbital frontal cortex decreases, and the function of the reduced, orbital, frontal cortex soon becomes more aggressive. The orbital, frontal lobe is known to be related not only to aggression but, also, to the various functions, such as substance abuse, emotional processing, and decision-making. Francel et al. had used a proposer-receiver

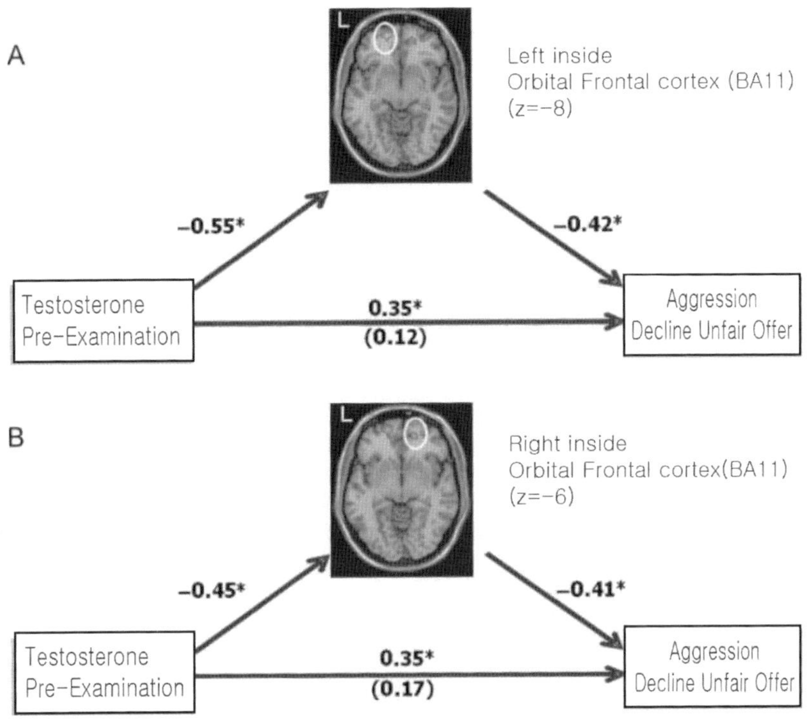

Figure 9-7. Testosterone, orbital frontal lobe, causal relationship model of aggression [17]

The above results are the average of 32 right - handed men and women. The number on the arrow table is the regression coefficient, and the star table on the number indicates statistical significance. The numbers in parentheses below the arrow table indicate the relationship between testosterone and aggressiveness after adjusting for brain activity. In Figure A, the causality of testosterone -〉 aggression was 0.35 in the statistics without the left orbital frontal lobe. This means that aggression increases by 0.35 when the testosterone level is increased by 1. However, if the causal relationship is set to testosterone -〉 left orbital frontal lobe -〉 aggression, the causal effect of testosterone -〉 aggression is reduced to 0.12 and there is no statistical significance. In other words, the effect of aggression on testosterone increases the aggressiveness through the orbital frontal lobe. In Figure A, the testosterone -〉 coefficient of the orbital frontal lobe is -0.55. This means that when testosterone is increased by 1, the activity of the orbital frontal lobe is reduced by 0.55. The value of the orbital frontal lobe -〉 aggressiveness is then -0.42. This means that if the activity of the orbital frontal lobe is increased by 1, the aggressiveness decreases by 0.42. Therefore, an increase in testosterone levels reduces the activity of the orbital frontal lobe, and the less active orbital frontal lobe increases aggressiveness.

model. This means that a certain amount of money is to be decided by the proponent and presented to the audience. If the recipient accepts the proposal even though the amount received is low, both the recipient and the proposer can receive the money, and, if the proposal is rejected, neither person will receive the money.

In most cases, the audience does not accept the proposal whatever the proportion and rejects the proposal, which means that the audience is aggressive to the proposer. During the course of the experiment, the changes in the brain activity were examined in real time on a monitor through an instrument called the 'echo-planar imaging (EPI)', and the testosterone levels were examined by acupuncture. The results were consistent with the hypotheses first established by these researchers. The increased testosterone had inhibited the activity of the medial, orbital, frontal lobe, and the inhibited orbital, frontal lobe had increased the aggressiveness, which is an instinctive characteristic (Fig. 9-6) [17].

9.10. Changes in the levels of the male hormones in the blood of the vegetarians

The most representative method to determine the effects of the dietary cholesterol intake on the steroid hormone level is to compare the vegetarian and non-vegetarian diets. There were several research reports on this.

Peter and Ernist noted the relevance between the high levels of some hormones and the high cancer incidence and had looked at the prevention and therapeutic potentials of the vegetarian diets. When 11 men had been fed a vegetarian diet for 2 weeks and the blood had been collected between 4 pm and 5 pm and the testosterone was measured, the concentration was 373±33 ng/100 ml for the vegetarians compared to 553±57 ng/100 ml for the non-vegetarians. And the difference was statistically significant [18].

The reduction of the testosterone by the vegetarian diet was, also, confirmed by a study by Kaaks et al. on postmenopausal women. They focused on the anticancer, nutritional elements of the vegetarian diet, notably the decrease in the total fat intake, the increased fiber and omega-3, the decreased omega-6 fatty acids, and the increased intake of the vegetable estrogen.

The researchers randomly divided 99 postmenopausal women into two groups, one being served a vegetarian diet and the other being served a diet containing normal meat. The test results showed that testosterone, a male hormone, and estradiol, a female hormone, were lower in the vegetarian group than in the non-vegetarian group, and the difference was statistically significant [9]. In particular, the sex hormone-binding globulin (SHBG) had increased by 25.2% in the vegetarians compared to 3.6% in the non-vegetarian group. The free testosterone and the free estradiol had decreased by 28.6% and 23.4%, respectively, compared to 8.2% and 6.8%, respectively, in the non-vegetarian group.

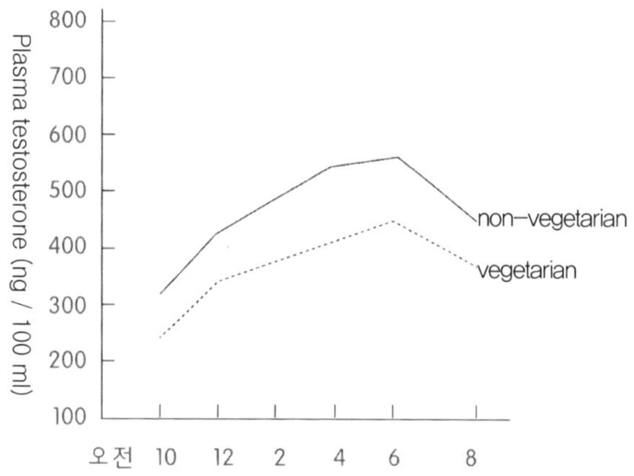

Figure 9-8. Differences in testosterone levels between vegetarian and non-vegetarian [18]

The average non-vegetarian phosphorus is 553 ng / 100 ml, while the vegetarian phosphorus is reduced by about 33% to 373 ng / 100 ml.

Table 9-9. Comparison of testosterone levels between vegetarian and non-vegetarian diets

Inspection items	vegetarian (number)	January	June	Change	p-value
SHBG (nmol/l)	vegetarian (50)	36.03	45.10	25.2% ↑	0.0001
	non-vegetarian (49)	36.32	37.61	3.6% ↑	
Testosterone (ng/ml)	vegetarian (50)	0.41	0.33	18.3% ↓	0.004
	non-vegetarian (49)	0.42	0.39	6.4% ↓	
Free testosterone (pg/ml)	vegetarian (50)	6	5	28.6% ↓	0.0001
	non-vegetarian (49)	10	10	8.2% ↓	
Free estradiol (pg/ml)	vegetarian (50)	0.23	0.17	23.4% ↓	0.05
	non-vegetarian (49)	0.22	0.21	6.8% ↓	

Sex hormone-binding globulin

9.11. The balance between insulin and glucagon

This is a unique organ that has both the endocrine and exocrine glands. The exocrine gland produces the digestive enzymes and releases them into the digestive organs through the ducts to aid the digestion. The endocrine glands of the species are called "the Islets of Langerhans", which are divided into the exocrine cells. There are the three types of the cells: The alpha, beta, and delta. The alpha cells make the glucagon, the beta cells make the insulin, and the delta cells synthesize the somatostatin.

The human cells use the glucose as a fuel source. The glucose concentration in the human body should be between 80 mg/dL and 115 mg/dL, as the body must be fueled steadily to achieve a constant rate. The higher is called the "higher blood sugar", and the lower is called the "lowering blood sugar."

Insulin is released from the pancreas when the postprandial glucose is absorbed into the blood, which binds to the insulin receptors of the cells, allowing the blood glucose to enter the cell. And it converts the glucose into the cell and, again, into an efficient storage form of the glycogen, and then it converts itself into fat.

Glucagon stimulates the hepatocytes when the sugar levels in the blood are lowered, converting the stored glycogen to glucose and releasing it into the blood. Somatostatin inhibits the secretion of insulin and glucagon as a buffer when the glucose and the

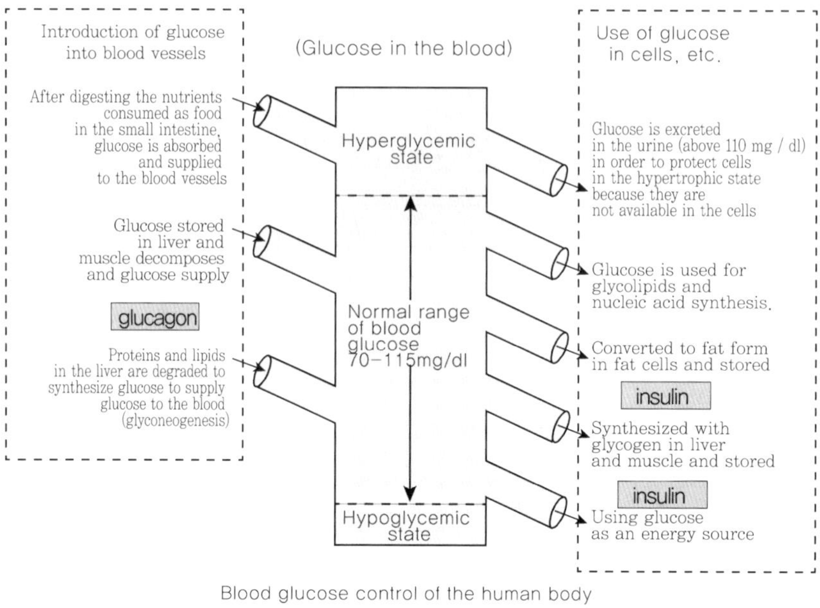

Figure 9-9. Regulation of blood sugar through glucose inflow and outflow

amino acids increase rapidly, while slowing down the rate of the absorption of the nutrients from the digestive tract.

There are two ways in which the body can amplify the actions of the hormones. One is to increase the amount of the released hormone, and the other is to increase the number of the receptors in the target cell. However, when increasing the release of the

Table 9-10. glucose load (glucose index×Amount of carbohydrate per 100g) [19]

food	glycemic Index	glycemic load	food	glycemic Index	glycemic load
glucose	97	96.8	Peeled potato	85	19.5
cornflakes	88	77.3	Boiled 수수	71	16.8
Korean cake	82	66.9	Boiled kidney beans	79	15.5
Sugar	65	64.9	Sweet potato	54	13.1
Corn chips	73	46.3	banana	53	12.1
Bagel bread	72	38.4	grape	43	7.7
donut	76	37.8	carrot	71	7.2
White wheat bread	70	34.7	Apple	39	6.0
All whole grains	42	32.5	watermelon	72	5.2
Whole wheat bread	69	31.8	Orange	43	5.1
fruit sugar	23	22.9	peach	28	3.1

Am J Clin Nutr (1995) 62, 871S-890S

hormones, the effect is temporarily increased, but the target cells reduce the number of the receptors to maintain a homeostasis in the human body. This is called the "downregulation". One example may be a decrease in the insulin sensitivity due to a decrease in the number of the receptors of the cells in chronic hyperinsulinemia

9.12. Diabetes prevention and the diabetes index of the whole grains.

The rate of the blood glucose increase in the body is influenced by the type of the food it ingests and how it is consumed. For example, if you eat brown rice or whole wheat, which is rich in fibrin, the nutrients contained in the fibrin are slowly released and absorbed along the digestive tract by the sponge action of the fibrin, and the blood sugar in the blood slowly rises to the extent that it supplies the energy used by the human body. However, when the simple carbohydrates, such as refined rice and refined wheat, which have been depleted of fibrin, are eaten, they are concentrated at a high concentration, resulting in a rapid increase of the blood sugar. The rapid increases in the hyperglycemia and the hyperinsulinemia are primarily influenced by the glycemic index and the glycemic load (glycemic index × carbohydrates per serving size) [19].

Even if the index is high but the amount of the carbohydrates is low, the risk of the hyperglycemia in the human body is not so great. In analogy, no matter how high the concentration is, if the amount consumed is small, the actual, total amount becomes small. For example, in Table 9–10, the blood glucose level of the peeled potatoes is 85, which is high, but the blood glucose load is only 19.5 days.

Most fruits have the water content of more than 90%, so even though the sugar index is high, the blood glucose load is very low.

Table 9-11. Dietary features of vegetarian and non-vegetarian groups

	vegetarian group		non-vegetarian group	
	At start	12 weeks	At start	12 weeks
Total calorie intake (kcal/day)	1,683	1,409	1,430	1,526
protein (%)	20	14	23	18
carbohydrate (%)	46	75	46	51
Fiber (g)	14	26	12	20
Lipid (%)	34	11	31	31
Saturated fat (%)	10	3	11	8
cholesterol (mg)	289	4.4	310	122

Preventive Medicine (1999) 29, 87-91

Table 9-12. Changes in body after 12 weeks in vegetarian dietary pattern [20]

	vegetarian group		non-vegetarian group	
	At start	12 weeks	At start	12 weeks
weight (kg)	96.7	89.5	97.0	93.2
Fasting blood sugar (mmol/L)	10.74	7.75	9.86	8.64
Glycosylated hemoglobin (HbA1c(%))	8.3	6.9	8.0	7.0
cholesterol (mmol/L)	5.26	4.63	5.56	4.93
HDL (mmol/L)	1.15	0.95	1.12	1.10

Preventive Medicine (1999) 29, 87-91

However, when concentrated like a fruit juice, the blood sugar load is very high, and, thus, the risk of the hyperinsulinemia increases when the amount of the excess is taken into account. When the extracellular fluid is hyperglycemic, the water is released from the cells and is threatened by the normal cell metabolism, so the body rapidly produces and releases the insulin to protect itself. When this condition persists, it is called the "hyperinsulinemia". When the carbohydrates are mixed with the proteins and the lipids, the insulin response to the total sugar is low, but, if you continue to eat the foods with the high glucose levels, your blood glucose and insulin levels will increase.

When the insulin is increased, it is effective at first, but,through the downstream regulation, the target cells reduce the number of the insulin receptors. When the number of the insulin receptors is reduced, the rate at which the blood sugar enters the cell decreases when the food consumed increasesrapidly, and the insulin produces more insulin than before. Eventually, the vicious cycle is repeated, the interest is accelerated, and the function is lost. This process is the general progression of the Type 2 diabetes, which accounts for 90% of the diabetic patients, thereby, differentiating it from the 10% of the genetically-related, type 1 diabetes.

9.13. Vegetarian diet and the prevention of diabetes.

In 1999, Nicholson et al. noted that the epidemiologic studies report that people who eat the low-fat, vegetarian diets are less likely to have the type 2 diabetes and have the fewer complications. In fact, they experimented with the effect of a vegan diet on diabetes. Thirteen subjects with the type 2 diabetes were divided into two groups. One group had been fed a vegan diet, and the other group had been fed a normal, non-vegetarian diet. The veal menu included the lentil soup, the salad, and the rice crackers for lunch, and the chickpea stew, the flour food, and the leaf vegetables for dinner. From 10% to 15% of the calories were from the protein and 10% of them were from the lipids. The carbohydrates ingested the complex carbohydrates (whole grains) without any major nutrients removed. On the other hand, the control group had from 55% to 60% of the carbohydrates and 30% of the fats in the total calories, and the cholesterol had been about 200 mg per day [20].

After 12 weeks of the feeding, the vegan group had decreased by 28% regarding the fasting glucose, while the non-vegetarian group had decreased by 12% regarding the fasting glucose. The blood cholesterol had been lowered from 289 mg to 4.4 mg in the vegetarian group and from 310 mg to 122 mg in the non-vegetarian group. Even though the total calories consumed had not been limited, the weight of the vegetarian group had decreased by an average of 7.2 kg. The average reduction in the non-vegetarian

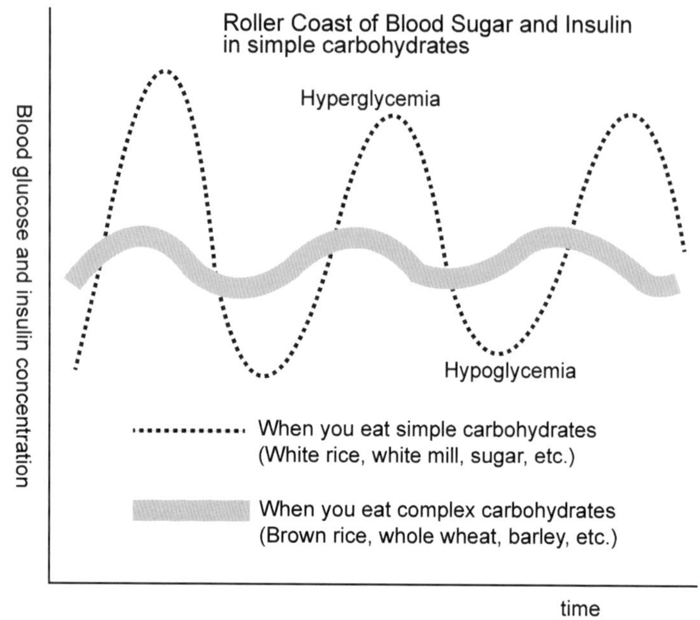

group was 3.8 kg. The mean, fasting blood glucose had decreased from 10.74 to 7.75 in the vegetarian group and from 8.86 to 8.64 in the non-vegetarian group [20].

The authors concluded that the vegetarian diets had been beneficial to diabetes because the fasting blood sugar levels, the weights, and the urinary proteinshad been reduced in the low-fat, all-vegetarians even though the number of the subjects had been small, but the medical treatment had been decreased for 12 weeks.

9.14. Hyperinsulinemia and the metabolic syndrome.

The side effects of the insulin elevation in the blood are the cascades, and they are diverse. As the insulin secretion increases due to the ingestion of the simple carbohydrates and the meat, the insulin receptor is regulated downstream in the peripheral organs, and the insulin production is increased again to compensate. At this time, the synthesis of the insulin–like growth factor–binding protein–1 (IGFBP–1) is decreased in the liver, and, at the same time, the free IGF–1 is increased to promote the cell proliferation and the secretion of the growth hormone .

The decrease in the growth hormone, also, decreases the amount of the IGFBP–3 that is synthesized. The IGFBP–3 inhibits the unwanted cell growths in a variety of the body tissues by allowing the retinoids to bind to the receptors in the nucleus and, thereby, induce an apoptosis.

Thus, when the IGFBP–3 levels are lowered in the plasma by the hyperinsulinemia, the normal growth of the epithelial cells is not restricted in the various tissues (Fig. 9–9). And this is manifested in the various disease patterns [21].

All organs of the human body are composed of the four basic tissues: The epithelial tissue, the connective tissue, the muscle tissue, and the nervous tissue. The epithelial tissue makes up the surface of the internal passage, such as the glands, the bladder, and the digestive tract. The glomeruli of the kidneys, the salivary glands of the mouth, the glands of the pancreas, the airways of the lungs, and the internal surface of the digestive tract are the locations of the epithelial tissues.

Therefore, the IGFBP production is reduced due to the hyperglycemia, and the resulting, apoptotic–function disturbance of the retinoids is likely to be applied to all of these epithelial tissues. The inability of the necessary apoptosis to occur can increase the likelihood that the abnormal cells, such as the cancer cells, are not controlled and may be associated with the cancer cells, such as breast cancer, prostate cancer, ovarian cancer, and colorectal cancer that do not die early and multiply.

On the other hand, hyperinsulinemia increases the production of the sex hormones and decreases the the synthesis of the sex hormone–binding globulins, thereby, increasing the amount of the free hormones circulating in the blood. Excessive sex hormone action causes the ovarian abnormalities,the male hair loss, and the loss of life. The increased sex hormones, the decreased sex hormone–binding globulin, and the uncontrolled cell proliferation increase the likelihood of myopia, ache, acanthosis, the polycystic ovarian syndrome, and skin papilloma.

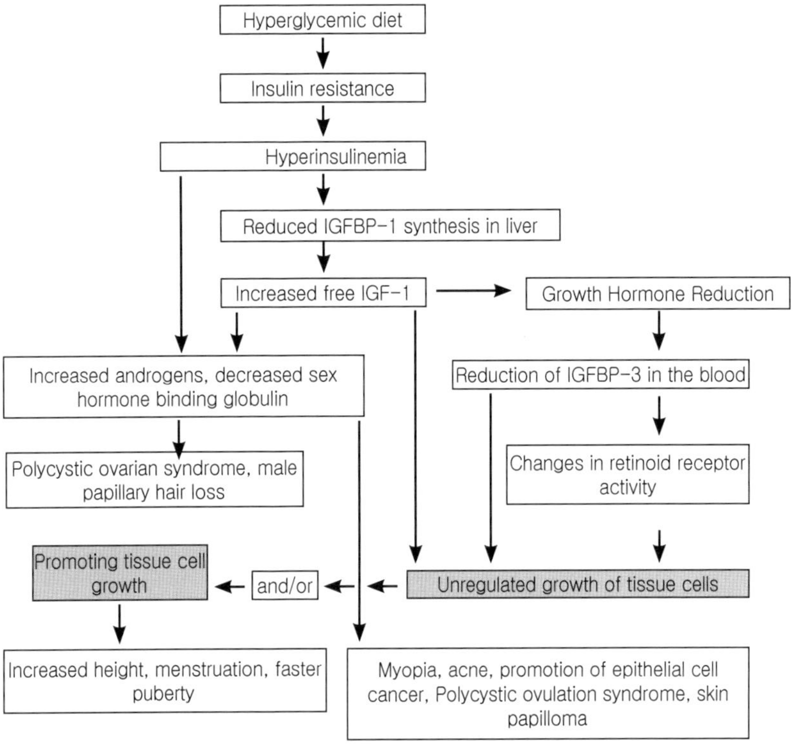

Figure 9-10. The role of hormones and the development of metabolic syndrome

9.15. The adrenocorticotropic,hormone–releasing hormone (CRH) and the drinking behavior.

The adrenocorticotropic, hormone–releasing hormone (CRH) is a hormone secreted from the hypothalamus and has a direct effect on the drinking behavior. For example, the mice treated with the CRH in the cerebral blood vessels of the rats were less likely to drink ethanol, but the ethanol consumption had decreased. The higher the CRH dose, the further the alcohol consumption had been reduced. At this time, the food intake for 24 hours had been, also, slightly decreased, but the weights of the rats had not changed. The influence of the CRH on the drinking is clear, so that the mice whose CRH production had been completely blocked by the removal of the CRH genes are twice as likely to drink alcohol than the normal mice. And the mice that had been crossed for the alcohol pReferences usually have the significantly–reduced CRH levels in the central nervous system, compared to the other mice [22].

The alcohol intake and the HPA axis.

Excessive alcohol consumption changes some hormone levels in the plasma, especially, the hormones in the hypothalamus–pituitary–adrenal (HPA) axis. The major thrust in the HPA axis is the hypothalamic, adrenocorticotropic, hormone–releasing hormone (CRH). Together with the CRH, the vasopressin signals the

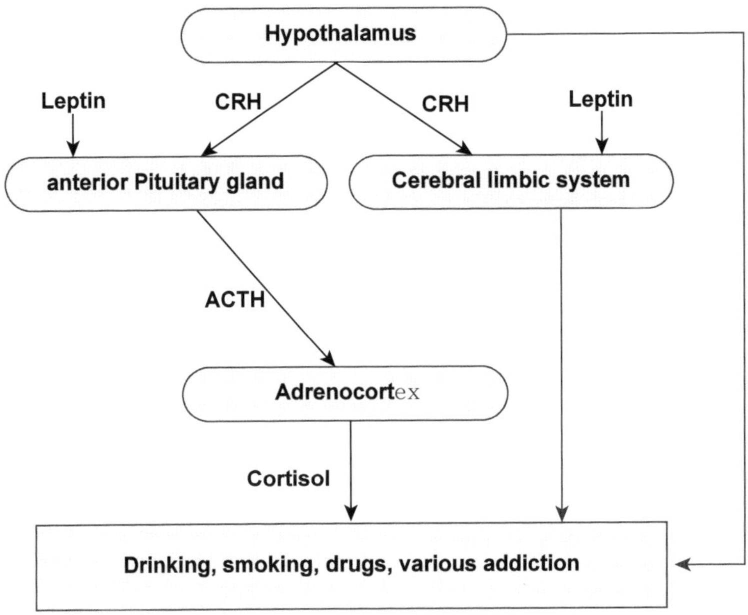

Figure 9-11. Relationship between hypothalamic-pituitary-adrenal cortical hormone axis and drinking

pituitary gland to release the adrenocorticotropic hormone (ACTH) and the endorphin (Fig. 9-10).

ACTH stimulates the cortex to release the cortisol (glucocorticoid). The increased cortisol acts on the negative feedback, weakening the activity of the HPA system, so that the entire HPA is regulated in a constant state. All the hormones released from the HPA system regulate the alcohol–related behavior, which occurs independently of the effects of stress and anxiety [23].

In addition to the CRH, the various hormones are associated with the drinking behavior. For example, when the ACTH or its analog is added to rats, the mice consume less alcohol under the free–choice condition. In addition, the leptin, which is a neuroendocrine hormone that is secreted from the adipocytes, increases the alcohol consumptions when administered to the rats. It seems that the leptin increases the secretion of the alcohol by decreasing the secretion of the CRH in the hypothalamus. The blood of the alcoholics had the high leptin levels. After 14 days of the treatment, their plasma leptin level had decreased significantly and showed no need for alcohol any more.

A study on the relationship between the cortisol and the alcoholics was, also, reported. The average age of the 12 male alcoholics was 42.9 years old. The first addiction was in the year 22.1, the average duration of the addiction was 20.7 years, and, on the average, they had consumed 256g of alcohol a day. The mean age of the normal subjects was 38.5 years old. The beginning of this week had been the last 0.5 day of the alcohol consumption. The concentration of the cortisol in the alcoholics had decreased from 806 nmol/ L(nano(10^{-9}) mol/L), for the first time, to 512 nmol/L for 3 weeks after the alcohol withdrawal. The mean value for the normal people was 453 nmol/L. The prolactin, also,had decreased from 7.4 ng/mL at the beginning of the week to 4.9 ng/mL after 3 weeks of the lactation and the average of the healthy men was 3.9 ng/mL [24].

Alcohol addiction, anxiety, and depression.

The symptoms of anxiety and depression, which often occur among the alcoholics, are said to be related to the control disorders in the HPA axis. Anxiety and depression have the commonality of the CRH elevation, but the pathophysiology is different.

Patients with depression have an increase in the pathological CRH and the subsequent elevation of the plasma ACTH and the cortisol (Fig. 9–11). Pathological anxiety, on the other hand, is caused by the stress–induced desensitization of the active HPA axis, which, in turn, leads to the loss of the ACTH when the CRH is released when the stress is repeated. Therefore, the blood cortisol concentrations in the patients who are pathologically unstable are chronically low. In other words, the HPA control disorder, alcohol addiction, anxiety, and depression can interact with each other and have a causal relationship with each other [25].

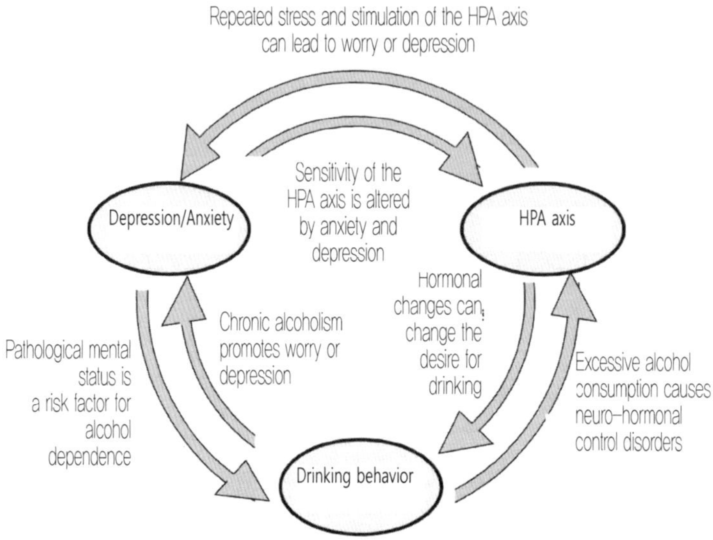

Figure 9-12. Drinking, HPA axis, triangle axis of anxiety depression [13]

Table 9-13. Effects of drugs on hypothalamus – pituitary – adrenal axis [26]

Kinds	term	ACTH · Cortisol
Nerve stimulation	Acute	increase
	Chronic	no tolerance
Alcohol	Acute	increase
	Chronic	tolerance
nicotine	Acute	increase
	Chronic	tolerance

Pharmacol Rev (2001) 53:209-243

9.16. Nicotine, alcohol, drugs, and the HPA axis.

Smoking is one of the major causes of death in the developed and developing countries. The first addictive substance in the cigarettes is the nicotine. In addition, the nicotine has the effect of stimulating the various psychological states, such as anxiety, depression, stress, and emotion, via the dopamine. Some studies have shown that nicotine can reduce anxiety and stress. This phenomenon is related to the nicotine stimulating the hypothalamus–pituitary–

Table 9–14. Psychiatric incidence of addicts and non–addicted readers (%) [27]

	Non–addiction	Nicotine addiction	Alcoholism	Drug addiction
No psychosis	87.8	77.6	70.4	54.8
One mental illness	10.9	18.8	12.5	33.0
More than one mental illness	1.3	3.6	6.2	12.2

British Journal of Psychiatry (2001) 179: 432–437

Table 9–15. Comparison of types of mental illness among addicts and non–addicts (%)

	Non–addiction	Nicotine addiction	Alcoholism	Drug addiction
No psychosis	87.5	77.0	69.4	52.9
Mixed anxiety	6.2	10.2	9.9	16.3
General anxiety	2.4	4.1	5.3	7.3
depression	1.2	3.7	7.3	9.1
phobia	0.8	1.5	1.0	5.4
Panic disorder	0.5	1.5	2.7	2.5

British Journal of Psychiatry (2001) 179: 432–437

adrenal axis to increase the level of the cortisol in the circulatory system. For example, the administration of nicotine increases the cortisol mRNA levels in the donor cells that are important for the emotional formation and increase the CRF and ACTH levels in the plasma.

The hormones in the HPA axis seem to be associated with a variety of the addictions because the cortisol and the ACTH are equally increased when there is the acute administration of the alcohol and the drugs, as well as the nicotine [26]. The acute doses of the alcohol, nicotine, and drugs share the same phenomenon of the elevated ACTH and cortisol, and, if these hormones affect the neurotransmission, there is likely to be a link between these drugs and the mental phenomena (Fig. 9-12).

Addiction and psychosis

In the UK, there had been a nationwide survey of the mental illness rates in 1995. A total of 10,018 adults between the ages of 16 and 64 had responded to the interview. Of the total samples, 67% were non-weighted and 33% were classified as the drugs, the nicotine (tobacco), and the alcohol. The incidence of the psychiatric illnesses among the independent and addicted people was different: 12% of the respondents had the mental illnesses, while 22% of the nicotine addicts, 30% of the alcoholics, and 45% of the drug addicts had the mental illnesses [27].

The psychotic outbreaks of the addicts and the non-addicts

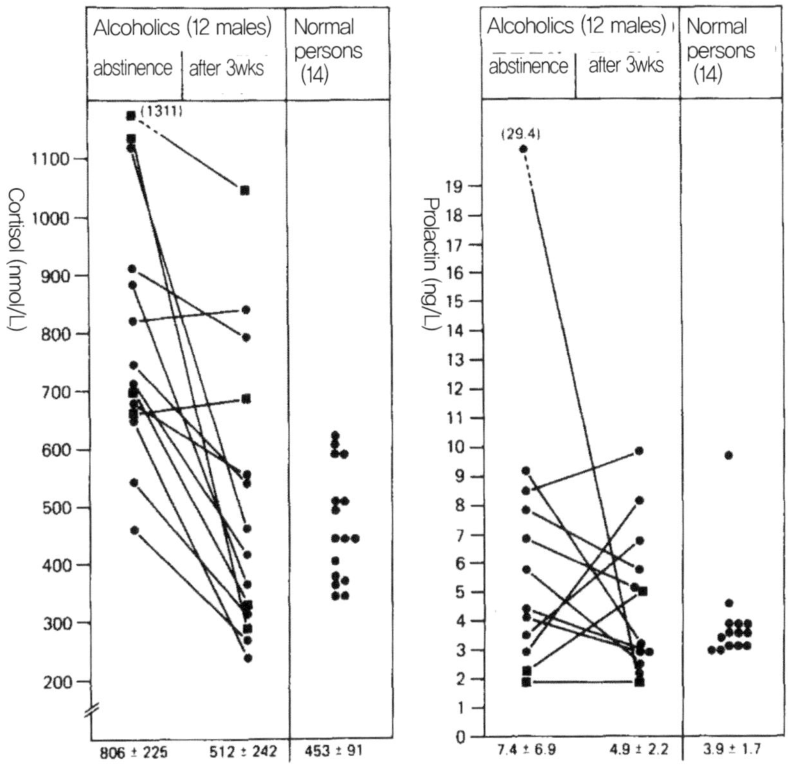

Figure 9–13. Difference of cortisol and prolactin hormone in alcoholics and normal people

had, also, been examined. In all types of the psychiatric disorders, including mixed anxiety, generalized anxiety, depression, phobia, and panic disorder, the addicts were more likely to develop them than the non–addicted, with the highest incidence occurring among the drug addiction group

9.17. Drinking and smoking by the vegetarians.

An Adventist mortality study recruited the participants at 198 meetings in California in 1960.The Healthy Food Buyers Study had been conducted in 1974 through the Healthy Food Store in the UK and through the Vegetarian Diet Adventist Health Study in 1976. AHeidelberg study recruited through a German vegetarian magazine in 1978. The Oxford Vegetarian Study recruited in 1981 through the British Vegetarian Association and the vegetarian magazines.

Table 9-16 shows the smoking and drinking rates of the vegetarians and the non-vegetarians. The Adventist mortality studies have shown that the non-vegetarians smoke at 7.2% less than the half, while the vegetarians smoke at 2.9% less than the half. In terms of drinking alcohol, the non-vegetarians were 2.0% less than the half, while the vegetarians were 0.7% less than the half.

These patterns were similar in other studies, such as the health food purchase research, the Adventist health research, the Heidelberg research, and the Oxford vegetarian studies. That is, in the five independent studies that had been conducted atthe different times and the regions, the smoking and drinking rates of the non-vegetarians were lower than those of the vegetarians. Compared to the other studies, the Adventist Mortality Study and the Adventist Health Study, especially, the low smoking and drinking rates seem

Table 9-16. Smoking and drinking rates of vegetarian and non-vegetarian people

Study name	diet type	participants	mean age	smoking (%)	Drinking (%)
male					
Adventist mortality rate	non-vegetarian	5,023	49	7.2	2.0
	vegetarian	3,971	51	2.9	0.7
Health food buyer	non-vegetarian	2,462	46	30.6	-
	vegetarian	1,519	41	20.1	-
Adventist Health	non-vegetarian	9,045	52	8.5	14.0
	vegetarian	3,169	51	0.2	0.4
Heidelberg	non-vegetarian	304	45	9.9	29.4
	vegetarian	408	43	4.2	14.1
Oxford vegetarian	non-vegetarian	2,572	34	29.1	86.0
	vegetarian	1,603	33	17.5	63.2
female					
Adventist mortality rate	non-vegetarian	9,257	50	1.2	1.6
	vegetarian	6,287	54	0.1	0.7
Health food buyer	non-vegetarian	3,626	45	18.0	-
	vegetarian	2,271	47	12.3	-
Adventist Health	non-vegetarian	11,904	52	2.7	4.8
	vegetarian	4,834	54	0.2	0.2
Heidelberg	non-vegetarian	370	49	3.2	24.9
	vegetarian	603	53	2.2	7.3
Oxford vegetarian	non-vegetarian	3,801	34	18.5	76.3
	vegetarian	3,071	32	13.4	56.5

Am J Clin Nutr (1988) 48:739S-48S, Am J Clin Nutr (1982) 36:873-7
Cancer (1989) 64:570-81, Nutr Cancer (1988) 11:117-26
BMJ (1994) 308:1667-71, by Am J Clin Nutr (1999) 70:516S-24S

to be due to the Adventists, who recommend quitting drinking. However, the commonality of all these studies, whether they are targeted at the Adventists or not, is that the vegetarians have the lower smoking and drinking rates than the non–vegetarians [28–32]. In response to these results, some argue that vegetarian diet is what people originally look for in health. However, the causality is more likely to be the opposite. The difference in the smoking and drinking rates between the vegetarians and the non–vegetarians suggests that the concentration of the hormones in the HPA axis, which affects the smoking and drinking trends, may change because of the dietary patterns.

9.18. The cortisol levels of the vegetarians and the non–vegetarians.

Experiments had been conducted on six healthy adults to determine whether a short–term, whey, vegetarian diet affects the adrenal corticoid activity and the adrenal androgens. The participants had been three women aged from 24 to 25 and three men aged from 31 to 49. They started with a diet that starts with a normal diet (95 g of protein per day, 700 g of the fruits and the vegetables) and went onto a slightly protein–rich diet (protein– 120 g, fruits and vegetables– 230 g). The first regular diet had been repeated for 5 days, but the interval was set at 9 days without any dietary restrictions.

Experimental results showed that the plasma steroids had been almost unchanged, but the amount of the cortisol released into the urine had decreased from 218 nmol/day to 159 nmol/day (Fig. 9–13). The DHEAS had, also, been very low for the vegetarians [33].

9.19. The vegetable,female hormones and the cortisol.

It is, also, reported that certain components of food affect the cortisol secretion. In a study of 18 postmenopausal women with an average age of 56.9 years, the cortisol levels were lower as more isoflavones had been consumed [34] (Table 9–17). The associations

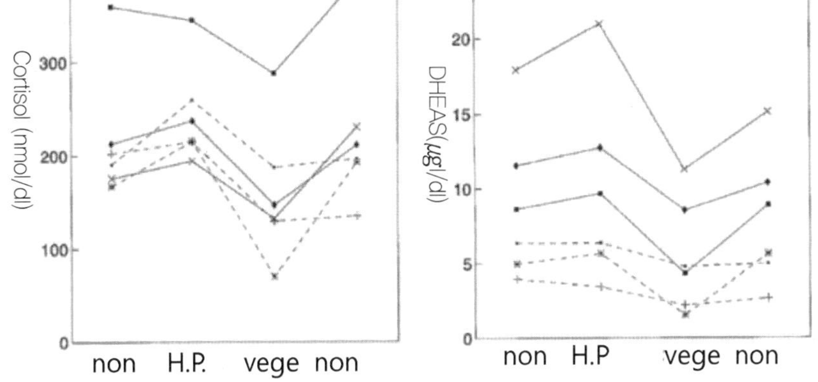

Figure 9–14 Changes in cortisol and DHEAS hormones according to dietary patterns

non:non–vegetarian diet, H.P.:high protein diet, vege:vegetarian diet

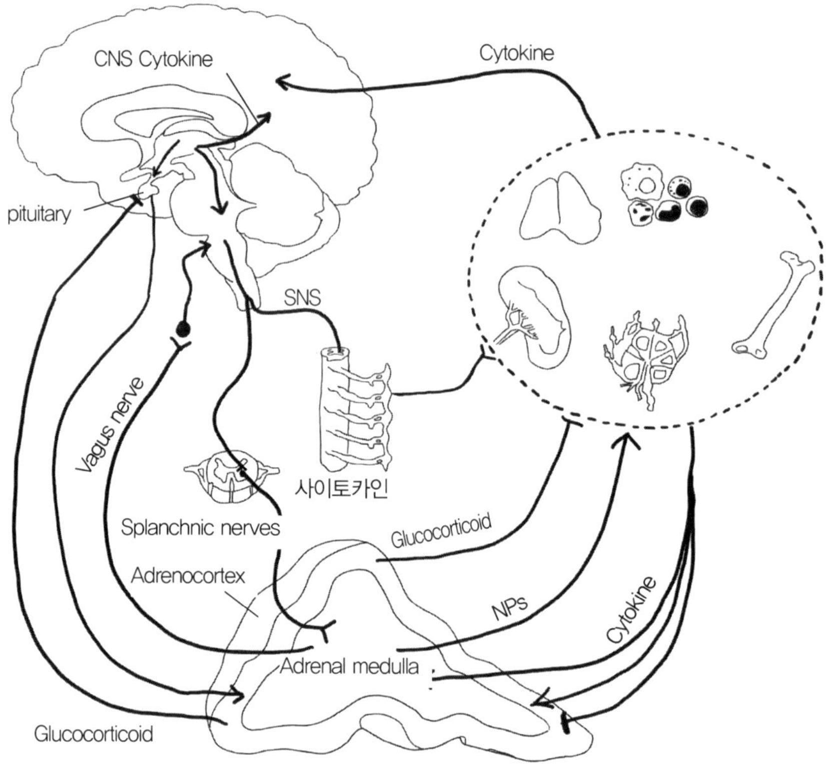

Figure 9–15. Interaction of hypothalamic–pituitary–adrenal hormone axis with autonomic nervous and immune

of the hormones and the alcohols that are associated with the HPA axis,the nicotine,and the drug-related behaviors and mental functions, such as depression and anxiety, are not yet known to be directly causal, but they are known to be correlated.

The neuronal and hormonal actions are wide and complex, so the mechanismsare not clear yet. However, vegetarians have the lower rates of the alcohol consumption and the nicotine addiction than non-vegetarians. And, when you are vegetarian, the changes in the cortisol are clear, and the vegetable ingredients, such as the isoflavones, can lead to the changes in the hormones, such as the cortisol. The vegetarian diet certainly evokes many hormonal changes associated with the HPA axis and produces the healthy lifestyle of quitting and the abstinence. Healthy nutrition, also known as the vegetarian diet, can help turn an adaptive response into a normal physiological state through a variety of pathways.

Table 9-17. Decrease in plasma cortisol levels following consumption of isoflavones in postmenopausal female

	base (0g)	Low isoflavone	High isoflavone
Cortisol (nmol/L)	495.0	446.5	410.4

J Clin Endocrinol Metab (1999) 84:3479-3484

Isoflavones rich in soy and nuts decrease the levels of the human stress hormone Cortisol. High levels of cortisol are associated with depression and anxiety.

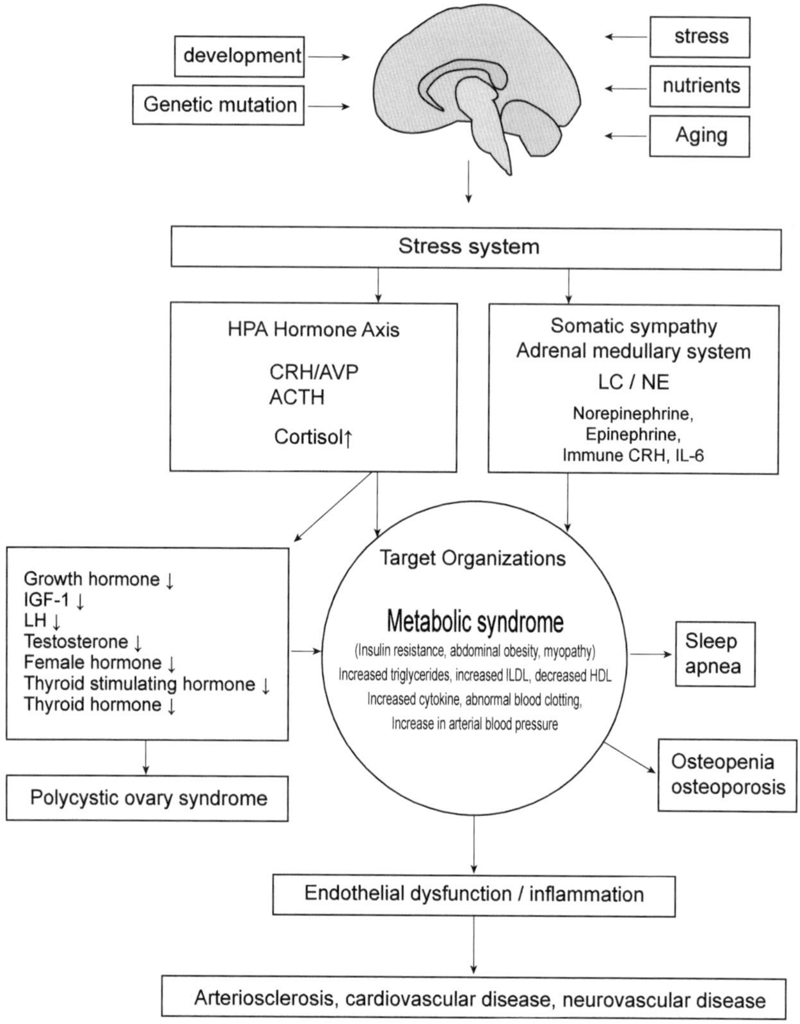
development
Genetic mutation
stress
nutrients
Aging
Stress system
HPA Hormone Axis
CRH/AVP
ACTH
Cortisol↑
Somatic sympathy
Adrenal medullary system
LC / NE
Norepinephrine,
Epinephrine,
Immune CRH, IL-6
Growth hormone ↓
IGF-1 ↓
LH ↓
Testosterone ↓
Female hormone ↓
Thyroid stimulating hormone ↓
Thyroid hormone ↓
Polycystic ovary syndrome
Target Organizations
Metabolic syndrome
(Insulin resistance, abdominal obesity, myopathy)
Increased triglycerides, increased ILDL, decreased HDL
Increased cytokine, abnormal blood clotting,
Increase in arterial blood pressure
Sleep apnea
Osteopenia osteoporosis
Endothelial dysfunction / inflammation
Arteriosclerosis, cardiovascular disease, neurovascular disease

9.20. The vegetarian diet single case study

In 2010, the effects of the vegetarian diets on the female college students in Korea were reported [35]. The participants in this program were close to the boundaries of obesity and were overweight compared to their height. So, I had tried a vegetarian diet for a week because of a recommendation.

The participants had been vegan for a week, before and after the blood was taken, and several biochemical components, including the hormones, were measured. I asked the analyst for the numerical results and the analyst answered as follows:

In Table 9-18, (1) first, the cortisol levels had been decreased

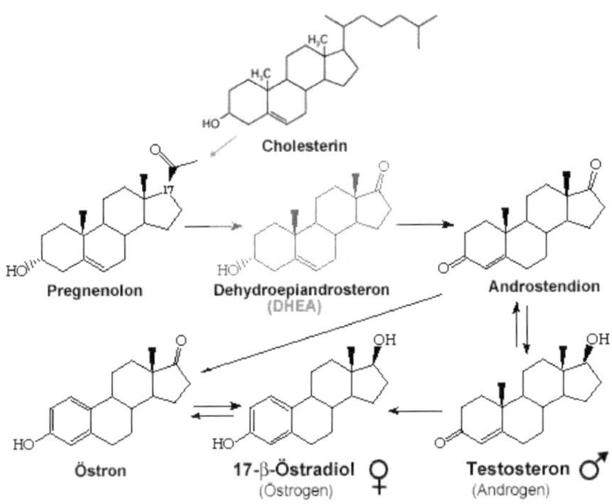

Figure 9-16. Biosynthesis of DHEA and steroid hormones

from 9.3 μg/dL before the vegetarian diet to 8.5 μg/dL after the vegetarian diet. Cortisol is known to be a stress hormone, and, when it is too high, its immune function is inhibited, and its immune system weakens [36]. In addition, since cortisol can inhibit the normal secretion of the other hormones [37], this declining trend seems desirable. The ACTH stimulating the secretion of the cortisol, also, decreases, indicating a tendency to coincide with the decreases in the cortisol levels.

(2) The total cholesterol level had decreased by 26% from 145 mg/dL to 107 mg/dL. The LDL–cholesterol is commonly known to be a bad cholesterol that causes a cardiovascular disease, dementia, diabetes, and gallstones [38], decreasing from 85 mg/dL to 57 mg/dL. On the other hand, the HDL–cholesterol, which is a good cholesterol, had remained almost unchanged. In addition, the triglyceride level had decreased from 98 mg/dL to 44 mg/dL by more than 55%. This indicates that the lipid causing the abdominal obesity had been reduced to the state of good health.

(3) Cholesterol is used as a precursor of the DHEAS, and the DHEAS is used as a sex hormone(female hormone and male hormone) precursor, and it had decreased from 326 μg/dL to 219 μg/dL. This is consistent with the decreases in the total cholesterol and the LDL–cholesterol. Although the DHEAS decreases with age, practically, it is important to reduce the cortisol/DHEAS ratio. In other words, a decrease in this ratio is beneficial in the various areas, such as the increased immune system activity, the prevention

Table 9-18. Changes in blood biochemistry table before and after a week vegetarian (21 year old female student)

Vegetarian Diet	Acidity (pH)	Total protein (g/dL)	Triglyceride (mg/dL)	Blood sugar (mg/dL)	Total cholesterol (mg/dL)
Before	5.0	7.6	98	76	145
After	5.5	7.6	44	78	107
Change	0.5 increase	no change	55%decrease	2%increase	26%decrease
Vegetarian Diet	**HDL-Chol (mg/dL)**	**LDL-Chol (mg/dL)**	**DHEA-S (μg/dL)**	**Testosterone (ng/mL)**	**Cortisol (μg/dL)**
Before	52	85	326	0.58	9.3
After	53	57	219	0.31	8.5
Change	1%increase	32%decrease	33%decrease	47%decrease	9%decrease
Vegetarian Diet	**ACTH (pg/mL)**	**Growth hormone (ng/mL)**	**Estradiol (pg/mL)**		
Before	22.8	0.07	115.7		
After	15.1	3.15	107.2		
Change	34%decrease	44 time increase	7%decrease		

DHEA-S: Dehydroepiandrosterone sulfate, Since it is difficult to measure DHEA directly, it is measured with sulfate (sulfate) attached instead.

of the metabolic syndrome, and the improvement of depression [39].

(4) Estradiol, a female hormone, had decreased from 115.7 pg/mL to 107.2 pg/mL, and estrodiol, on a high, premenopausal level, may promote the various cancers, including breast cancer[40]. The trend seems to be desirable.

(5) It is highly desirable that the growth hormone is increased from 0.07 ng / mL to 3.15 ng / mL. The growth hormone deficiency is very similar to the metabolic syndrome [41]. The growth hormone increases may be considered as a reduction in the likelihood of the metabolic syndrome.

(6) The pH of the blood had increased from 5.0 to 5.5, which meant the alkalization in the body. Although not investigated in this experiment, the calcium content in the body may have increased. That is, in order to prevent osteoporosis, it is preferable to alkalize the blood within this normal range. This is because, the more acidic the blood is, the worse the osteoporosis becomes.

(7) The blood sugar levels had ranged from 76 mg/dL to 78 mg/dL, with little difference between before and after the vegetation and the normal range.

(8) The total protein content was 7.6 g/dL, and there was no change in the body regarding this before and after the vegetarian diet. In other words, the protein deficiency due to vegetarianism was not a problem at all.

(9) The male hormone of testosterone had decreased by 47% from 0.58 ng/mL to 0.31 ng/mL. The decreased testosterone is known

to be responsible for the depression, the excess of the abnormal, sexual desire, the increased aggression, the baldness, and the hirsutism, so a reduction in the normal range appears to be beneficial to the human health.

Participants said that, after a week of vegetarianism, their minds became light and refreshing. And the fear of obesity, which seemed to be impossible because of the decrease in the weight and, especially, because of the decrease in the body fat, had disappeared. It seems that the confidence in life and the love for the family had also increased. These positive psychological changes are common in vegetarians.

9.21. The vegetarian diet patterns affect the psychology

A study on the relationship between the vegetarian diet patterns and the psychology was reported. Beezhold et al. compared the anxiety scores of 60 vegetarians and 78 non-vegetarians. As shown in Table 9-19, the vegetarians had an average of 8.32 versus 17.51 for the Depression Anxiety Stress Scale (DASS), which was less than a half for the non-vegetarians, and the difference was statistically significant [43]. And the POMS index showed that the vegetarian diet was healthy compared to the non-vegetarian diet regarding all the items, such as tension-anxiety, depression, anger-aggression, fatigue, confusion, and vitality. As I have inferred, the decline in

Table 9-19. vegetarian and non-vegetarian anxiety index

	normal value	non-vegetarian	vegetarian	p-value
		Mean (standard error)	Mean (standard error)	
DASS-total	18.38	17.51 (1.88)	8.32 (0.88)	0.000
DASS-D	5.55	4.81 (0.69)	1.67 (0.28)	0.000
DASS-A	3.56	4.31 (0.53)	1.53 (0.24)	0.000
DASS-S	9.27	8.40 (0.92)	5.12 (0.52)	0.024
POMS-total	14.8~20.3	15.33 (3.10)	0.10 (1.99)	0.007
Tension - Anxiety	7.1~8.2	6.04 (3.83)	3.83 (0.40)	0.031
Depression - discouraging	7.5~8.5	8.99 (0.80)	4.36 (4.10)	0.000
Angry - Aggression	7.1~8.0	7.08 (6.72)	4.28 (0.55)	0.010
fatigue	7.3~8.7	7.59 (0.66)	5.03 (0.47)	0.021
confusion	5.6~5.8	4.65 (0.43)	3.24 (0.38)	0.085
vitality	19.8~18.9	19.15 (0.71)	20.61 (0.71)	0.133

* DASS: Depression Anxiety Stress Scale
POMS: Profile of Mood States

* Significance If the p-value is less than 0.05, it is interpreted that there is a statistically significant difference between the two groups. In other words, vegetarian and non-vegetarian people have statistically significant differences in depression, fatigue, aggression and fatigue, and the vegetarian is more beneficial than non-vegetarian.

the cortisol level through the vegetarian diet and the depression, anxiety, loneliness, decreased testosterone level and the decreased aggressiveness may have been related. Of course, it, also, includes the intake of the high-quality, essential, fatty acids. Food and mind seem to have the deep, causal relationship.

9.22. The neuroendocrine nutrition

Epigenetics is associated with the phenotypic changes without altering the gene sequence. In other words, the structure, the function, and the amount of the proteins that are produced depend on how the switch, called "the regulatory gene", determines the expression of a gene into a protein. The range of the posterior sexes includes the DNA methylation, the histone modification, and the microRNA, which are related to the function of the neuroendocrine ganglion that is mediated by the nuclear receptor, a gene regulator, that is regulated by the ligand steroid hormone (Fig. 9–14). There are five steroid hormones in the body: The male hormone, the female hormone, the cortisol, the aldosterone, and the progesterone. Each of these hormones regulates the activity of the nuclear receptors in almost all cells of the body, and the nuclear receptors move into the nucleus to regulate the hundreds of the genes (Fig. 9–15).

The crawling caterpillar crawling on the ground changes into a beautiful butterfly.The tail of the tadpole that swims in the water disappear the legs appear, and the frog changes into a lungy breathing frog. However, the transformation is regulated by the signaling of the nutrients they ingest. That is, the origin of the hormones was the nutrients they ingested from the outside. Still, two of the nutrients that control the body's genes are vitamin A and vitamin D. And I estimate that many nutrients that have not yet

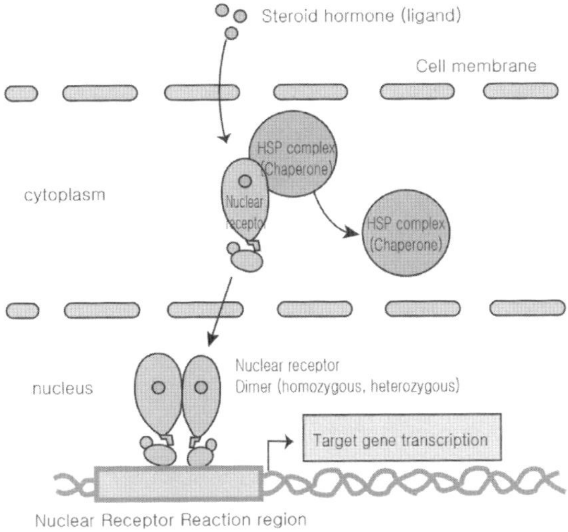

Figure 9–17. Genetic control of nuclear receptors.

When the steroid hormones pass through the cell membrane and bind to the nuclear receptors in the cytoplasm, the nuclear receptors are activated as they separate from the chaperone. The activated nuclear receptors, either alone or after the binding of the two nuclear receptors, pass through the nuclear membrane and bind to the nuclear receptor response site of the gene in the nucleus, thereby regulating the transcription of the target gene. Many metabolites in the body and the nutrients from the food are thought to act as the ligands for the nuclear receptors. One nuclear receptor regulates over 200 genes.

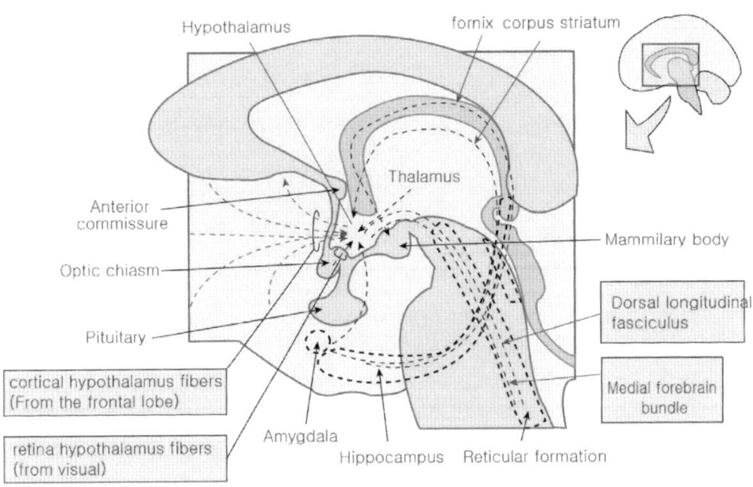

Figure 9–18. The afferent circut of the hypothalamus

been revealed are controlling the genes of the human body. These nutrients can change the form and function of life.

Abzhanov et al. reported the cause of the difference in the phenotype of the beaks of the Galapagos Island finches that had inspired the Darwinian evolution. Due to the isolation of the Galapagos Islands, the beak size and sharpness of the finches were different. This was related to the difference in the BMP4 protein levels through a molecular analysis [44]. The BMP4 is affected by the various hormones,the lipid-soluble vitamins, and the regulation of its expression level. Thus, it is possible to speculate that the Galapagos finches differ with regard to their prey, that the nutrient differences in their diets had altered the endocrine system, and had, subsequently, changed the beak of the finches by affecting the expression of the BMP4.

In the 'Philosophie Zoologique', published in 1809, Lamarck (1744-1829) states that the living organisms are capable of responding to their environment and that the response of an organism adapts the structure and function of the organism in relation to the environment. The genesis of the trait of the Lamarck had been forgotten by Darwin's "The Origin of Species" for 50 years after Lamarck's claim, but, studies on the heritability of the recent trait features are underway. Duncan has two recent discoveries in this regard. The first is that, under certain circumstances, the environmental conditions can influence the epigenetic programming, and the second is that such information is likely to be transmitted

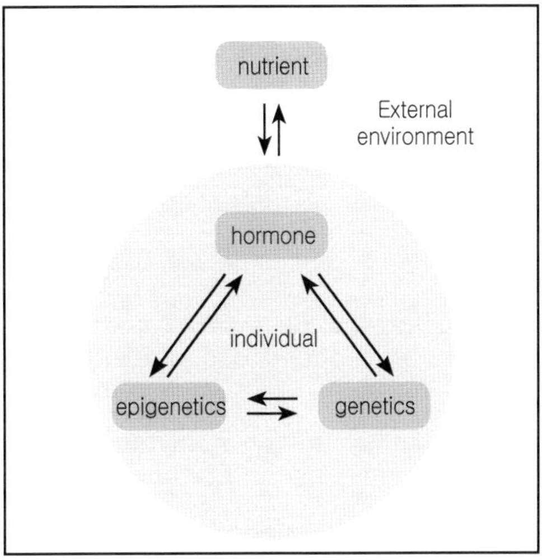

Figure 9–19. Mechanism of epigenetic characteristics of nutrients via endocrine system

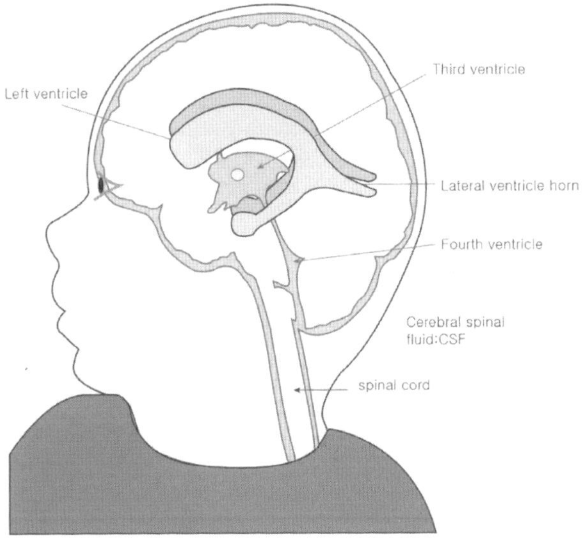

Figure 9–20. Structure of the ventricle

The ventricles are connected to the spinal cord and circulate about twice a day. Nutrients, like hormones, can act as ligands, affecting receptors in brain cells, affecting psychology and gene expression,.

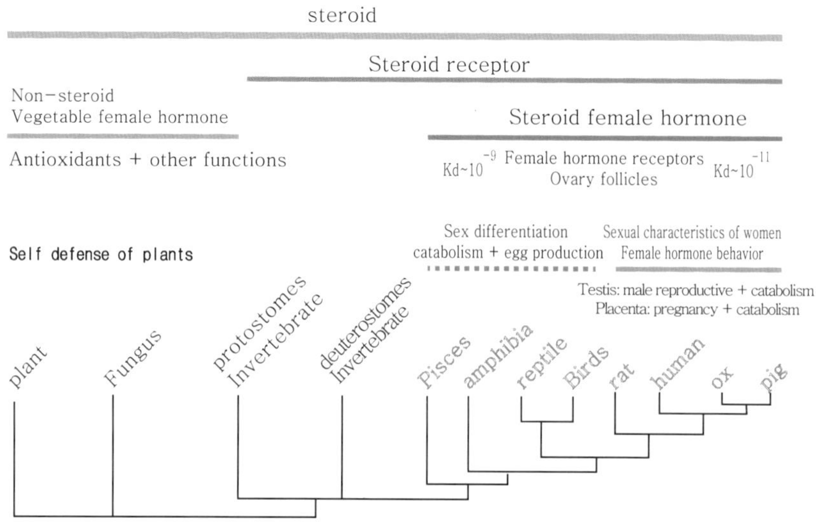

Figure 9-20. The process of evolution of steroid hormones and receptors

to the next generation through the germ cells [45]. It is necessary to further study how the changes in the nutrients according to the dietary patterns, including the vegetarian and the non–vegetarian, may be related to the epigenetic mechanisms through the endocrine systems (Fig. 9–15, Figure 9–16) [46].

References

1. Ben–Shlomo A, S M: Hypothalamic Regulation of Anterior Pituitary Function. In THE PITUITARY. 3th edition. Edited by S M: Elsevier; 2011

2. C K, J W, E A: Neuroscience. Maryland USA: Wolter kluwer. Lippincott Williams & Wilkins; 2012.

3. Chrousos GP: Stress and disorders of the stress system. Nat Rev Endocrinol 2009, 5:374–381.

4. Chrousos GP, Gold PW: The concepts of stress and stress system disorders. Overview of physical and behavioral homeostasis. JAMA 1992, 267:1244–1252.

5. Miller AE, Heyland A: Endocrine interactions between plants and animals: Implications of exogenous hormone sources for the evolution of hormone signaling. Gen Comp Endocrinol 2010, 166:455–461.

6. Miller WL, Bose HS: Early steps in steroidogenesis: intracellular cholesterol trafficking. J Lipid Res 2011, 52:2111–2135.

7. Repa JJ, Mangelsdorf DJ: Nuclear receptor regulation of cholesterol and bile acid metabolism. Curr Opin Biotechnol 1999, 10:557–563.

8. Kliewer SA, Lehmann JM, Milburn MV, Willson TM: The PPARs and PXRs: nuclear xenobiotic receptors that define novel hormone signaling pathways. Recent Prog Horm Res 1999, 54:345–367; discussion 367–348.

9. Kaaks R, Bellati C, Venturelli E, Rinaldi S, Secreto G, Biessy C, Pala V, Sieri S, Berrino F: Effects of dietary intervention on IGF–I and IGF–binding proteins, and related alterations in sex steroid metabolism: the Diet and Androgens (DIANA) Randomised Trial. Eur J Clin Nutr 2003, 57:1079–1088.

10. Nagel SC, vom Saal FS, Welshons WV: The effective free fraction of estradiol and xenoestrogens in human serum measured by whole cell uptake assays: physiology of delivery modifies estrogenic activity. Proc Soc Exp Biol Med 1998, 217:300–309.

11. Keinan–Boker L, Peeters PH, Mulligan AA, Navarro C, Slimani N, Mattisson I, Lundin E, McTaggart A, Allen NE, Overvad K, et al: Soy product consumption in 10 European countries: the European Prospective Investigation into Cancer and Nutrition (EPIC) study. Public Health Nutr 2002, 5:1217–1226.

12. Pino AM, Valladares LE, Palma MA, Mancilla AM, Yanez M, Albala C: Dietary isoflavones affect sex hormone–binding globulin levels in postmenopausal women. J Clin Endocrinol Metab 2000, 85:2797–2800.

13. Allen NE, Appleby PN, Davey GK, Key TJ: Hormones and diet: low insulin-like growth factor-I but normal bioavailable androgens in vegan men. Br J Cancer 2000, 83:95–97.

14. Nelson RJ: An Introduction to Behavioral Endocrinology. 2nd edn; 2000.

15. Zitzmann M, Nieschlag E: Testosterone levels in healthy men and the relation to behavioural and physical characteristics: facts and constructs. Eur J Endocrinol 2001, 144:183–197.

16. Baars BJ, Gage NM: Cognition, Brain, and Consciousness. MA, USA: Elsevier; 2010.

17. Mehta PH, Beer J: Neural Mechanisms of the Testosterone Aggression Relation: The Role of Orbitofrontal Cortex. Journal of Cognitive Neuroscience 2009, 22:2357–2368.

18. Hill PB, Wynder EL: Effect of a vegetarian diet and dexamethasone on plasma prolactin, testosterone and dehydroepiandrosterone in men and women. Cancer Lett 1979, 7:273–282.

19. Foster-Powell K, Miller JB: International tables of glycemic index. Am J Clin Nutr 1995, 62:871S–890S.

20. Nicholson AS, Sklar M, Barnard ND, Gore S, Sullivan R, Browning S: Toward improved management of NIDDM: A randomized, controlled, pilot intervention using a lowfat, vegetarian diet. Prev Med 1999, 29:87–91.

21. Cordain L, Eades MR, Eades MD: Hyperinsulinemic diseases of civilization: more than just Syndrome X. Comp Biochem Physiol A Mol Integr Physiol 2003, 136:95–112.

22. Bell SM, Reynolds JG, Thiele TE, Gan J, Figlewicz DP, Woods SC: Effects of third intracerebroventricular injections of corticotropin-releasing factor (CRF) on ethanol drinking and food intake. Psychopharmacology (Berl) 1998, 139:128–135.

23. Kiefer F, Wiedemann K: Neuroendocrine pathways of addictive behaviour. Addict Biol 2004, 9:205–212.

24. Heinz A, Rommelspacher H, Graf KJ, Kurten I, Otto M, Baumgartner A: Hypothalamic-pituitary-gonadal axis, prolactin, and cortisol in alcoholics during withdrawal and after three weeks of abstinence: comparison with healthy control subjects. Psychiatry Res 1995, 56:81–95.

25. Kiefer F, Wiedemann K: Neuroendocrine pathways of addictive behaviour. Addiction Biology 2004, 9:205–212.

26. Sarnyai Z, Shaham Y, Heinrichs SC: The role of corticotropin-releasing factor in drug addiction. Pharmacol Rev 2001, 53:209–243.

27. Farrell M, Howes S, Bebbington P, Brugha T, Jenkins R, Lewis G, Marsden J, Taylor C, Meltzer H: Nicotine, alcohol and drug dependence and psychiatric comorbidity. Results of a

national household survey. Br J Psychiatry 2001, 179:432–437.

28. Snowdon DA: Animal product consumption and mortality because of all causes combined, coronary heart disease, stroke, diabetes, and cancer in Seventh–day Adventists. Am J Clin Nutr 1988, 48:739–748.

29. Beeson WL, Mills PK, Phillips RL, Andress M, Fraser GE: Chronic disease among Seventh–day Adventists, a low–risk group. Rationale, methodology, and description of the population. Cancer 1989, 64:570–581.

30. Frentzel–Beyme R, Claude J, Eilber U: Mortality among German vegetarians: first results after five years of follow–up. Nutr Cancer 1988, 11:117–126.

31. Thorogood M, Mann J, Appleby P, McPherson K: Risk of death from cancer and ischaemic heart disease in meat and non–meat eaters. BMJ 1994, 308:1667–1670.

32. Key TJ, Fraser GE, Thorogood M, Appleby PN, Beral V, Reeves G, Burr ML, Chang–Claude J, Frentzel–Beyme R, Kuzma JW, et al: Mortality in vegetarians and nonvegetarians: detailed findings from a collaborative analysis of 5 prospective studies. Am J Clin Nutr 1999, 70:516S–524S.

33. Remer T, Pietrzik K, Manz F: Short–term impact of a lactovegetarian diet on adrenocortical activity and adrenal androgens. J Clin Endocrinol Metab 1998, 83:2132–2137.

34. Duncan AM, Underhill KE, Xu X, Lavalleur J, Phipps WR, Kurzer MS: Modest hormonal effects of soy isoflavones in postmenopausal women. J Clin Endocrinol Metab 1999, 84:3479–3484.

35. Seo Ha–Na (Jung–Won): (2011) Seoul National University, Winter Training of Bechelor Degree. Department of Social Wellfare. Korea: Korea Medical Life Corp.

36. Jefferies WM: Cortisol and immunity. Med Hypotheses 1991, 34:198–208.

37. Tsigos C, Chrousos GP: Hypothalamic–pituitary–adrenal axis, neuroendocrine factors and stress. J Psychosom Res 2002, 53:865–871.

38. Patsch W, Gotto AM, Jr.: High–density lipoprotein cholesterol, plasma triglyceride, and coronary heart disease: pathophysiology and management. Adv Pharmacol 1995, 32:375–426.

39. Goldman N, Glei DA: Sex differences in the relationship between DHEAS and health. Exp Gerontol 2007, 42:979–987.

40. Dorgan JF, Stanczyk FZ, Kahle LL, Brinton LA: Prospective case–control study of premenopausal serum estradiol and testosterone levels and breast cancer risk. Breast Cancer Res 2010, 12:R98.

41. Burt MG, Gibney J, Ho KK: Characterization of the metabolic phenotypes of Cushing's syndrome and growth hormone deficiency: a study of body composition and energy metabolism. Clin Endocrinol (Oxf) 2006, 64:436–443.

42. Arnett TR: Extracellular pH regulates bone cell function. J Nutr 2008, 138:415S–418S.

43. Beezhold B, Johnston C, Daigle D: Vegetarian diets are associated with healthy mood states: a cross-sectional study in Seventh Day Adventist adults. Nutrition Journal 2010, 9:26.

44. Abzhanov A, Protas M, Grant BR, Grant PR, Tabin CJ: Bmp4 and morphological variation of beaks in Darwin's finches. Science 2004, 305:1462–1465.

45. Duncan EJ, Gluckman PD, Dearden PK: Epigenetics, plasticity, and evolution: How do we link epigenetic change to phenotype? J Exp Zool B Mol Dev Evol 2014, 322:208–220.

46. Zhang X, Ho SM: Epigenetics meets endocrinology. J Mol Endocrinol 2011, 46:R11–32.

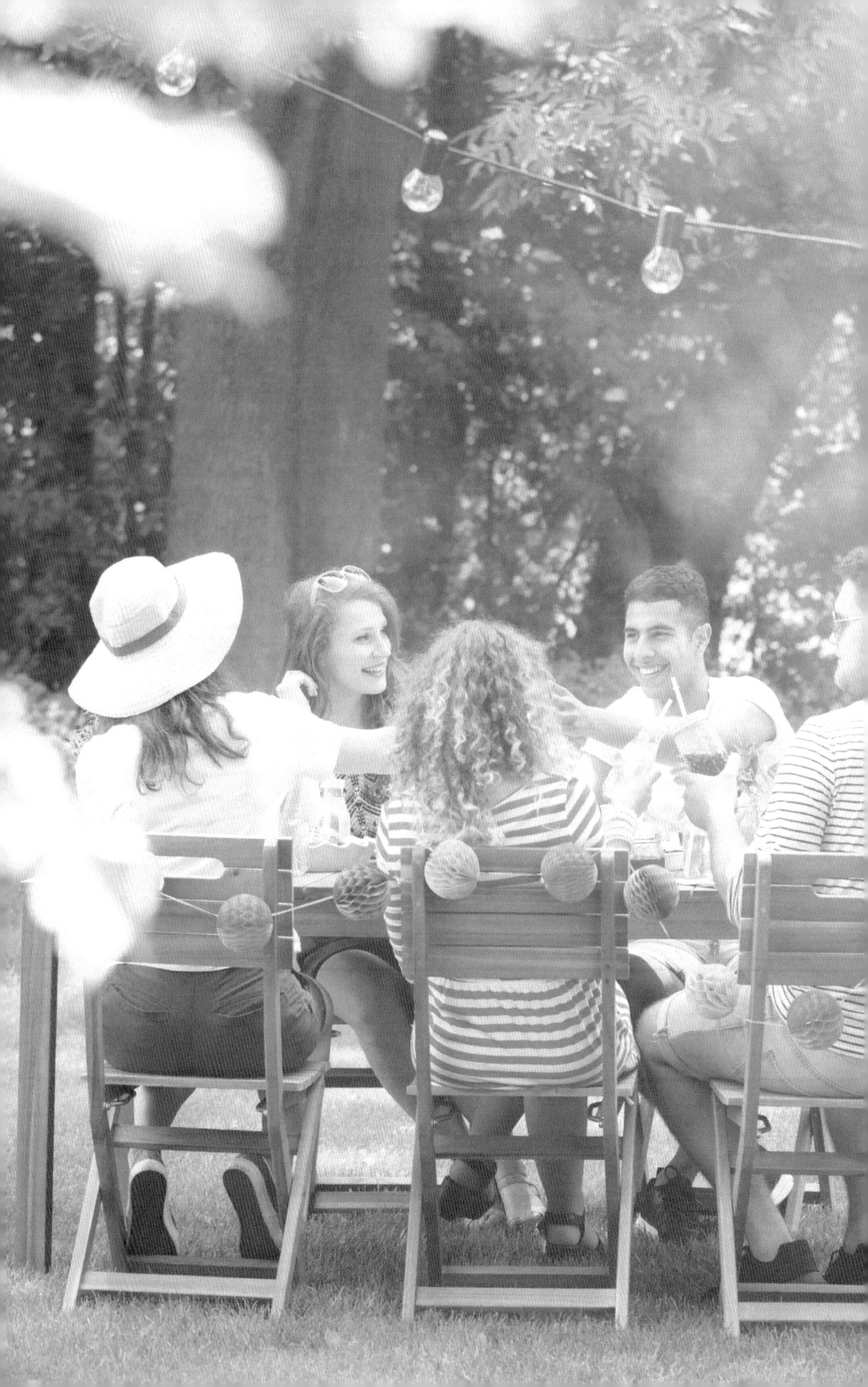

Chapter 10. Integumentary System and Vegetarian Diet

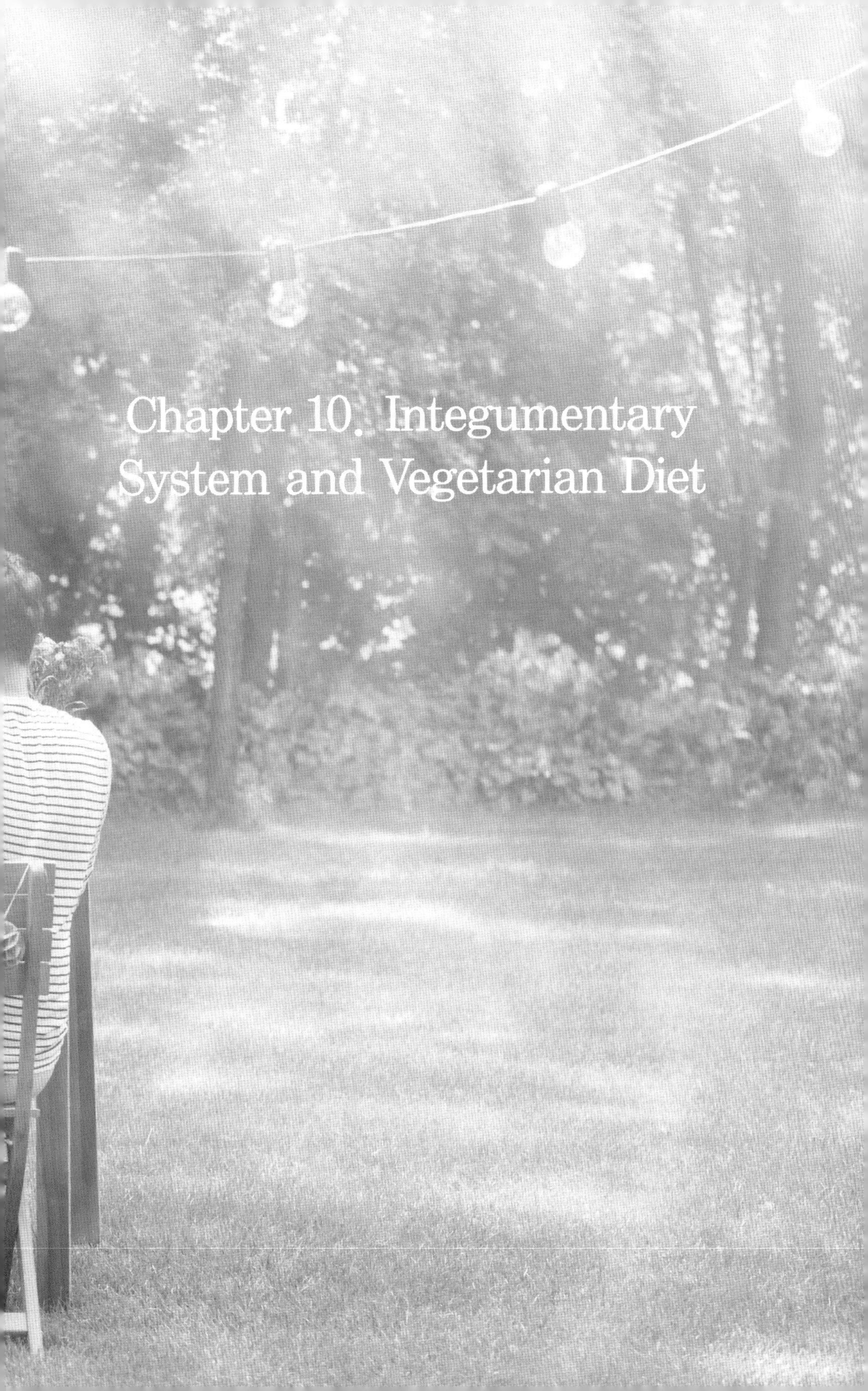

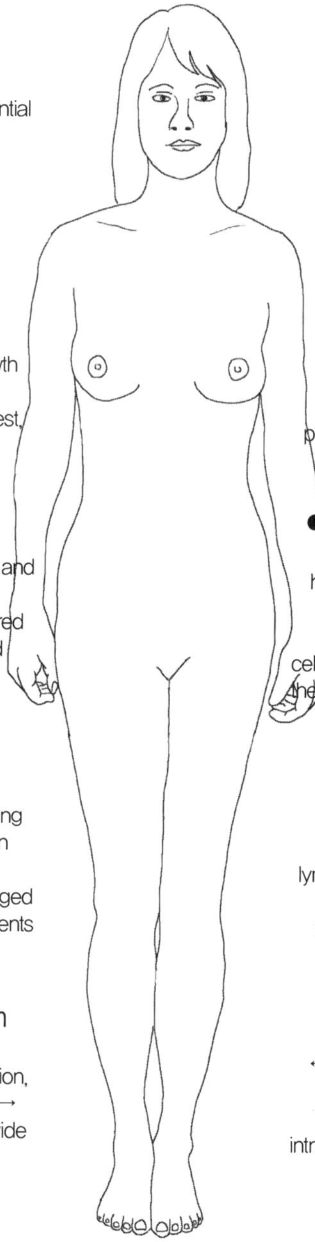

● Skeletal system

Provide structural support →
Synthesizes vitamin D3 essential for calcium and phosphorus absorption ←

● Endocrine system

Growth Hormone, Thyroid Hormone Control Bone Growth →
Endocrine system (brain, chest, pelvis) protection ←

● Digestive system

Provides nutrients to all cells and fat for fat cells →
Synthesis of vitamin D_3 required for absorption of calcium and phosphate ←

● Urinary system

Excretion of waste and keeping the body's normal pH and ion concentration →
Water and solute are discharged by sweat. Horny dermis prevents liquid loss in skin←

● Reproductive system

Sex hormones help hair distribution, fat tissue distribution, and development of hairline →
Cover external genitalia. Provide a sense to stimulate sexual activity ←

● Muscular system

← skeletal muscle contraction is pulled on the face skin to express the doctor's face Make it possible
→ synthesis of vitamin D_3 is essential for normal calcium absorption

● Nervous system

← Control blood flow and sweat gland activity for body temperature control
→ The dermis and Table B receptors provide contact, pressure, vibration, temperature, and pain information.

● Cardiovascular system

← Provide nutrients, oxygen, hormones and immune cells to eliminate CO_2, waste products
→ The stimulation of the mist cells changes the blood flow and the permeability of the capillaries.

● Immune / lymphatic system

← Macrophages and lymphocytes help skin defenses
→ Physical barriers block toxin entry Mast cells stimulate inflammation and immune responses

● respiratory system

← Supply oxygen and remove CO_2
→ The nose hair protects the intrusion of the foreign substance into the nasal cavity.

Chapter 10. The skin system and the vegetarian diet.

10.1. The structure and the function of the skin system.

The skin system is a large, highly complex organ that accounts for 16 percent of the total body weight. Its surface area is from 1.5 square meters to 2 square meters, and the average thickness is from 1 mm to 4 mm. It prevents the attack of the microorganisms that are outside the body, the solar radiation, and the surrounding chemicals. As with many other organs, the skin system has a variety of the other structures (Table 10–1).

Like other body organs, the skin system does not function alone, but the dermis has the extended branches of the blood vessels and the sensing information, such as the contact, the pressure, the temperature, and the pain, which is transmitted to the central nervous system. The skin system consists of two components: The skin membrane and the accessory structure. The skin membrane is composed of the epidermis of the surface and the dermis of the lower surface, and the sub–structure includes the outer glands that are composed of the hair, the nails, and the multicellular cells.

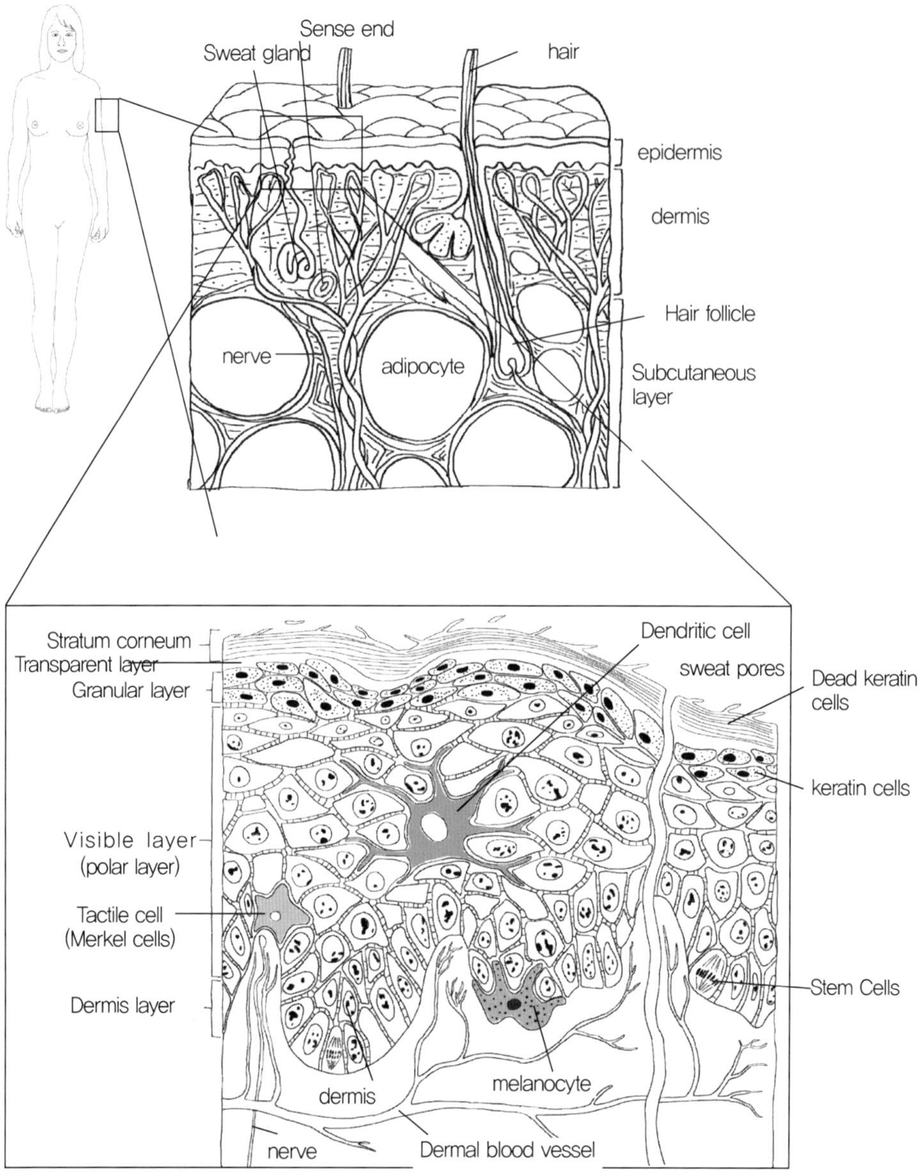

Figure 10-1. Structure of skin system

Table 10-1. Various functions of the skin system

Kinds	function
Protection	Protect the following organizations and organizations against impacts, abrasions, and chemical attacks.
secretion	It secretes salts, water and organic wastes by skin line.
maintain	If necessary, keep the body temperature normal by cooling by evaporation of heat or sweat.
synthesis	A vitamin D3 steroid is converted to calcitriol hormone. This substance is important for normal calcium metabolism.
storage	Lipids are stored in adipose cells in the dermis and subcutaneous layer.
detection	Contact, pressure, pain, temperature stimuli, etc. are detected and transmitted to the nervous system.

These dermis-based structures penetrate the epidermis and come to the surface of the skin

The skin color

The skin color is the result of the interaction between the epidermal pigment and the dermis circulation. The epidermis contains the two pigments, carotene and melanin, the amounts of which vary from time to time. Carotene is an orange-yellow pigment, which usually accumulates in the epidermal cells and appears to be a phenomenon called "the skin stratum corneum of the bright skin". This pigment is also distributed in the adipose tissue of the dermis. Carotene is found in the various orange vegetables, such as the carrots and the amber. The vitamins and the minerals are the most common carotenoids in the world. Carotene can be converted to vitamin A. Vitamin A is required for the synthesis of the photoreceptor pigment in the eye for the normal maintenance of the epithelial cells

The melanocytes.

Melanin is produced by the melanocytes, which is a brown, yellow–brown or black pigment. The melanocytes are located in the stratum germinative under or between the epithelial cells. The melanocytes produce the melanin from the amino acid, tyrosine molecule and store it in the intracellular vesicles called the "melanosomes". When the melanin pigment is transferred from a melanocyte to a keratinocyte, the color of the keratinocyte changes. When the melanosomes are fused with the lysosome and are destroyed, the color change disappears.

For blacks, the melanoma is large, and the pigmentation becomes darker and more persistent. The melanin in the keratinocytes can protect the epidermis and the dermis from the harmful effects of sunlight, which contains a significant amount of the infrared light. As is well known, some of the sun's infrared rays are very beneficial by promoting the synthesis of the dermis, but the excessive, infrared rays damage the DNA and cause the mutations and cancer. The melanocytes are concentrated in the nuclear, surrounding areas of the keratinocytes and prevent the attack of the infrared.

The synthesis of the melanin starts slowly at first and accelerates

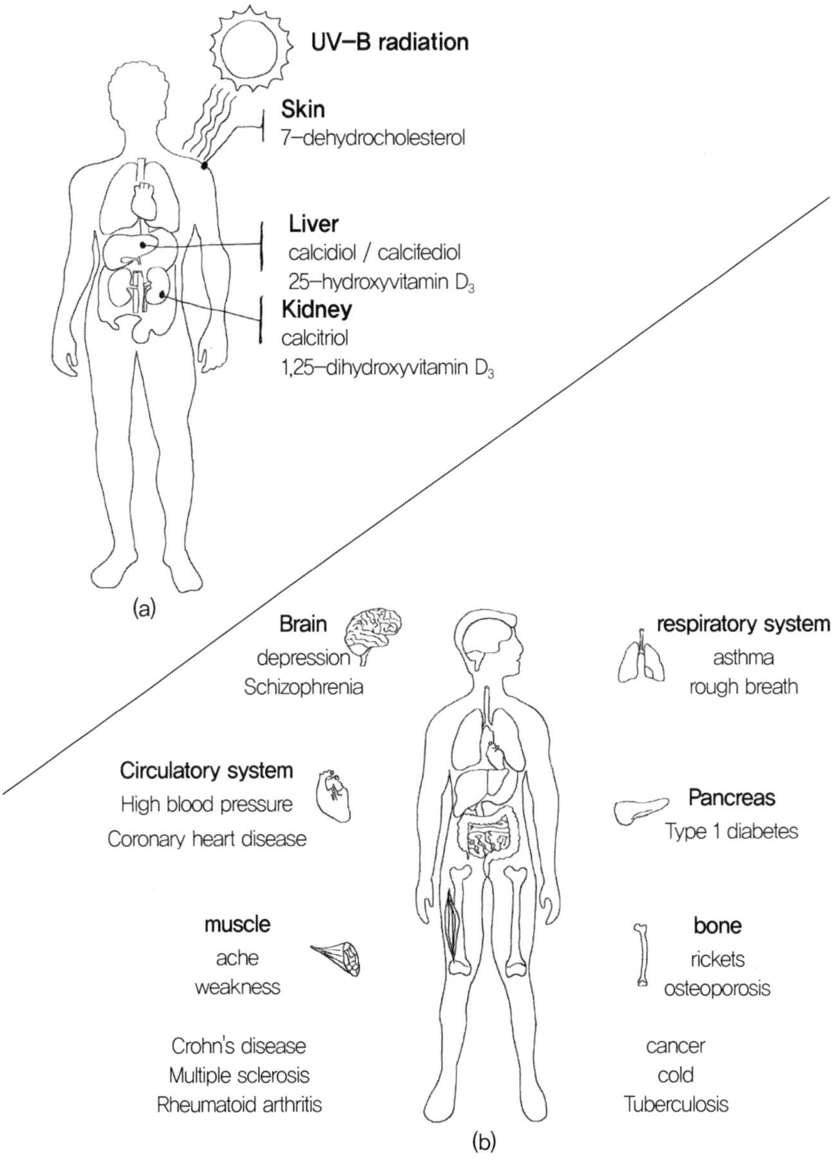

Figure 10–2. Synthesis of vitamin D (a) and deficiency (b)

later. It reaches the maximum peak 10 days after the exposure to the sunlight for the first time. A rich variety of the vitamins in the fresh veggies brightens the skin by removing the melanoma cotton around the keratinocytes when there is no sunlight stimulation.

In some cases, the stratum corneum is weakly acidic (pH 5.45) and inhibits the bacterial growth. The melanocytes suppress the free radicals through the ultraviolet light, while the keratinocyte corneocytes are flattened. It is a double layer in the form of a physical defense against the external attacks. And the intercellular seizure between the stratum cornea is beneficial with the neutral lipids and the ceramides retaining the adequate moisture. All of

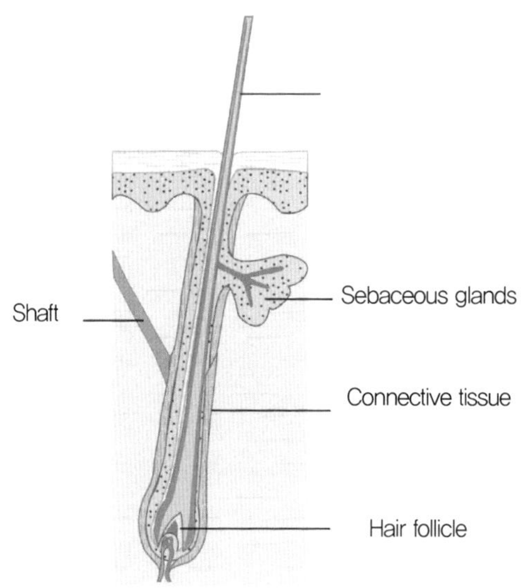

Figure 10-3. Structure of hair

these functions are done normally due to the regular and smooth keratinization and elimination. If the skin is abnormally keratinized, it appears as itching, acne, eczema, and dryness.

Each hair is a long, cylindrical structure that extends outward beyond the surface of the skin. The hair root is the part where the hair is anchored to the skin and becomes the base of the hair. The hair section has a three-layered structure consisting of the cortex and the mosophy, with the water at the center. The part of the hair inside the skin is called the "hair root", and the part coming out of the skin is called the "hair shaft" (Fig. 10-1).

The hair follicle is surrounded by the other hair follicles, which are called the"hair bulbs", like a tray at the bottom, and a concave-shaped, connective tissue at the bottom of the follicle nourishes the hair with a hair papilla. The hair follicles are formed by the intrusions of the skin. The inner layer is connected to the epidermis, and the outer layer is connected to the dermis. On the slope of a hair follicle, there is thesebaceous gland, which secretes fat. Between the follicular part and the dermal papilla layer, it makes the hair stand straight and shrinks the sebaceous glands when shrinking

.

Hair

Each hair is a long, cylindrical structure that extends outward beyond the surface of the skin. The hair root is the part where the hair is anchored to the skin and becomes the base of the hair. The hair section has a three–layered structure consisting of the cortex and the mosophy, with the water at the center. The part of the hair inside the skin is called the "hair root", and the part coming out of the skin is called the "hair shaft" (Fig. 10–1).

The hair follicle is surrounded by the otherhair follicles, which are called the"hair bulbs", like a tray at the bottom, and a concave–shaped, connective tissue at the bottom of the follicle nourishes the hair with a hair papilla. The hair follicles are formed by the intrusions of the skin. The inner layer is connected to the epidermis, and the outer layer is connected to the dermis. On the slope of a hair follicle, there is thesebaceous gland, which secretes fat. Between the follicular part and the dermal papilla layer, it makes the hair stand straight and shrinks the sebaceous glands when shrinking.

10.2. Baldness and androgen.

The growth cycle of hair is divided into three stages: The growth phase, the regenerator phase, and the rest period phase. In the case of baldness, the growth cycle is shortened and the hair follicles become smaller, so the hair loss in baldness progresses rapidly. An important part of the effect of the various hormones on hair growth is related to androgen. The activity of the androgens is mediated by the androgen receptors and plays an important role in the progression of baldness.

Testosterone, a representative of the androgens, is converted to dihydrotestosterone (DHT) by the specific enzymes by the reductase. The DHT binds the androgen receptor from 5 times to 10 times more strongly than testosterone and is, also, associated with the pathogenesis of the several diseases, such as malignant, prostatic hyperplasia, prostate cancer, acne, and alopecia.

Estestosterone, on the other hand, is a naturally–occurring analogue of testosterone that competes with testosterone at the same receptor to inhibit the effects of testosterone and prevent testosterone from converting to the DHT.

In 2004, a journal called 'Skin Science' reported how androgens induce the development of baldness. A team of researchers from the Kyunghee University and the Yonsei University collected the blood from 13 normal male subjects, aged from 26 years old to 43 years old, and had examined the progress of the baldness. According to

Table 10-2. Hormone levels in normal and bald

	upper head boldness		back head boldness	
	bald	Normal	bald	Normal
DHT	2.94	1.25	2.94	1.88
Epi-testosterone(E)	0.71	0.82	0.71	0.73
testosterone(T)	8.59	9.12	8.59	12.23
T/E ratio	18.2	6.70	14.44	14.40
DHT/T ratio	0.26	0.16	0.37	0.16

their survey, the bald patients had the higher DHT levels and more DHT / ep testosterone baldness than the healthy controls.

The testosterone levels in the blood of the bald group ranged from 3.19 ng/ml to 4.36 ng/ml, with an average of 4.36 ng/ml, while those of the normal group ranged from 2.06 ng/ml to 4.36 ng /ml, with an average of 3.05 mg/ml. The DHT concentration was 71.84 ng/ml (20.50 ng/ml ~ 221.08 ng/ml) in the bald group and 1.41 ng/ml (0.45 ng/ml ~ 2.40 ng/ml) in the normal group (Table 10-2).

In the case of baldness, the prostate cancer, also, occurs because, while the free testosterone acts on the hair,it acts on the prostate gland to promote the cancer cell proliferation. Testosterone is synthesized from the cholesterol, and the sex hormone changes depending on the dietary type. As we have seen in the endocrine system in Chapter 9, the vegetarian diet reduces the level of testosterone

10.3. Acne and androgen

About from 23% to 50% of the teens suffer from acne. Men are twice as likely to have acne as women, and 15% of men have acne, which is more than 9% for women. Severe acne can be an emotional and behavioral problem, and women have more serious mental problems than men.

Causes of acne can be divided into four broad categories, including the increased sebum, the blockage of the sebaceous follicle entrance due to the excessive keratinization of the sebaceous glands, the proliferation of the bacteria called the "pyrophosphoric bacteria", and inflammation. The androgens, the male hormone, and the action of the cytokines released by the immune cells are involved.

Acne is caused by the action of the androgens on the adipose and the keratinocytes of the skin. When the androgen acts on the receptor, the adipose cells of the acne patient begin to secrete the excess sebum, which, when deficient in the essential fatty acids, such as the linoleic acid and the linolenic acid, causes the excessive keratinocyte proliferation and the accumulation of the keratinocytes on the skin surface. The sebum outlet is clogged. With the surface of the skin blocked, the sebum continues to form and build up under the skin, eventually causing the hair follicles to expand.

This air-blocked environment is an ideal environment for the propagation of the bacterium called "Propionibacterium". This

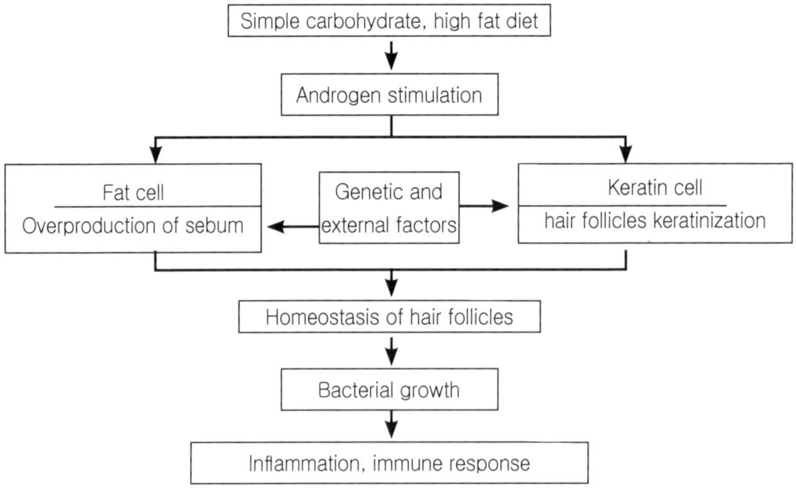

Figure 10–4. Simple carbohydrate and high–fat acne–causing process

bacterium, which grows well in the absence of oxygen, causes the cell wall, itself, to promote the inflammation and lead to the white blood cell migration, destroying the hair follicle. When the hair follicles are destroyed and the contents of the hair follicles are released into the dermis, the inflammation becomes worse, and the scarring acne progresses. This process can be summarized in Figure 10–2 [4].

The release of the androgen hormone is, also, affected by the type of the food it ingests and the way it is eaten, which involves the insulin. Insulin affects the whole of the androgen axis, including the pituitary gland, the ovaries, the production of the SHBG in the

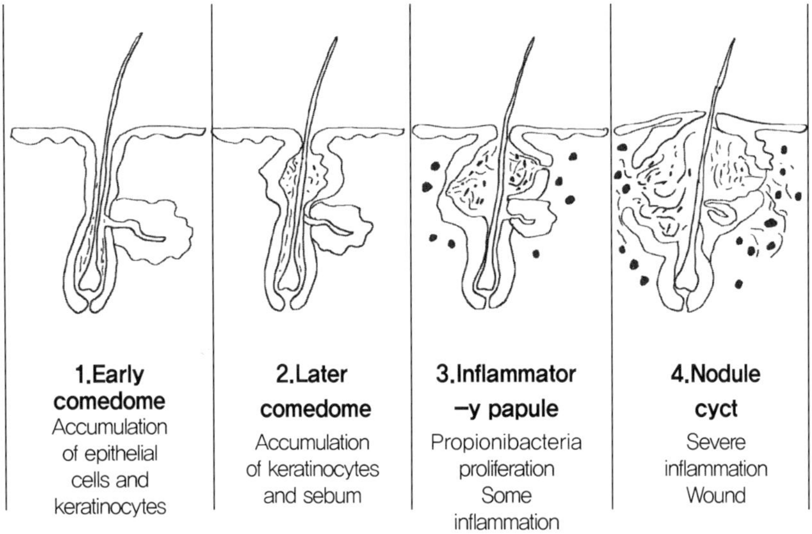

Figure 10–5. Progression of acne

liver, and the hair follicles themselves. In other words, when eating the refined and simplified foods, such as the cereal grains and the sugars, it is easy to develop acne. As a representative example, in Okinawa, before World War II, the traditional diet had been vegetarian, and the acne had been rare. With the introduction of the diet that was the same as the diet of the industrialized society of the West, the number of the acne patients began to increase in Okanagawa. The same was true for Peru's rural villages and the Eskimos.

The secondary sex is affected by the hormones and is, therefore, also, associated with acne. Globally, in the early 1900s, the age of the menarche was 14, but, in 1973, it was 12.76, and, in 1990, it was 12.54, the aging of which has been getting faster and has been getting 3.2 months less every decade. Girls with such a quick start of the menstrual cycle and the early maturing boys have been developing more severe acne later on.

The various types of the hormones are involved in the development of acne, but, especially,the androgens play a central role. The high-fat, high-carbohydrate diets increase the sebum production. On the other hand, the healthy vegetarian diets, such as those including the whole grains, the legumes, the nuts, the vegetables, and the fruits, prevent all of these causes.

The bacterium Pyrophosphonium, which makes the acne inflammation, is killed by sunlight, so sunbathing is recommended for 15 minutes or more every day.

The significant evidences that the androgens stimulate the sebum production.

1. In the early stages of the acne development during puberty, the DHEAS, the precursor of the testosterone in the serum, rises.
2. Without the androgen receptor, the sebum is not produced, and acne is not developed.
3. People with uterine cancer or the adrenal tumors associated with androgen often develop acne.
4. The prescription of testosterone and the DHEAS increases the size and secretion of the sebaceous glands.
5. In severe acne, the sebaceous androgen levels are often elevated

10.4. Hirsutism and the androgen

Hairy hyperhidrosis is divided into two types– focal hyperhidrosis and systemic hyperhidrosis. 'Firs hirsuties' refers to the growth of the hairs on the face and the body of men after puberty. At first, the hair starts to appear on the lips, then,it appears on the chin and the cheeks, and, finally, the hair grows to the shins, the thighs, the arms, the belly, the hips, the chest, the back, the arms, the shoulders, and so on.

Systemic hypertrichosis is a uniform hair growth disorder throughout the body, which manifests as a metabolic disease, such as anorexia nervosa, hypothyroidism, or the side effects of drugs. In general, the subject of interest is focal hirsutism, with a distribution of the morbidity ranging from 6% in Italy to 17% in the United States. However, hirsutism is closely related to the hormone levels.

A team of medical researchers from Turkey studied the blood constituents in 32 hirsutism women and 17 healthy women. The average age of the women with hirsutism was 24.8 years, and the average age of the healthy women was 25.8 years. Estradiol, afemale hormone, was 57.3 pg/ml in the patients with hirsutism, while it was 85.6 pg/ml in the normals, and while the testosterone, a male hormone, was 2.2 pg/ml in the women with hirsutism and 1.6 pg/ml in the normal women (Fig. 10–3).

The higher insulin levels in the blood are known to stimulate the androgen release, and the basic insulin dose is 10.9 mU/L in the patients with hyperhidrosis, which is higher than 5.7 mU/L in the normal women [5]. The free state of the testosterone is less than 1%, and most of it is associated with the transport protein, 70%–80% of which is bound to the sex hormone–binding globulin (SHBG) and 20%–30% of which is bound to the albumin. The SHBG, together with the sex hormone–binding function, finds the receptors on the surface of the specific cells for the SHBG and delivers the sex hormones. All androgen precursors (such as the DHEA) are converted to testosterone and dihydrotestosterone (DHT).

Most androgens interacting with the androgen receptors are the testosterone and the DHT. The DHT is the conversion of the testosterone to the action of the enzymes, which is 5 to 10 times more potent than the androgen receptor and the testosterone.

Acne starts in adolescence and reaches its maximum at about 18 years of age and is relieved by the mid–20s. Hirsuties is hairy on the face and the chest, like men, among women. It appears between 20 years of age and 40 years of age. On the surface, these two things appear to be the quite different phenomena, but we can see that the male hormones are involved in the working principle in common.

Table 10-3. Hormone levels in patients with hirsutism and in the general population [5]

	Hirsutism	Normal
estradiol (pg/ml)	57.3	85.6
Free male hormone (pg/ml)	2.2	1.6
estradiol/Free male hormone	36.3	81.8
Basal insulin (mU/L)	10.9	5.7

* Patients with hirsutism have lower female hormone levels compared to normal, while male hormones and insulin levels are higher

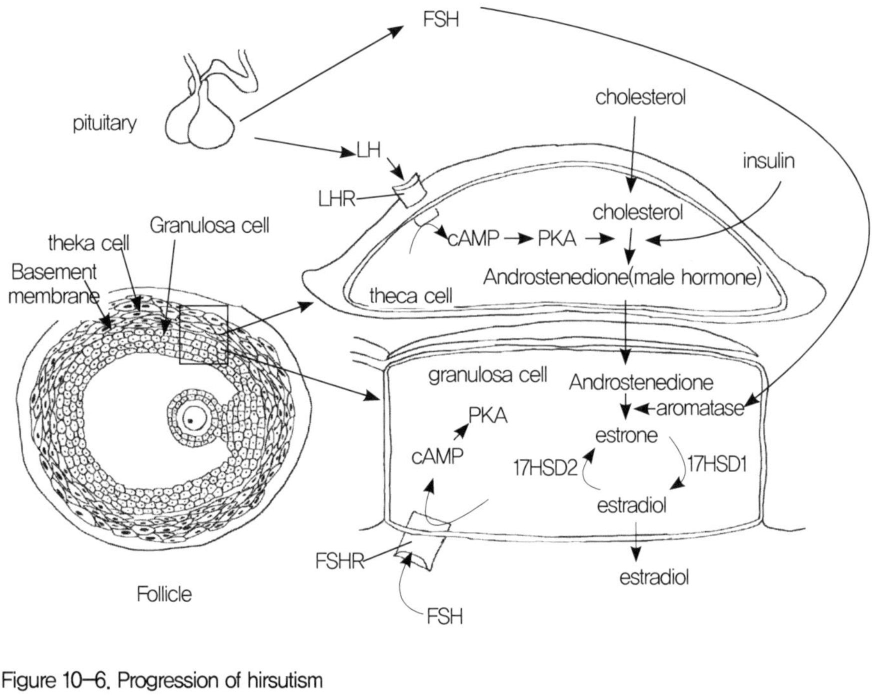

Figure 10-6. Progression of hirsutism

FSH released from the pituitary stimulates granulosa cells to convert male hormones into female hormones. On the other hand, LH stimulates Seka cells and increases the production of male hormone. The intake of refined carbohydrates (white, white rice) increases the level of insulin drastically, and insulin promotes male hormone production. At the same time, the synthesis of sex hormone-binding globulins is inhibited to increase the level of free male hormone, and eventually to promote hyperhidrosis.

10.5. Vitamin C and the aging of the skin.

Collagen is the most abundant and unique synthesis of the animal proteins. The biggest cause of the wrinkling as you age is the increasing thinning of the collagen layer and the decreasing amount of the skin that is produced. Vitamin C is involved in the process of making the collagen. The most widely-known function is to hydrate the collagen materials—the lysine and the proline, which is the process of stabilizing the collagen fibers. Vitamin C also activates the collagen synthesis gene to allow the collagen synthesis.

Vitamin C plays an important role in the skin health as an antioxidant. This is because the active oxygen oxidizes and damages the skin. The UV rays, theozone, and the other environmental factors accumulate the damages and can, eventually, lead to skin cancer, skin inflammation, and skin aging.

Skin inflammation can be induced by the active oxygen. The neutrophils release the peroxidic radicals to kill the microorganisms, which add to the burden of the reactive oxygen, which leads to the skin irritation due to the tissue damage caused by the autoxidation. The skin diseases associated with this process include the skin-vascular inflammation, the vesicular disease, the acne, the redness, the psoriasis, and the like.

Vitamin C removes the active oxygen that is generated by the ultraviolet rays, the ozone, the tobacco smoke, and the dietary quinone. The DNA is attacked by the active oxygen several thousand times a day, and it is repaired by using the enzyme in the cell. However, by attacking beyond its ability to repair, the cells die or mutate. Vitamin C initially reduces the mutations of the cells by removing the active oxygen.

The half-life of vitamin C in the cell ranges from one week to 20 days. 20 mg per kg of the body weight corresponds to the maximum saturation dose of 0.9 mg per 1 dl of the plasma. In the digestive tract, the absorption efficiency decreases as the intake increases, but the maximum absorption is 3 g at a time. After three hours, the plasma level becomes 3.5 mg.

For humans, the vitamin C concentration in the epidermis is 3.8 mol per gram of skin and 0.72 mol per gram of dermis. These differences reflect the difference in the antioxidant activity of the epidermis and the dermis. The US recommended dose is 60mg per day. To increase the serum levels, 50 mg to 100 mg per day is required. Smokers are recommended to eat 140mg per day. It is not recommended to consume it too much regarding the pregnant or lactating women.

Vitamin C promotes the iron absorption in the intestines. It, also, has the effect of treating the wounds, preventing cancer, preventing the cataracts, preventing atherosclerosis, and enhancing the immune system. Especially, it is important for the normal

Table 10-4. The benefits of vitamin C as an antioxidant
1. Can be used in many organizations and can be fully supplied.
2. Can accumulate in specific tissues or cells
3. Reduced in the oxidized state and can be reused
4. Can act on various types of rayleurs
5. Overdose (100 times the recommended amount) is toxic even if ingested.
6. Reduce oxidized tocopherol to regenerate

treatment after the surgery. Vitamin C levels are low in the patients who have the sutures after a surgery.

10.6. Skin cancer, the ultraviolet rays, and the dietary patterns.

Skin cancer development and the progression of the skin-aging process share a similar process. Skin cancer is divided into the melanoma and non-melanoma skin cancers. Melanoma is a melanoma cell that has developed into a malignant cell. In other words, the melanocytes are the cells that produce the pigments, and they are in the epidermis. The UV rays weaken the skin immune system, generate the active oxygen, attack the melanocyte DNA, inhibit the apoptosis, and, eventually,generate the cancer cells.

Apoptosis is a mechanism that acts when a cell is infected with a harmful bacterium or a virus or when the whole health is threatened or when the cells between the fingers of a fetus, such as the webbing, are no longer needed. If apoptosis occurs at the inappropriate times, or, if the necessary apoptosis is suppressed, the likelihood of developing the various diseases, such as cancer, increases.

Far infrared UV-A of 320-400 nm and UV-A of 290-320 nm are particularly important. Melanoma has increased 15 times in the United States over the past 40 years. In Australia, melanoma has increased to 22% of the males and 12% of the females over the past decade. In addition, the incidence of melanoma in the elderly people who are over 65 years old is increasing (Table 10-5) [6].

Table 10-5 Number of Melanoma Deaths and Increase Ratio

		Number of occurrences	Number of deaths	10-year growth rate
Australia (2001)	male	41.4	5.1	22%
	female	31.1	2.6	12%
USA (2001)	male	21.4	3.9	31%
	female	13.8	1.8	25%
Netherlands (1998)	male	11.5	3.1	21%
	female	14.8	2.1	11%
England (2000)	male	9.7	2.7	59%
	female	11.2	1.9	41%

The progression of the melanoma proceeds to the radioactive growth stage and the vertical growth stage. In the radioactive phase, it remains mostly in the epidermis but it spreads more rapidly in the next stage of the vertical growth. In the vertical phase, it penetrates into the dermis, digs into a deeper structure, and there are the transitions to the other parts of the body. Melanoma mainly transforms into the brain, the lungs, and the liver to produce a new cancer. The transition phase is a six-step process.

(1) Release of the cancer papules from the primary carcinoma.

(2) Intrusion into the blood vessels or the lymph vessels.

(3) The adhesion to the epithelial cells of the organ to be attacked

(4) The ejection of the cancer cells outside the blood vessels.

(5) The survival in a new, organizational environment.

(6) Finally, the full-scale proliferation after the incubation period of the cancer cells progresses to the secondary cancer.

The previous four steps are easy, but the latter two steps are not easy [7].

10.7. The three dietary factors to prevent skin cancer.

Non-melanoma skin cancer, like the melanoma, is the main cause of the ultraviolet rays of the sun. The difference is related to the characteristics of the sun irradiation. That is, the risk of the melanoma is associated with the strong solar irradiation, even if intermittent, and the non-melanoma is a major cause of the long-term, accumulated, solar irradiation.

Non-melanoma skin cancer is the most prevalent malignant disease of the White people, and it is said that about one million new cases occur annually in the United States. Due to this seriousness, in 2004, the American Cancer Society had surveyed 200 populations and found the cause. The result was the free radicals mediated by the sunlight.

There are the three dietary factors that reduce the incidence of the cancer caused by the free radicals in relation to the skin cancer: The decreased caloric intake, the decreased polyunsaturated fatty acid intake, and the increased intake of the dietary antioxidants. The first reason is that you need to reduce your calorie intake.

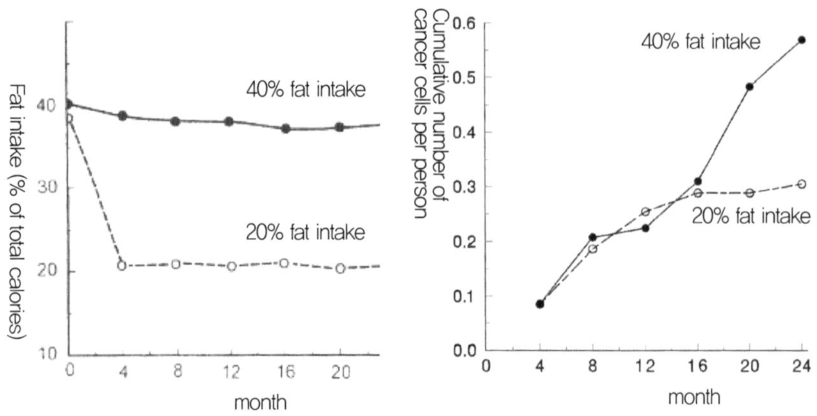

Figure 10–7. Relationship between skin cancer and fat intake

Table 10–6. Fat intake and skin cancer incidence

Group	Person number	Early 8 months	8 months later
40% fat intake	58	0.21	0.26
20% fat intake	57	0.19	0.02

Under the normal conditions, only 1% to 2% of the oxygen consumed changes to the active oxygen species. However, when the body is stressed, it rises to around 10%. Excessive calorie intake is a stress to the human metabolism, which causes a lot of the reactive oxygen species and attacks the human body.

Second, the reason for the reduction of the fat intake has been proven by many experiments. Jaax and colleagues divided 115 groups into two groups and had fed the calories of the fat intake up to 40% in one group and up to 20% in another group for two years. The surveys had been conducted every 8 months, with little difference between the first 16 months, but there was a significant difference in the skin cancer incidence during the last 8 months (Fig. 10–3, Table 10–6) [8]. That is, the skin cancer incidence per patient was not significantly different by being from 0.21 to 0.26 for each 40% fat intake group, but the 20% fat intake group had decreased significantly from 0.19 to 0.02. This is about 9 times the difference of the skin cancer incidence [8].

10.8. The kinds of the fatty acids are also important for the skin cancer prevention.

There are, also, the debates on the types of the fatty acids in relation to the skin cancer prevention and the fat intake. It was presumed that the polyunsaturated fats would be more easily oxidized than the saturated fats in the molecular structure, and, therefore, the excessive intake of the unsaturated fats would be problematic. As expected, the polyunsaturated fats were easily oxidized by the ultraviolet light. However, among the polyunsaturated fatty acids, omega–3 and omega–6 have the different effects on the skin cancer development. The omega–6 fatty acids promote the development of the skin cancer, while the omega–3 fatty acids inhibit the development of cancer, although

Table 10-7. Types of lipids ingested and cancer incidence

Lipid Source (Dietary%)	Cancer latency period (week)	Cancer incidence (number)
Corn oil (Omega-6) (0.75)	21.88	0.47
Corn oil (Omega-6) (4.00)	19.00	1.43
Herring Oil (Omega-3) (4.00)	23.21	0.41
Herring Oil (Omega-3) (12.00)	26.14	0.23

both groups are oxidized by the ultraviolet light.

The reason for this difference is that the oxidation of the omega-6 fatty acids slows down the immune response and slows the response of the immune system, while the omega-3 fatty acids keep the immune response high. Corn oil is the main component of the Omega-6 family. The rats that had been fed with the corn oil with 0.75% of the dietary caloric intake had a latency period of 21.99 weeks and a cancer cell count of 0.47 per mouse. When the intake had been increased to 4.0%, the cancer latency period had been shortened to 19 weeks, and the number of the cancer cells had been increased to 1.43. However, when 4% of the omega - 6 fatty acid-rich, herring oil had been supplied, the duration of the cancer latency was longer than omega - 6 at 23.21, while the number of the cancer cells had decreased to 0.41 or less. Increasing the intake by 12% leads to a longer cancer latency and further decreases the cancer incidence [9].

The third is the intake of the dietary antioxidants. The biologically active antioxidants can be divided into the enzymatic and non-enzymatic systems. First, the enzymatic antioxidants include the vitamin C, the tocopherol, the beta carotene, the reducing coenzyme Q, the bithiquinol, and the reduced glutathione, which actively block the active oxygen in the cell and which stop the chain reaction of the free radicals.

The non-enzymatic antioxidants are the small molecules that act in the intracellular and extracellular spaces, which are important in the intravascular and connective tissue spaces. The non-enzymatic antioxidants are, again, divided into the liposoluble and the water-soluble. The tocopherol (vitamin E) and the beta-carotene (vitamin A precursor) are the important, lipid-free, non-enzymatic antioxidants, and they are mainly located in the cell membrane and the LDL. The alpha tocopherol, the most active form of vitamin E, acts in the early stages of the lipid oxidation, and the beta carotene primarily removes the oxygen.

Beta-carotene had already been shown to have a significant effect in preventing the development of cancer through the ultraviolet light in the 1970s and in the 1980s. Beta-carotene not only acts directly on the reactive oxygen but, also, it acts indirectly to help the action of the vitamin E and the vitamin C. Beta-carotene is especially effective in the development of the lung cancer that is caused by smoking. Ninety percent of the lung cancer patients are due to smoking.

The American Cancer Society's conclusions on the skin cancer development are as follows:

1. The free radicals are produced when the skin is exposed to the ultraviolet light.
2. The oxidation of the sterols in the skin by the ultraviolet rays produces the cholesterol epoxide, which is presumed to be carcinogenic.
3. The dietary antioxidants prevent the oxidation of the cholesterol.
4. The ultraviolet rays produce the lipid peroxides in the skin.
5. The dietary antioxidants prevent the production of the lipid peroxides.
6. The dietary compounds that are susceptible to the attack by the free radicals, such as the polyunsaturated fats, promote the process of the cancer development that is caused by the ultraviolet light.

The problem of the over-consumption of the omega-6 fatty acids is a problem that is caused by consuming a lot of the refined oil on the part of the modern humans. The vegetarians who do not consume the animal foods are more likely to use the vegetable oil. Therefore, the problem of overeating the omega-6 fatty acids is no exception for the vegetarians. The approximate intake ratios of the omega-6 fatty acids to the omega-3 fatty acids are recommended from 1: 1 to 2:1 and to 3: 1, with the modern intake of about from 10: 1 to 15: 1. According to some studies, regarding this, the vegetarians are higher than this, ranging from 15: 1 to 20: 1. The healthy vegetarians use the nuts, seeds and legumes rather than the refined oils. The perilla is rich in the omega-3 fatty acids from the plants, and the flaxseed is used in the Western countries. Next to this, the walnuts and the legumes are the omega-3 sources that can be easily ingested. The natural foods have an outer protective layer and are safe for the human body because they contain the natural antioxidants, such as vitamin C and vitamin E, inside to protect the seeds themselves.

References

1. Bang H-J, Yang YJ, Lho D-S, Lee W-Y, Sim WY, Chung BC: Comparative studies on level of androgens in hair and plasma with premature male-pattern baldness. Journal of dermatological science 2004, 34:11–16.

2. Giltay EJ, Toorians AW, Sarabdjitsingh AR, de Vries NA, Gooren LJ: Established risk factors for coronary heart disease are unrelated to androgen-induced baldness in female-to-male transsexuals. J Endocrinol 2004, 180:107–112.

3. Kaaks R, Bellati C, Venturelli E, Rinaldi S, Secreto G, Biessy C, Pala V, Sieri S, Berrino F: Effects of dietary intervention on IGF-I and IGF-binding proteins, and related alterations in sex steroid metabolism: the Diet and Androgens (DIANA) Randomised Trial. Eur J Clin Nutr 2003, 57:1079–1088.

4. Krautheim A, Gollnick HP: Acne: topical treatment. Clin Dermatol 2004, 22:398–407.

5. Unluhizarci K, Karababa Y, Bayram F, Kelestimur F: The investigation of insulin resistance in patients with idiopathic hirsutism. J Clin Endocrinol Metab 2004, 89:2741–2744.

6. Thompson JF, Scolyer RA, Kefford RF: Cutaneous melanoma. Lancet 2005, 365:687–701.

7. Chambers AF, Groom AC, MacDonald IC: Dissemination and growth of cancer cells in metastatic sites. Nat Rev Cancer 2002, 2:563–572.

8. Jaax S, Scott LW, Wolf JE, Jr., Thornby JI, Black HS: General guidelines for a low-fat diet effective in the management and prevention of nonmelanoma skin cancer. Nutr Cancer 1997, 27:150–156.

9. Orengo IF, Black HS, Kettler AH, Wolf JE, Jr.: Influence of dietary menhaden oil upon carcinogenesis and various cutaneous responses to ultraviolet radiation. Photochem Photobiol 1989, 49:71–77.

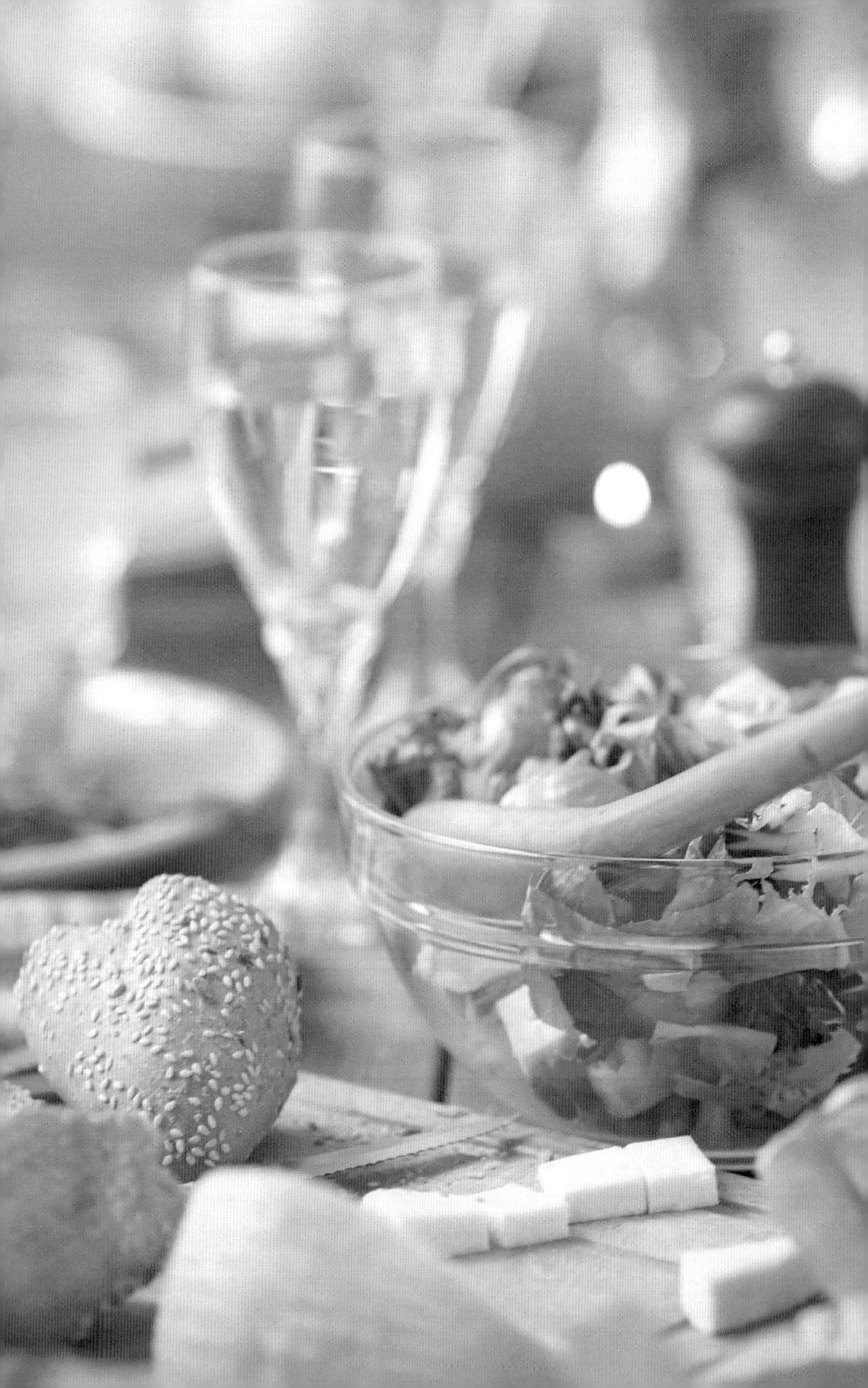

Chapter 11. Recommended Dietary Allowances

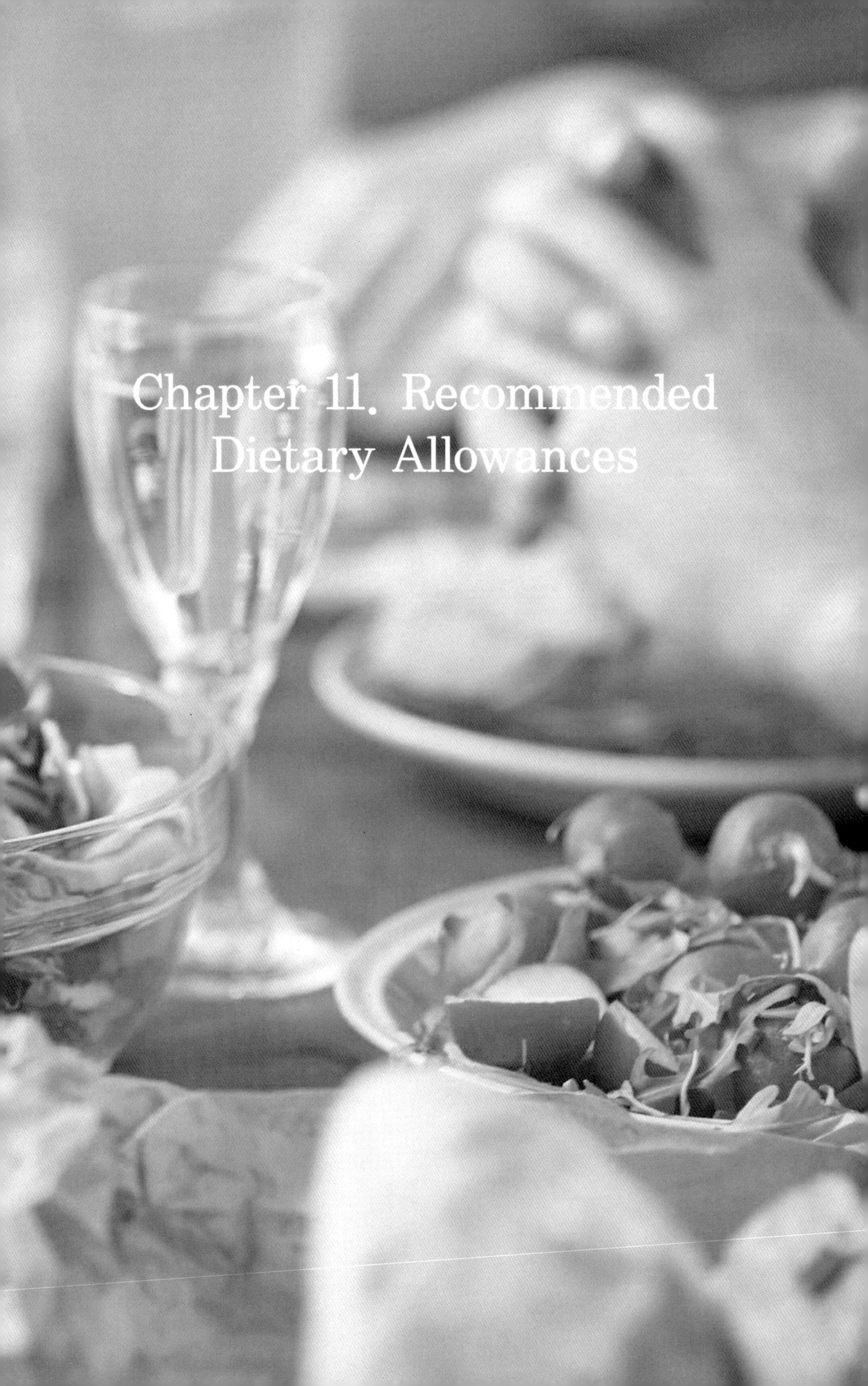

11장. Understanding the nutritional recommendations.

"One day, suddenly on my plate,
I realized that it was a living, breathing life.
I could not pretend to know it anymore. "
– Ellendeznur –

11.1. Introduction.

The amount of the nutrients needed for our daily life is often set based on the nutritional recommendation. However, to avoid the risk of deficiency, the nutritional recommendation is set so that 97% of the population, twice the standard deviation of the mean value, can be met with (see Figure 1–13), rather than the average of the population needs. Therefore, the nutritional recommendation is not a standard for any individual. That is, it does not say that even if an individual has been consuming less than the nutritional recommendation, it is a problem. This is because subtracting approximately from 20% to 30% of the nutritional recommendation means averaging, and the addition and the subtraction of twice the standard deviation of the mean are included in the normal distribution.

Rather than the concern about the deficiency, as in the case of the fat–soluble vitamins or the iron, the nutrients needed for the human body are too toxic to be over–consumed.

A vegetarian perspective was a diet with a high likelihood of a deficiency, which was before the 1970s. However, since 1980, the vegetarian diet has been replaced by a diet that is less likely to be toxic due to the over–consumption of the nutrients, and, in recent years, it has attracted the attention as an ideal, nutritional supplement with the fewer deficiencies and excesses.

This chapter focuses on the diseases caused by the deficiency and examines how the "vegetarian paradigm" has changed in the background of the history of the nutrition that reveals the nutrients one by one and the increase of the chronic diseases caused by the excess of nutrients in the modern times. And what is the message to the modern society where the aging and the chronic diseases increase?

11.2. The discovery of the proteins and the minerals as the essential nutrients.

In 1816, Magendie of France found that the body's protein had decreased significantly when he had fed only a carbohydrate or a lipid to a dog. Then, in 1827, the British Prout said that the nutrition of the higher animals could be the proteins, carbohydrates, and fats.

By 1850, the six trace elements of calcium, phosphorus, sodium, potassium, chlorine, and iron were found to be necessary for the survival of the animals. The German chemist Liebig suggested that the carbohydrates, lipids, proteins, and a few minerals are the essential nutrients that are enough to be ingested and that the nutritional values of the foods are based on their total chemical

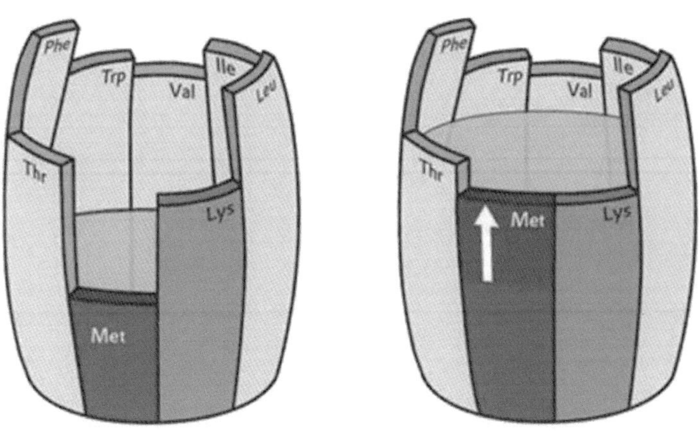

Figure 11-1. Libby's Law

composition. It is widely known as the Libhich barrel. In other words, the nutrients should be balanced as a whole, and, if one of the essential ingredients is not enough, the balance of the body is broken as if a part of a barrel is broken and the water flows out from there

.

11.3. Discovering the vitamins as the essential nutrients.

In 1847, Pereira of the United Kingdom claimed that a wide range of the foods were needed for human health and that a lack of the food intake could be associated with the diseases, such as scurvy. is the vitamins are the nutrients needed by the human body in addition to the previously-known nutrients. Ivanovich Lunin and C.A. Socin then discovered that rats were unable to survive for more than five weeks when they had been fed the previously-known nutrients, including the proteins, fats, carbohydrates, and some minerals.

11.4. The Japanese sailors' disease and brown rice.

In the 1880s, Kanehiro Takaki discovered that the Japanese sailors'disease was widespread. The illness is "beriberi" in English, which means "I cannot". The symptoms are the weight loss, the muscle weakness, and pain, as well as the irregular heartbeats, the poor sensory perception, and the emotional disturbance.

The British Navy did not have these symptoms, so a comparison with the Japanese Army was made about the difference in the food supply between the two groups. Takaji focused on the more protein intake of the British Navy, replaced the barley with milk, meat, and some of the white rice in the Japanese Navy sailors' diet, and the symptoms of the angina in the Japanese Navy had been improved. However, in fact, it was not due to the lack of the protein, but it was because of the lack of vitamin B1 (thiamin), and this was included in the barley, which is an uncleaned, whole grain [1].

11.5. Rice bran.

In the 1880s, the Dutch East Indies (now Indonesia) had been infected by the local settlers and the criminals imprisoned in the prisons in the Java Island (Figure 11–2). Especially, by the European settlers. The East India Company dispatched a medical team to find out the cause. Christiaan Eijkman, a military surgeon who was a member of the dispatched team, had investigated the patients' blood, drinking water, and food through a microscope [2].

He accidentally saw the chickens showing the symptoms that were similar to herpes. He immediately analyzed the blood of the chickens, but could not find any bacteria. After all, he assumed that the diet consisting mainly of the white rice had been chronically deficient in some nutrients and that this was the cause of the angina. He collected the food from the soldiers at the hospital and confirmed that the chickens had the similar neurological symptoms. However, when he fed the remaining shells to the chickens, they did not develop any symptoms, such as the angelic disease, and were healthy. He concluded that the high carbohydrate intake led to the toxic substances in the digestive tract, and that the rice bran detoxified the toxicity

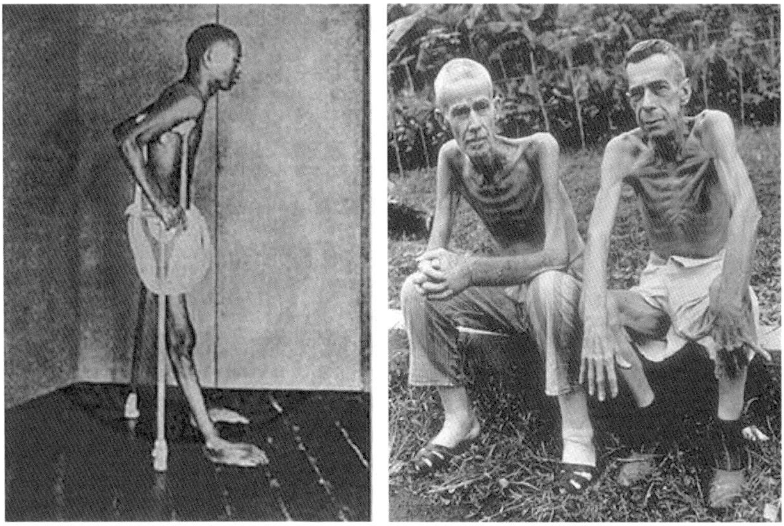

Figure 11–2. Symptoms of beriberi

http://en.wikipedia.org/wiki/Beriberi

11.6. Discovering the fat–soluble vitamins and the water–soluble vitamins.

Between 1909 and 1913, E.V. McCollum and Margaret Davis found that rats that had been fed with the butterfat had grown well but had replaced the growth with the pig oil or the olive oil. They extracted the active substance from the milk fat and then added it to the olive oil. Then, after making the mice ingest it, the mice had grown again. The researchers call this substance the "fat–soluble A".

McArthur and Davis had further advanced the study and found that the growth was still halted when the purified white rice and the fat solubility A that were used in Eckman's angular disease studies were taken together, and this was called the "water–soluble B" [1]. Until 1915, four kinds of amino acids, three vitamins, and six minerals were identified as the essential nutrients. By 1950, almost all of the essential nutrients had been identified, including the nine amino acids, the essential fatty acids, 12 vitamins, and 11 minerals.

Table 11-1. Deficiency and hyperplasia of fat-soluble vitamins

Kinds	Food Sources	Internal function	Deficiency	Hyperplasia
vitamin A (Retinol)	Green-yellow vegetables	Dark red, Epithelial cell protection	Night blindness, blindness, dry eye syndrome	Headache, vomiting, loss of appetite, Pain in muscles and bones
vitamin D	Sunlight, yeast, corn, Oats, plants and plants	Bone growth, Calcium absorption enhancement	Rickets (children) Osteoporosis (adult)	Vomiting, diarrhea, weight loss, Kidney damage
vitamin E (Tocopherol)	Seeds, green and yellow vegetables	antioxidant (Anti-cancer effect)	Red blood cell hemolysis, anemia	Almost non-toxic
vitamin K	Green, yellow, vegetables, grains, Fruits, Nuts	Blood coagulation	Bleeding (internal bleeding)	Almost non-toxic

11.7. The criteria of the essential nutrients.

Alfred E. Harper has set the benchmark for the essential nutrients as follows:

1. The substances required for the diet for the growth, health, and survival.
2. If the diet is missing or deficient, the characteristic deficiency symptoms will appear, and the person will, eventually, die.
3. The characteristic signals of the growth retardation or deficiency can only be prevented by a nutrient or its precursor.
4. The growth response or the severity of a deficiency at any given intake is dependent on the amount ingested.
5. The substance is not synthesized in the body and is necessary for the certain functions throughout life

11.8. Setting the nutrition recommendation criteria.

By 1950, as the presence and the functions of the essential nutrients became known, the diseases caused by a nutrient deficiency had disappeared, at least in the developed countries. In the United States, in 1940, the National Research Council established the Food and Nutrition Commission and set the standards for the allowable levels of the nutrients that should be consumed to prevent the exacerbation of the health of the population.

And, in 1941, the Recommended Dietary Allowance (RDA) for the Americans was first created. However, these recommended doses were based on the short-term animal growth trials and were not intended for the long-term human life. In 1939, Clive McCay at the Cornell University found that the mice had been slower in growth but had survived longer [3], although the mice were nutritionally well-tolerated and were given a limited amount of the free intake

The recognition of the side effects due to the excessive nutrient intake.

The term Recommended Dietary Allowance (RDA), which has been used since 1943, was replaced by the 1997 Dietary References Intakes (DRIs). And before 1997, if the focus had been on preventing the nutrient deficiency, then there had

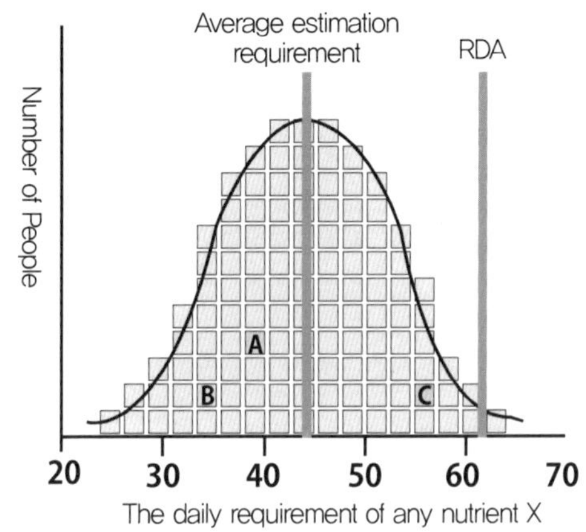

Figure 11–3. Comparison of nutritional recommendation (RDA) and mean estimator

1. One square represents one person. A requires an amount of 40, B requires 35, and C requires an amount of 55 or more. Thus, A, B, and C are less than RDA, but not necessarily deficient. There are the most people around the average and all are within normal range.
2. The recommended amount of nutrients (RDA) is set higher than the average estimated requirement. RDA is standardized so that 95% of people are not shortages. In the case of energy, the average is RDA.

been an added interest in the side–effects from an overdose. It should include the purpose of reducing the chronic diseases that are associated with overeating. For example, in Australia, the recommended nutrient intake (RDI) of vitamin C had been based on the following four criteria [2].

"The amount to prevent scurvy, the amount to prevent the saturation on the skin, the amount to maximize the absorption of the nonhemmetal iron, and the amount to minimize the occurrence of stomach cancer."

The four nutrition standards.

The Dietary References Intakes (DRIs) are planned and measured for the healthy people and are a References to the nutrient intake. There are the following four criteria for the nutritional intake of the modern nutrition: The Recommended Nutrient Intake (RNI), the Adequate Intake (AI), the Tolerable Upper Intake Level (UL), and the Estimated Average Requirement (EAR).

The Recommended Nutrient Intake (RNI) had been previously referred to as the Recommended Dietary Allowance (RDA) and has the same meaning as the RDA. Although these nutrient References values are based on the data obtained through the experiments and the observations, some of these data have not yet been clarified and may be based on a limited range of the results. The nutrition intake standards are constantly being revised and should, therefore, be understood as the References values rather than accepting them in absolute terms.

Understanding the four criteria for the nutritional intake can be helpful for the proper application and References procedures for the healthy nutrient intake. First, let's look at the EAR. The EARs are defined by the life cycle and the gender according to the age, which means that enough of the healthy population consumes. In the References Nutrient Intakes (RNI), the life cycle groups are divided into 16 groups and the average values are determined for each group [3]. For example, the 20-year-old men may vary in height from very short to very tall, and this can be represented by a symmetrical bell. In other words, a person with a very tall or short height has a small number of the people at the extreme left and right, with the largest number of the people gathering near the average. Likewise, even if they are of the same sex or gender, the distribution of the amounts of the nutrients needed for the different people, according to the height, weight, constitution, or genetic factors, is shown on the graph. And the median of the quantity is the EAR. If the shape of the distribution is symmetrical to the left or right, the median is the same as the mean.

The RDA is based on the amount of the daily, average dietary intake that is sufficient for almost all the healthy people based on the age and the gender. The basis for setting the RDA is the EAR. That is, the standard deviation is made based on the EAR, and the value obtained by adding 2 times the standard deviation to the average is the RDA. Therefore, in the case of the nutrients without the EAR, the RDA cannot be determined.

RDA = EAR + 2 × SD (standard deviation)

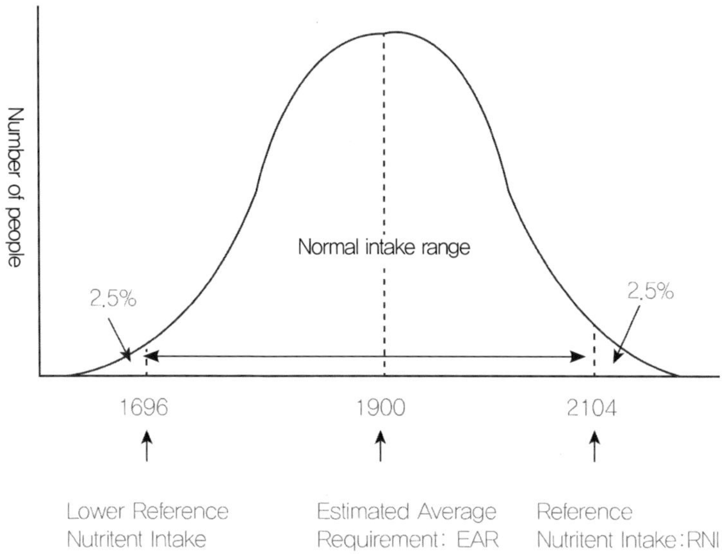

Figure 11–4. Normal distribution of nutrients and recommended intake

Deviation = Variance – Average

Variance = sum of the squares of the deviations / number of variances

Table sub–variance = square root of variance

	A	B	C	D	E
Amount required	1400	1800	1900	2000	2400
Quantity Needed – Average	1900–1400	1900–1800	1900–1900	1900–2000	1900–2400
	500	100	0	–100	–500
(Required amount – average)^2	25000—	10000	0	–10000	–250000
Sum value/5	(500)+(100)+(0)+(–100)+(–500) =520000/5=10400				
(sum/5) root	√(10400) =102				

11.9. How to find the standard deviation of the nutrients.

It is important to understand the standard deviation. Because the average and the standard deviation can be known, it is possible to know the approximate distribution.

(1) Obtaining the average.

Let's say that the nutrients needed by the five people A, B, C, D, and E are 1400, 1800, 1900, 2000, and 2400, respectively. The average of these five is (1400 + 1800 + 1900 + 2000 + 2400) / 5 = 1900.

(2) Find the difference between the mean and the variance.

(1900−1800), 0 (1900−1900), −100 (1900−2000), and −500 (1900−1900), respectively, when the mean value is 1900 and the difference of the five required nutrients is 1900−2400.

(3) Squaring the difference and dividing it by the number of the variances.

If the difference values are all summed, 500 + 100 + 0 + (−100) + (− 500) = 0 is obtained. In order to know the degree of the distribution of these values, the difference value is squared. In other words, each difference is squared, then all the differences are added, and then they are divided by the number of the variances, 5, to be distributed. That is, (500) + (100) + (0) + (−100) + (− 500) =

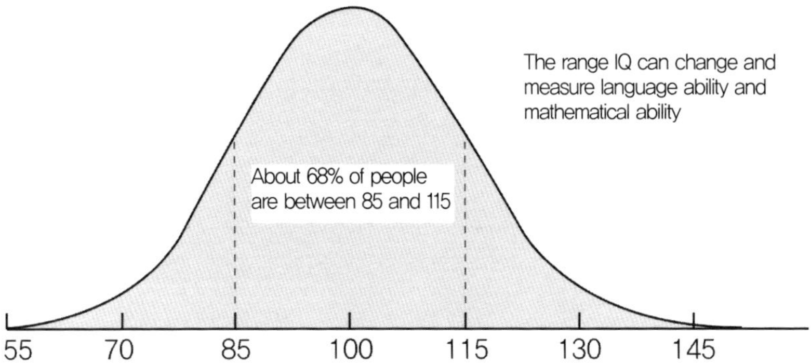

Very low intelligence 2.3%	Low intelligence 13.6%	Average 34.1%	Above average 34.1%	High intelligence 13.6%	Very high intelligence 2.1%	Genius 0.13%

Figure 11–5. Included ranges of samples according to standard deviation (IQ example)

The range obtained by adding and subtracting 1Table quasi-deviation (1σ) around the average includes approximately 68.2% of the samples. 95.4% of the samples are included in the range obtained by adding and subtracting the 2Table sub-deviation from the average. In nature, this range is generally regarded as the normal range. The average vegetarian child's average IQ is 119, which is within the top 10% on average.

520000/5 = 10400.

(4) Find the standard deviation with the square root of the variance.

If you multiply the variance by the square root, it is 10400 = 102, which is called the "standard deviation".

(5) Creating a distribution chart.

When the average value of 1900 is added to twice the standard deviation, it is 1900 + 2 × 102 = 2102. That is, the value of 2102 is

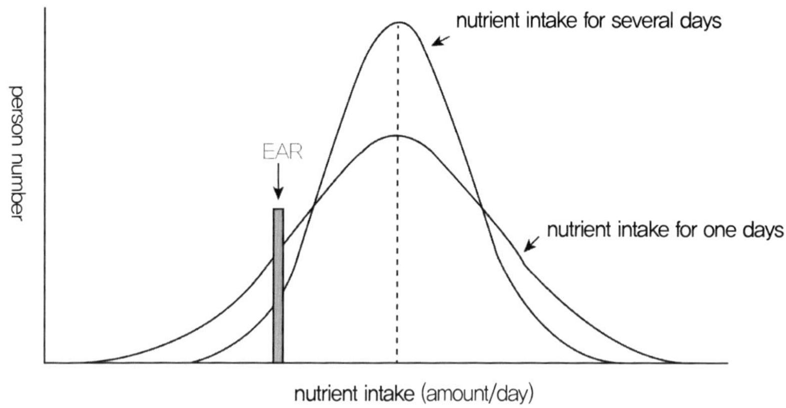

Figure 11-6. Distribution of nutrient intake for one day and several days

Appropriate translation of Dietary References Intakes (DRIs)

§ Recommended Dietary Allowance (RDA)

-) recommended nutrition tolerance

§ Estimated Average Requirement (EAR)

-) Estimated average requirement

§ Tolerable Upper Intake Level (UL)

-) Upper limit intake that can be tolerated

sufficient to be insignificant to 97.5% of the people in any group. If the data is insufficient to obtain the standard deviation, the RDA is determined by multiplying the EAR by a certain number according to the estimated variance. For example, if the estimated variance is 10% of the EAR, then RDA = 1.2 × EAR. Assuming that the estimated variance is 15% of the EAR, then RDA = 1.3 × EAR. .

If there is not enough scientific evidence to obtain the EAR and, therefore, the RDA cannot be calculated, it is sufficient to use it instead of the intake AI. The sufficient intake AI is obtained by observing, or experimenting with, the amount of the nutrients ingested by a healthy group of people. A typical example is the nutrition standard for the infants based on the nutrients contained in the breast milk that is drunk by the healthy babies who only consume the breast milk and do not eat other foods or drink other milk. In the nutritional intake standard for Koreans, the AI has been set to include vitamin E and vitamin K at 10 places (Table 11-2).

The 'upper limit of intake' (UL) means the maximum daily intake without any side-effects for almost all of the members of a population. If the intake of the AI is exceeded, the risk of a side-effect increases. The reason that the term 'tolerable' is used is to emphasize that the AI criterion is the most biologically tolerable rather than the beneficial effect [3]. In other words, if the nutrients that most healthy people consume are above the RDA or the full-dose AI, there is no health benefit. The upper limit of intake (UL) value can be usefully used as a References value when the foods that were fortified with the certain nutrients or the food additives are frequently eaten. For the foods that are particularly chronically used, the Referencess to the upper limit of intake (UL) are needed for the nutrients that accumulate. The estimated average intake (EAR) may differ between the amount observed during the day and the observed amount over several days. In other words, some people eat less nutrients on some days, but, the next day, they can eat a lot. Thus, as shown in Figure 11–6, the intake of the nutrients observed over the course of one day has a wider distribution, but averaging over several days will narrow the range of the distribution and reduce the number of the people with an excess or a deficiency.

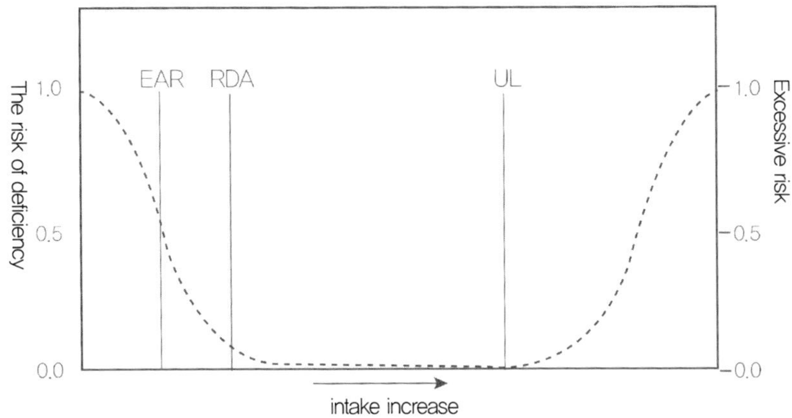

Figure 11–7. Assumptions of nutritional intake criteria and the risk of deficiency and overdose

Estimated average demand (EAR) is an intake with a 50% risk of deficiency. RDA is an amount that 97.5% of people consume enough, and the risk of deficiency is only 2.5%. The intake between RDA and UL is in the range of absence of deficiency and excess. Increased intake beyond UL is associated with increased risk of overdose.

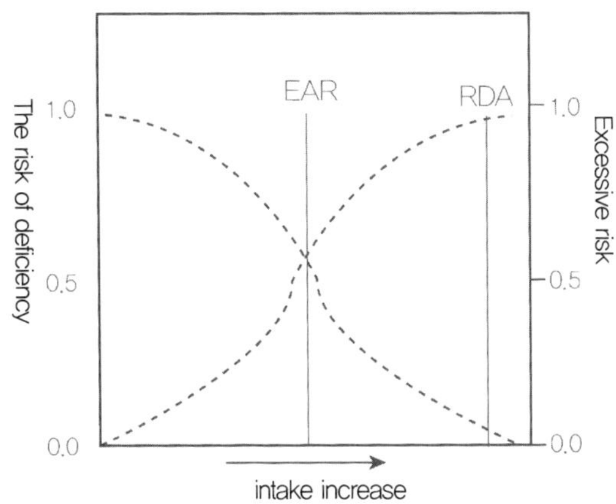

Figure 11–8. Deficiency and overage risk of accumulated nutrients

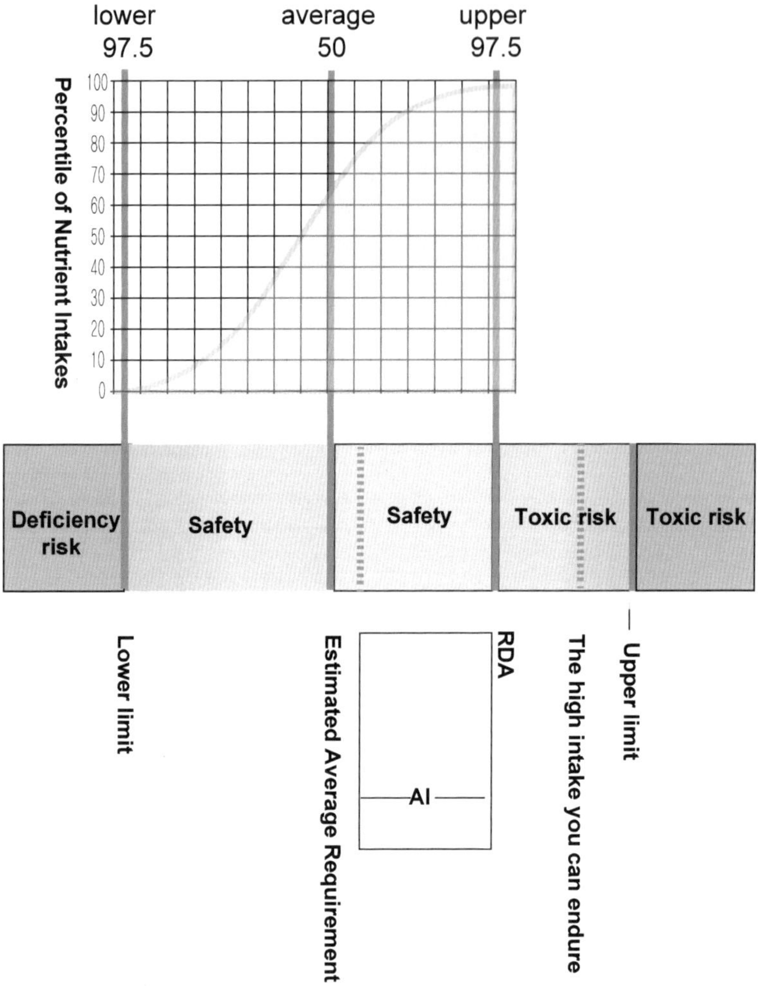

Figure 11–9. A simple viewpoint (a) and an accurate viewpoint (b)

Table 11-2. Korean Nutrition Standards

	Average requirement and recommended intake	Sufficient intake	Upper limit intake
calorie	O		
Macronutrient			
protein	O		
Dietary Fiber	O		
water		O	
Water-soluble vitamin			
vitaminC	O		O
vitaminB1 (Thiamin)	O		
vitaminB2 (riboflavin)	O		
vitaminB3 (niacin)	O		O
vitaminB6 (Pyridoxine, etc.)	O		O
folic acid	O		O
vitaminB12	O		
vitaminB5 (Pantothenic acid)		O	
vitaminB7 (Biotin)		O	
Fat-soluble vitamin			
vitaminA	O		O
vitaminD		O	O
vitaminE		O	O
vitaminK		O	
A large amount of minerals			
calcium	O		O
phosphorus	O		O
sodium		O	O
chlorine		O	
potassium		O	
magnesium	O		O
Trace mineral			
iron	O		O
zinc	O		O
cupper	O		O
Fluorine		O	O
manganese		O	O
iodine	O		O
Selenium	O		O
Molrebden			O

11.10. The risks of the excessive nutrient intake.

Until only a few decades ago, the history of mankind had always been in a time in which the nutrition had lacked. Naturally, the scientific and social view of nutrition had focused on preventing the problems caused by a lack of the nutrients. However, with the increase of the chronic diseases worldwide, the standard of the nutritional intake had changed. In other words, the criteria for the nutritional ingestion had included not only the deficiency but, also, the prevention of the problem of the toxicity due to an overdose. The Recommended Nutrient Intake (RNI) is based on the average needs of the age-specific population plus the two standard deviations, which were set at 97.5%. This is the standard. In other words, the nutrition standard is not tailor-made to the individuals in the groups of the people with the different heights, the different weights, and the different genetic and environmental characteristics.

In addition, setting the recommended intake is not based solely on the physiological needs. That is, after calculating the necessary amount that is not scientifically insufficient, it can be readjusted by adding an extra margin considering the incomplete utilization rate and the individual difference of the living body. Therefore, if the nutrients are consumed in accordance with the recommended amounts of the intake, a certain percentage of the individuals will inevitably have an excess over their actual needs. Professor

Campbell, on his website, NutritionAdvocate.com, says, in the article, "One day's recommendation: Time to remove the label."

"Daily nutritional recommendations are not the minimum requirements. They are much more than the amounts that are needed to avoid the risk of a deficiency."

Oxygen or water, which is absolutely necessary for our lives, can become toxic to the human body if we eat too much of any

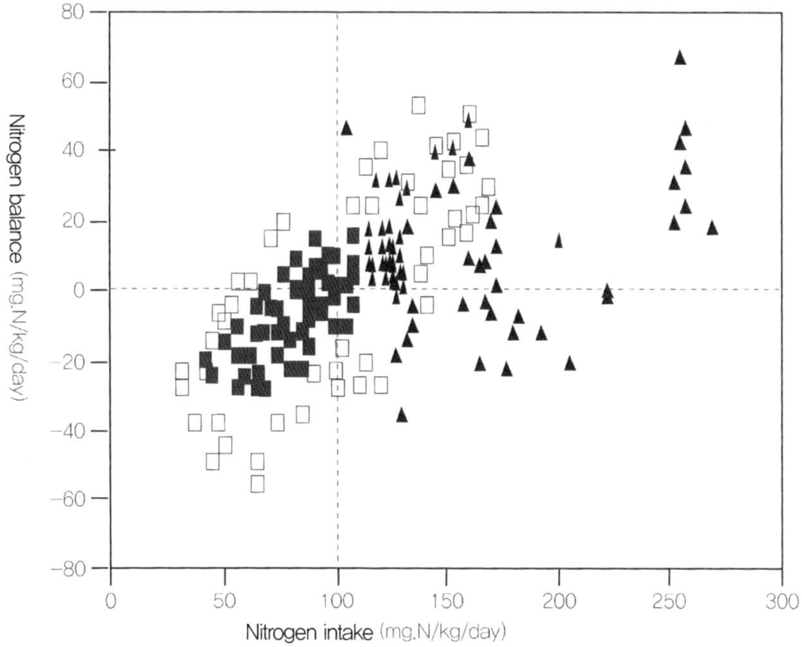

Figure 11-10. Balance of Nitrogen Intake and Nitrogen Loss in Healthy Adults

The average nitrogen demand is the point where the nitrogen balance is zero

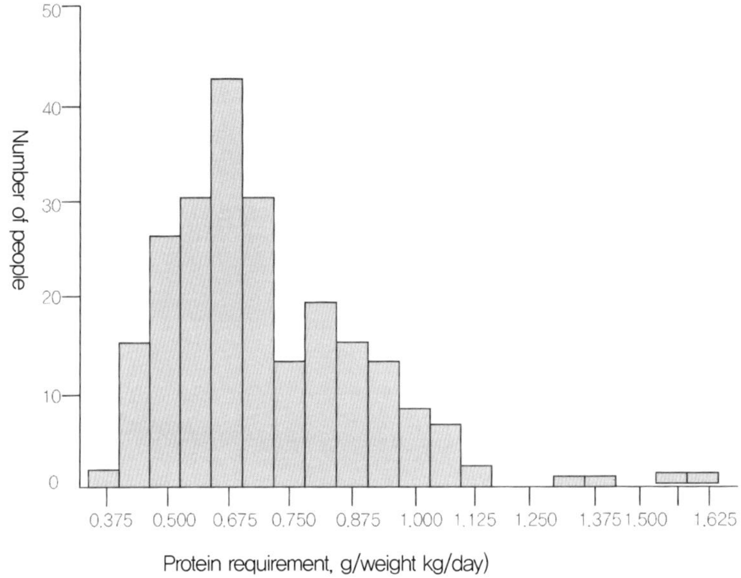

Figure 11–11. Estimated protein requirement for 225 adults (Rand et al., 2003)

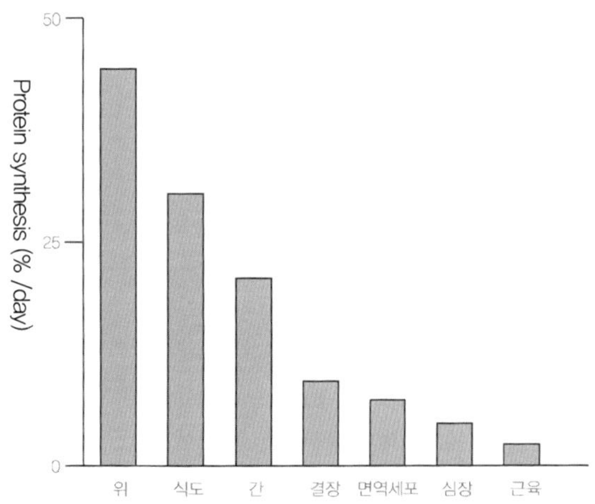

Figure 11–12. Fraction of Protein Synthesis in Human Tissue

The rate of protein synthesis was measured by adding L– [^{13}C] leucine or L– [^{2}H] phenylalanine to tissue proteins. Protein fractions represent proteins that are synthesized daily.

Table 11-3. Change of urine composition by diet [7]

Measurement variables	base	Western diet	non-vegetarian	lacto-ovo vegetarian	p
Urine volume (L/24hr)	1.29 ± 0.49	1.48 ± 0.38	2.30 ± .39	2.45 ± 0.76	〈0.001
pH	6.01 ± 0.47	5.95 ± 0.34	6.51 ± 0.22	6.80 ± 0.21	〈0.001
sodium (mmol/d)	159 ± 75	176 ± 40	146 ± 13	102 ± 48	0.045
chlorine (mmol/d)	164 ± 66	169 ± 39	139 ± 17	106 ± 43	0.024
ammonium (mmol/d)	30.8 ± 12.2	38.7 ± 5.1	25.6 ± 6.4	18.7 ± 5.9	〈0.001
Phosphate (mmol/d)	32.6 ± 8.1	35.4 ± 5.5	29.4 ± 3.5	25.2 ± 6.3	0.043
Sulfate (mmol/d)	18.5 ± 9.2	22.5 ± 3.1	18.1 ± 1.9	16.1 ± 3.7	0.004
Creatinine (mmol/d)	16.1 ± 4.4	16.9 ± 2.00	15.3 ± 1.3	13.8 ± 3.2	0.183
Uric acid (mmol/d)	3.59 ± 0.94	3.91 ± 0.67	2.93 ± 0.32	2.58 ± 0.52	〈0.001
RS Uric acid	2.90 ± 2.70	2.71 ± 2.82	0.41 ± 0.41	0.18 ± 0.15	0.009

RS Uric acid: relative supersaturation with respect to uric acid. Eur J Nutr (2003) 42:332-337

Table 11-4. Percentage(%) of Koreans' intake of nutrient intake by 2013

nutrient	male	female
Calory	106	96
protein	176	144
calcium	76	66
phosphorus	176	138
iron	207	145
vitaminA	115	108
Thiamin	208	171
riboflavin	112	107
Niacin	120	102
vitaminC	97	101
sodium	333	241
potassium	95	78

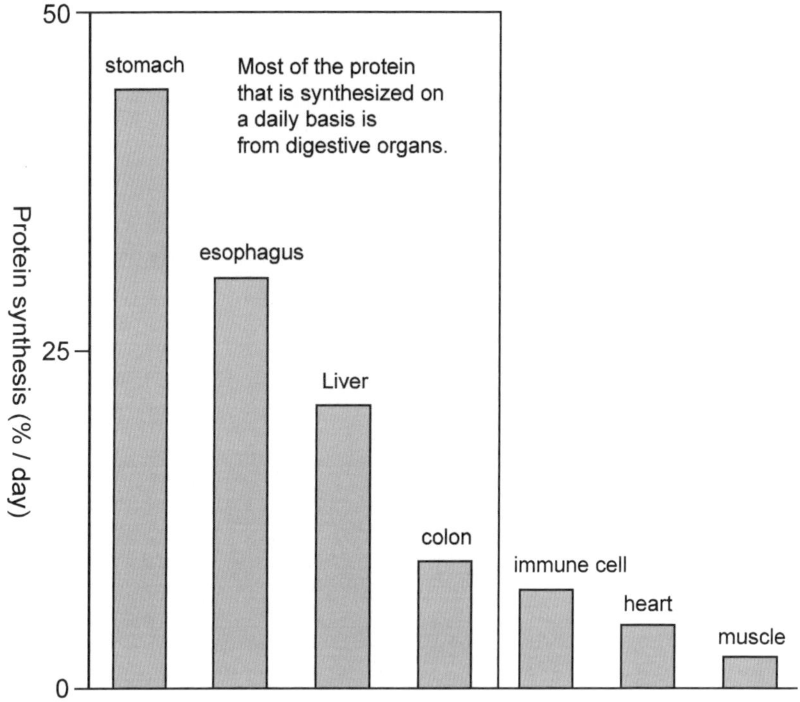

Fraction of protein synthesis in human tissue.
The rate of protein synthesis was measured by adding
L- [13C] leucine or L- [2H] phenylalanine to tissue proteins.
Protein fractions represent proteins that are synthesized daily.

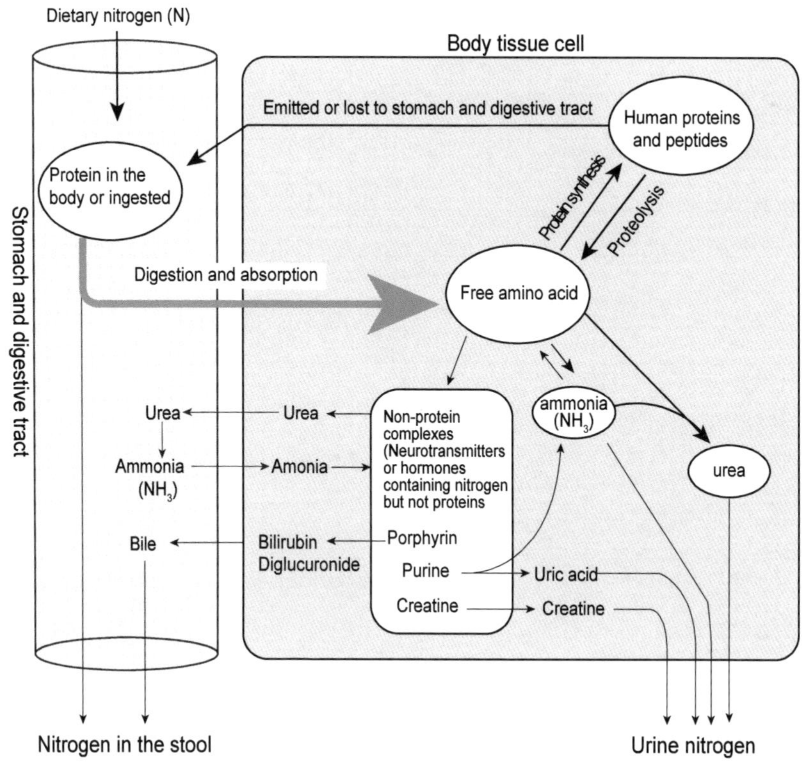

Figure 11–13. Circulation of nitrogen in the human body

nutrient, as can be seen from the fact that the excessively high concentrations or high doses may pose a life threat. Along with the surge of the diseases due to over–nutrition, studies on nutrition have revealed that the nutrients have the problems not only with regard to the risk of a deficiency but, also,with regard to the excessive intake and accumulation in the body. In relation to this, the concept of the upper limit of intake appears in the nutrition standard. In addition, a variety of the settings are set in the nutritional standards for a healthy life.

11.11. protein and the risk of overeating protein among the Koreans.

The protein requirement is estimated based on the current nitrogen balance. That is, by calculating the amount of the nitrogen excreted from the human body, the necessary protein is calculated. The amount of the nitrogen in the total protein is about 16%, and, when it is inversely calculated, the amount of the nitrogen released into the human body is multiplied by 6.25, which is the protein requirement. In Figure 11–9, the point where the nitrogen balance is zero is 105mg nitrogen/kg/day, which means that the protein intake is balanced. Multiplying the 6.25 g nitrogen–protein conversion factor results in the estimated, average requirement

(EAR) of 0.66 g/kg/day (105 mg×6.25) for the adults aged from 19 years old to 50 years old. In other words, if a woman weighs 57kg, on the average, 38g of protein per day is enough, and, even if a woman weighs 70kg, on the average, 47g of protein per day is enough. If the RDA is used, multiply the EAR by 25.7%, which is sufficient for 97.5% of the population (Figure 11–10 and Fig. 11–11).

According to the data published in the National Health and Nutrition Examination Survey, in the year of 2013, the Koreans had over–consumed with the protein, 176% for the males and 144% for the females [5]. Proteins are not stored in the body when they are over–consumed as compared to the carbohydrates or the fats. Because the nitrogen is toxic, the body removes the nitrogen from the protein and turns it into ammonia, which is then taken to the liver, making it a nontoxic element. The element is then moved to the kidney and excreted in the urine (Fig. 11–12).

Excess nitrogen cannot be converted into a source element and travels around the blood, which is called "hyperammonemia". The high–grade cancer mononemia is caused by a deficiency of, or a damage to, the urea synthase in the hepatocytes, but, it can, also, occur due to protein excess. Increased ammonia concentration in the blood is dangerous to the human body, especially in the nervous system, causing the brain encephalopathy or even a death by being severe. As shown in Table 11–3, the urinary ammonium and uric acid levels in the urine had been significantly reduced when compared to the Western diets. Table 11–4 shows the results

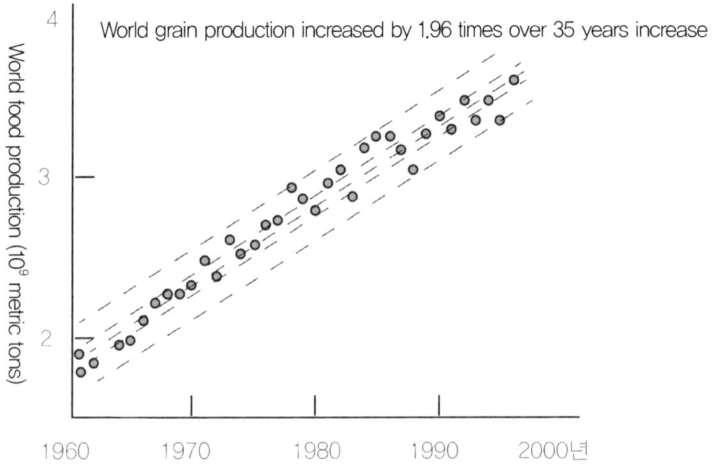

(a)

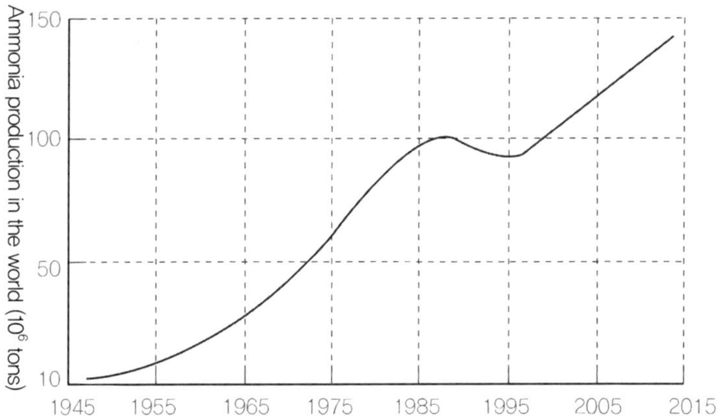

(b)

Figure 11–14. World food production (a) and nitrogen fertilizer production by FAO data (b)

According to the FAO data, world food production, measured as the sum of cereals, grains and root crops, nearly doubled between 1961 and 1996. The figure above shows 95% confidence interval and 99% confidence interval in regression.

of a National Health and Nutrition Examination Survey. As a result, it can be seen that the Korean adults had already consumed 176% of the recommended amount of protein and 144% of the women had already been overdosed. However, these figuresare based on the upper 97.5%, and, if they are compared with the average value, it is interpreted that they consume twice as much as the average.

11.12. Basal metabolism.

Metabolism is the process by which organisms generate and use energy, and the metabolic rate is the rate at which they produce and use energy. In other words, when there is no activity or growth, the animals require energy for blood circulation and respiration, protein synthesis, and ion pump operation, such as brain cells, and this is called basal metabolic rate. Historically, the initial basal metabolic rate (BMR) is defined by the minimum metabolic rate as measured by Rabwaj and is required even after resting after meals [6, 7].

Evolutionary evolution to fish, reptiles and mammals increases the basal metabolic rate, which inevitably has to pay for the increase in oxygen consumption. Mammals fulfill their needs by varying body structure and cell differentiation, and various changes in the level of molecules within the cell.

In Table 11-5, the human body's metabolic rate is 45% of the total energy used by a 10-kg infant in the brain. On the other hand, the heart is only 6%, kidney 5%, liver 19%, lung 4%. Even in adults with completed physical development, the brain accounts for only 2% of body weight, but uses 21% of energy, much more than 10% of the heart and 7% of the kidney [8]. Compared to the entire body, the energy used by the brain is 13% for chimpanzee and 7% for rats.

Basal metabolic rate is often used synonymously with the resting

Table 11-5. The metabolic rate of infants and adults [10]

Organ	10kg infant				70kg adult			
	OMR/Kg	weight	OMR	%	OMR/Kg	weight	OMR	%
	kcal/kg/day	kg	kcal/organ/day		kcal/kg/일	kg	kkcal/organ/day	
brain	260	0.92	240	45	260	1.4	365	21
heart	600	0.05	30	6	600	0.3	180	10
kidney	400	0.07	28	5	400	0.3	120	7
liver	350	0.30	105	19	350	1.6	560	32
lung	200	0.12	24	4	200	0.8	160	9
sum		1.46	427	79			1385	79
total BMR			540				1780	

BMR: Basal Metabolic Rate, OMR: Organ Metabolic Rate

metabolic rate, which means the energy needed to maintain basic human function while lying down quietly against the back. The left-wing activity accounts for approximately 60 to 75% of the energy expenditure per day [9]. The basal metabolic rate is higher in male than in female and decreases with age. Approximately 70% of the total energy expenditure of the human body is estimated to be consumed for the organs to function. 20% of the rest is used for physical activity, and 10% is used to keep the temperature constant for body temperature or baking [10]. It is important to control the body weight and body composition. Therefore, the need for clinical studies and research on the general public is increasing. There are several formulas for determining basal metabolic rate..

Table 11-6. Energy use of cells [11]

Contents	ratio		
Mitochondria and others	~10%		
Proton leak	~20%		
ATP produce	~70%	Na^+-K^+-ATPase activity	20-25% liver 10% / brain & kidney 60%
		Protein synthesis	20-25%
		Ca^{2+}-ATPase activity	~5%
		Gluconeogenesis	~7%
		Actin-myosin ATPase	~5%
		Other ATP process	~6%

The early Harris-Benedict formula

male: P = 13.7516 × body weight (kg) + 5.0033 × height (cm) -6.7550 × age (years) +66.4730 kcal

female: P = 9.5634 × body weight (kg) + 1.8496 × height (cm) -4.6756 × age (year) +655.0955 kcal

The modified Harris-Benedict formula

male: P = 13.397 × body weight (kg) + 4.799 × height (cm) + 5.677 × age (years) + 88.362 kcal

female: P = 9.247 × body weight (kg) + 3.098 × height (cm) -4.3306 × age (years) + 447.593 kcal

Mifflin St Jeor Equation

$P = 10.0 \times$ body weight (kg) $+ 6.25 \times$ height (cm) $+ 5.0 \times$ age (years) + s (kcal)

S = +5 (male), −161 (female)

Catch−McArdel Formula

P = 370 + 21.6 x LBM

LBM: lean body mass, female is 30%, and 1262kcal is the basal metabolic rate.

According to a report of 120 Korean college students, 1257.2 ± 147.9 kcal / day for REE, 1373.3 ± 45.4 kcal / day for WHO / UNU and Cunningham, and 1280.0 ± 61.7 kcal / day and 1187.6 ± 49.2 kcal / day [11]

The baseline metabolic rate varies from person to person, according to a study of 150 adults in Scotland, ranging from 1027 kcal (4301 kJ) to 2499 kcal (10455 kJ). Analysis showed that 62.3% of these differences were explained by the difference of fat free mass. Other factors were age (1.7%) and fat mass (6.7%) and the rest were unknown [12]. Another study found that the upper 5% of the basal metabolism was 28−32% higher than the lower 5%, even though the same lean body mass (body weight without fat) was observed [13]. According to another study, the same mean body mass was 43 kg and the difference was 715 kcal, with 1075 kcal for one person and 1790 kcal for another [13].

Modern people are mostly living in left-lane dining, and even the activity through walking is rapidly decreasing due to the development of transportation means. On the other hand, the supply of calories became easier than ever before. Unlike in the past, when fiber was abundant, excessive supply of refined calories inevitably led to various diseases such as obesity, diabetes, cardiovascular disease, and cancer. It is necessary to discuss the definitions and criteria of nutritional recommendation.

11.13. Until recently, the history of mankind had been a history of hunger.

The evolution of the animals depends on food. The animals in nature are constantly searching for food. As can be seen from the pointed fangs and the sharp claws of the predators, not only the appearances of the animals but, also, their biochemical functions are focused on the efficient acquisition and use of food. Based on Darwin's theory of natural selection, the lack of food is essentially the basic device of evolution.

The natural selection theory follows the order of overproduction → individual variation → survival competition → survival of the fittest → natural selection. In other words, creatures produce more offsprings than nature can support, and many offsprings are genetically different. It is easy to survive if the genetic mutation is valid according to the natural environment, and what is not so is removed. After all, the genes adapted to the natural environment are transmitted through the generations, and this is the natural choice and the engine of evolution.

Looking back at the history of mankind, until the 1960s, the food of the world had always been in short supply. The novel, "The Earth", which received the Nobel Prize for Literature, made the farmers from Mainland China as the characters for over 100 years. In Korea, there had been some people who had starved to death even a few decades ago, and many of the population now have such memories.

The reason for the limited production of food was that it required nitrogen for the protein synthesis. Nitrogen in the atmosphere chemically has three covalent bonds and is very stable. It is not readily decomposed and enters the biosystem through the lightnings or through the spikes of the bacteria. However, the amount had been limited, and the food produced by the plants had always been lacking.

Nitrogen fertilizer synthesis, the grain production increase, and the plant–based livestock.

The hunger situation has improved since the technology for artificially synthesizing the nitrogen fertilizers has been developed. This method, called the "Harbor method" or the "Harbor–Bosch method", can produce ammonia at about 200 atmospheres and from 400 degrees to 500 degrees using a catalyst. When this ammonia is mixed with the nitric acid or the sulfuric acid, it becomes a nitrogen fertilizer, such as the ammonium nitrate or the ammonium sulfate.

Harbor, in 1918, and Bosch, in 1931, received the Nobel Prize for Chemistry through this study. The chemical plants that had been built to make the weapons during the war began to turn into the nitrogen fertilizer plants after World War II, and the grain production had doubled in 35 years after 1960 with the mass production of the nitrogen fertilizers (Figure 11–14).

Grain production has increased, but poor people in the Third World have not been able to afford grain. The developed countries pay attention to the animal husbandry as a way to utilize the remaining grains. In other words, there had been a way of raising the livestock by feeding the grains to the dense space that was previously planted. And the growth of the livestock had been possible because of the increase of the meat consumption. At the same time, there had been the metabolic syndrome, such as obesity, diabetes, hypertension, cardiovascular disease, cancer, osteoporosis, etc.

11.14. The vegetarian paradigm revolution.

The vegetarian paradigm of the 1970s.

There had been a few studies on vegetarianism in the 1970s when the memories of the hunger had been vivid and when the nutritional deficiencies had been prevalent even in the industrialized countries. Thus, the topic of vegetarian nutrition had inevitably focused on the "diseases associated with a deficiency". A research report on vegetarianism centered on the case reports of the vegetarians visiting the hospital and focused on the short-term, nutrient deficiencies, not the chronic diseases like the present. These studies had been the animal experiments or the in vitro experiments targeting the specific nutrients under the controlled conditions. In this environment, the vegetarian diet is a model of the nutrient deficiency, suggesting that the diets based on the animal foods are rich in the nutrients (Figure 11-15).

The vegetarian paradigm in 1980 had beena diet that prevented overeating.

However, as the diverse degenerative diseases, including the cardiovascular disease, diabetes, and cancer, had been increasing rapidly in the wealthy countries around the world, the discussions had been made on the Westernmeat-based diets [6]. There had been, also, the new perspectives on the vegetarian diet. Noting that the diseases that are not well-known to the people in the

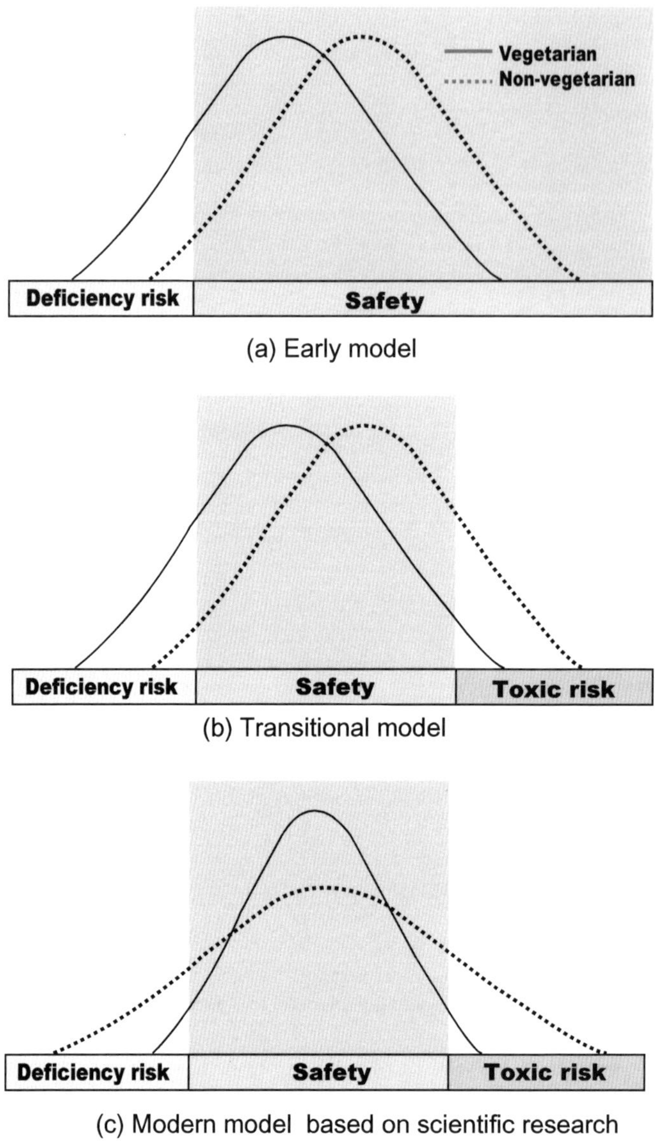

Figure 11–15. paradigm shift of vegetarian model

poor countries had been increasing in the wealthy nations of the West, the researches on the vegetarians in the rich countries had increased.

The recent vegetarian paradigm is an ideal diet that minimizes the excess and the deficiency.

The plant-based diets had not only lacked the nutrient diversity and abundance, but, also, the beneficial results in the chronic diseases, such as the cardiovascular disease, diabetes, and obesity. The whole grains, such as the whole wheat and the brown rice, had served the rich fibers and the various nutrients, and the nuts had supplied the high-quality, essential fatty acids, including the omega 3 fatty acids.

On the other hand, the animal food, that is, the meat consumption, had been very directly related to all the diseases. In many areas, such as the total fat intake, the saturated fats, the cholesterol, the protein, and the salinity, the animal foods had been the cause of overeating, and the excess of these nutrients had resulted in the development of the chronic diseases due to the risk of the toxicity. Thus, the vegetarian paradigm turns out to be that the risk of the deficiency is greater than that of meat, but the side-effects caused by an excess are less.

Recently, a research on the plant hormones has been going on. The modern vegetarian models are changing to a safe diet with the fewer risks and less risk of a deficiency

References

1. Jansen BC: Early nutritional researches on beriberi leading to the discovery of vitamin B1. Nutr Abstr Rev Ser Hum Exp 1956, 26:1–14.

2. Carpenter KJ, Sutherland B: Eijkman's contribution to the discovery of vitamins. J Nutr 1995, 125:155–163.

3. McCay CM, Maynard LA, Sperling G, Barnes LL: The Journal of Nutrition. Volume 18 July—December, 1939. Pages 1–13. Retarded growth, life span, ultimate body size and age changes in the albino rat after feeding diets restricted in calories. Nutr Rev 1975, 33:241–243.

4. Stipanuk MH: Protein and Amino Acid Requirements. In Biochemical, Physiological, Molecular Aspects of Human Nutrition. Edited by Stipanuk MH. PA. USA.: SAUNDERS ELSEVIER; 2006

5. 2013년 국민건강영양조사 [https://knhanes.cdc.go.kr/knhanes/index.do]

6. Hulbert, A. and P. Else, Basal metabolic rate: history, composition, regulation, and usefulness. Physiological and Biochemical Zoology, 2004. 77(6): p. 869–876.

7. Blaxter, K., Energy metabolism in animals and man. 1989: CUP Archive.

8. Lennie, P., The cost of cortical computation. Current biology, 2003. 13(6): p. 493–497.

9. Cooper, J.A., et al., Assessing validity and reliability of resting metabolic rate in six gas analysis systems. Journal of the American Dietetic Association, 2009. 109(1): p. 128–132.

10. McArdle, W.D., F.I. Katch, and V.L. Katch, Exercise physiology: nutrition, energy, and human performance. 2010: Lippincott Williams & Wilkins.

11. Chang, U.-J. and K.-R. Lee, Correlation between measured resting energy expenditure and predicted basal energy expenditure in female college students. Journal of the Korean Society of Food Science and Nutrition, 2005. 34(2): p. 196–201.

12. Johnstone, A.M., et al., Factors influencing variation in basal metabolic rate include fat-free mass, fat mass, age, and circulating thyroxine but not sex, circulating leptin, or triiodothyronine. The American Journal of Clinical Nutrition, 2005. 82(5): p. 941–948.

13. John R. Speakman, Elzbieta Krol, and Maria S. Johnson, The Functional Significance of Individual Variation in Basal Metabolic Rate. Physiological and Biochemical Zoology, 2004. 77(6): p. 900–915.

14. Sabate J: The contribution of vegetarian diets to health and disease: a paradigm shift? Am J Clin Nutr 2003, 78:502S–507S.

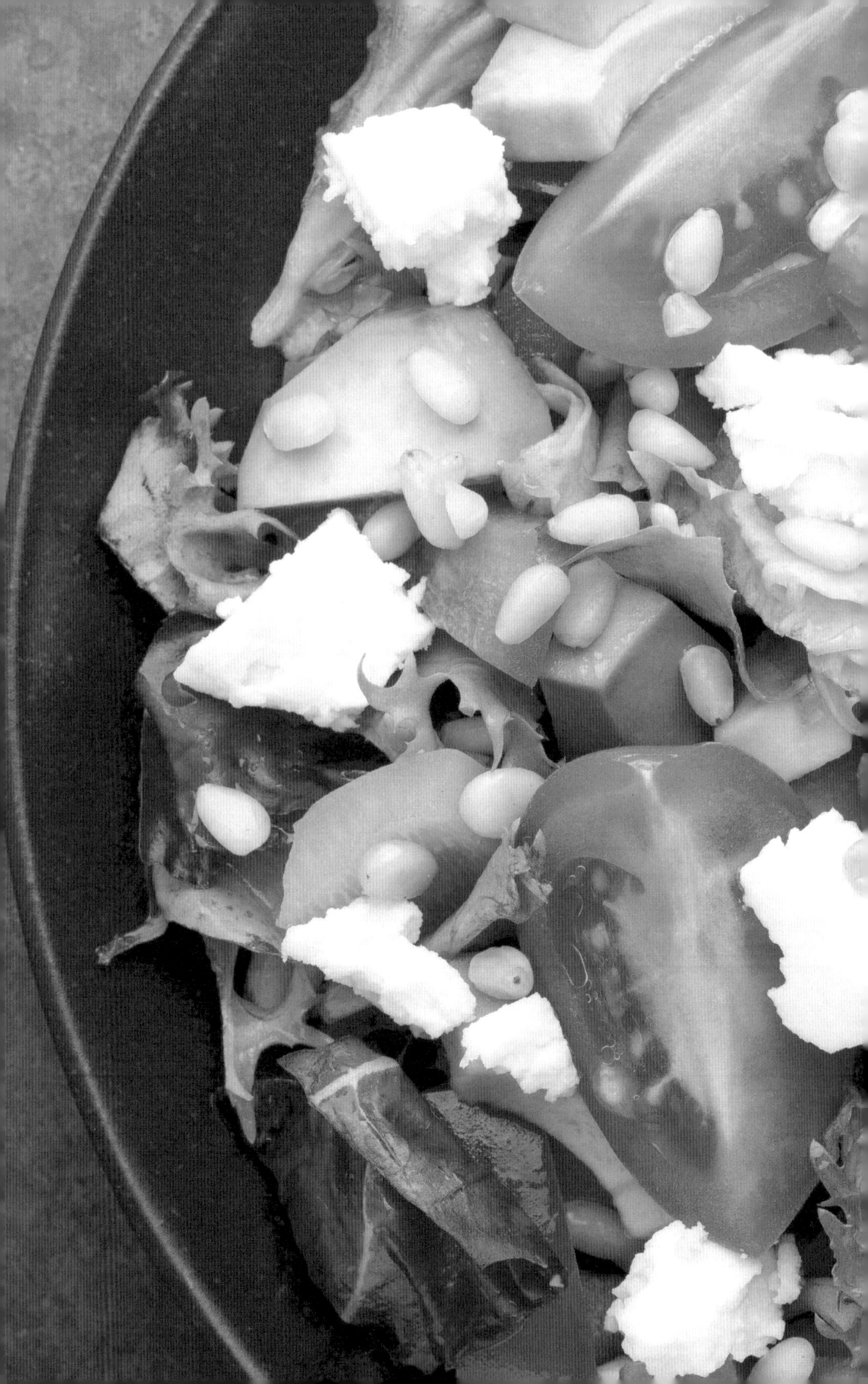

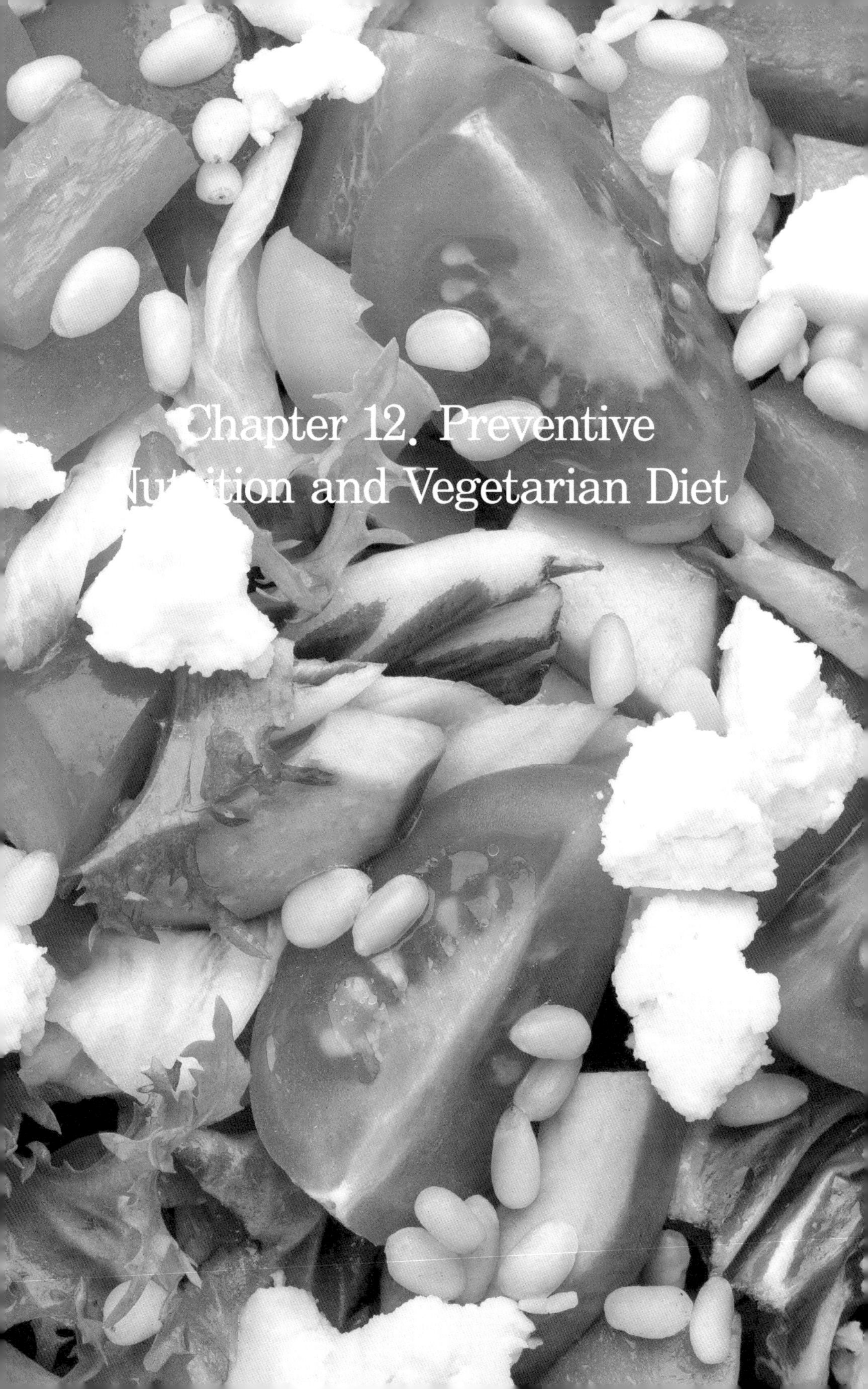

Chapter 12. Preventive Nutrition and Vegetarian Diet

12.1 Definition of vegetarianism.

The word 'vegetarian' was, first, used in England, where the first meeting of the vegetarians was held in 1839. The word is a combination of 'veget (able)' and '−arian'. 'Veget' comes from the Latin 'vegetus', which means 'vigorous', 'energetic', 'lively', 'move', and 'excite' (1). The influence of Pythagoras on the vegetarian diet has been very large in the Western history, as can be seen from the fact that the vegetarian diet before the word "vegetarian" was devised had been called the "Pythagorean diet" [2, 3]. The Pythagorean, vegetarian influences include Socrates, Plato, a number of the medieval mission theologians, Leonardo da Vinci, Newton, and others. For more information, see my "Vegetarian in History". The origin of the vegetarian diet in Korea is unclear, but, probably,it is the vegetables. The word 'vegetarians', which contains a strong sense of the word 'vegetable', can cause the nutritional misunderstandings. However, the vegetables include a wide variety of the plant foods. Based on the main nutrient content, the vegetarian food sector can be largely divided into three groups: The grains as the first carbohydrate source, the second as the protein,the lipid source, the soybean, the nuts, and the seeds, and the third as the source of the water−soluble vitamins and the phytochemicals, which are the fruits, the vegetables, and the seaweeds (Table 11−1). The range of the vegetarians can be divided into the semi−vegetarians, the pesco−vegetarian, the

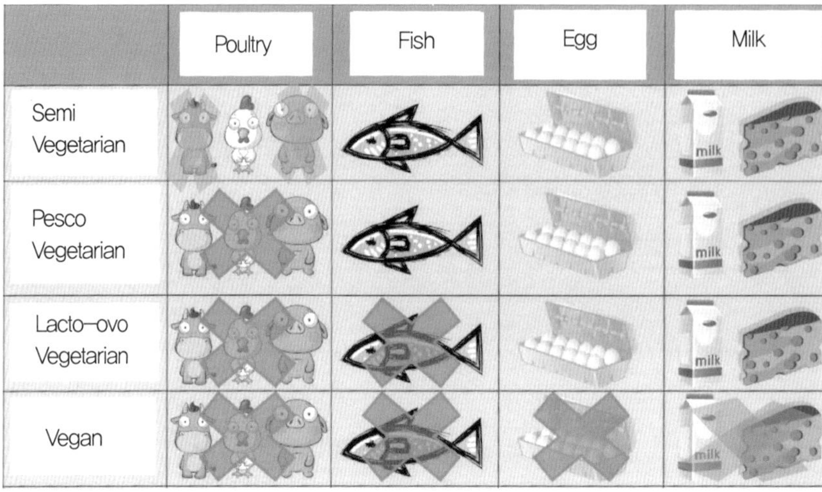

Figure 12-1. Various spectra of vegetarian

lacto-ovo vegetarians, and the vegans depending on the diets they consume. The semi-vegetarian eats the poultry but does not include the mammals, 'Pesco-vegetaria' eats the seafood that do not include the mammals, the chickens, and the poultry in their diet. The lacto-ovo vegetarian diet eats dairy products and the eggs. And the minimum standard of the vegetarian diet as defined by the International Vegetarian Union(IVU) is from the lacto-ovo vegetarian diet [4]. A vegetarian diet that does not include any dairy products and eggs is called the "vegan", which was originally proposed by Donald Watson in 1944 in the UK [5] (Table 12-1). As you can see, the vegetarians are very broad in the range of the diets and are not a uniform group. There are, also, the differences in the timing and the duration of the vegetarian initiation. As a result, in many vegetarian studies and researchs, the results, sometimes, do not show any statistical significance because of broad spectrum of vegetarian diet. However, in most health–related studies, the closer to the strictness or the completeness of the vegetarian diet and the longer the vegetarian period, the greater the beneficial effects on the health.

12.2. The Trinity vegetarian food group and the Trinity vegetarian diet.

In modern nutrition, the food group of the 5th group or the food group of the 6th group is used for the main nutrient intake method. The representative examples are the group 1 protein group, the group 2 calcium group, the group 3 vitamin, inorganic group, the group 4 carbohydrate group, and the group 5 fat group. The group 1 protein includes the meat and the beef, such as the beef and the chicken, and the calcium group includes the milk scabbard, the anchovies, and the dried laver. The minerals and the vitamins include the fruits and the vegetables, such as the apples, the grapes, the cabbages, the spinach, and the carrots. And the carbohydrate group includes the rice, the sweet potatoes, the potatoes, and the wheat corn. The fat group includes the sesame oil, the edible oil, and the walnuts.

Will they be able to meet these food groups with a vegetarian diet? The conclusion is that it is enough. However, based on the main nutrients of the vegetarian foods, there is no need to divide into the five food groups. There are several reasons: First, as described above, the recommended calcium intake is based on the highest intake of 97.5% of the subjects, so, it is sufficient to consume about 70% of the recommended intake regarding a certain group of people. Rather, the excess calcium can cause the cataracts, accumulate in the blood vessels, and cause atherosclerosis. Most

Table 12-1. Percentage of major nutrients in the vegetarian food group

Main nutrient	Food group	Kinds	carbohydrate	protein	Lipid
carbohydrate	Whole grains	Brown rice, whole wheat, barley etc.	70–75%	7–10%	1–2%
protein + Lipid	bean	Green beans, red beans, peas, etc.	20–50%	18–20%	20–30%
	Soybeans	Soybeans	18–20%	38–40%	15–17%
	Seedling	Perilla seeds, sunflower seeds	18–20%	18–20%	40–50%
	nuts	Walnuts, almonds, peanuts, cashew nuts	20–25%	15–18%	50–60%
Water-soluble vitamins	Vegetables	Root vegetables, leafy vegetables	5–6%	2–5%	0.1–1%
	Fruits	Apples, pears, plums, etc.	10–15%	0.1–1%	0.1–1%

**The vegetarian food group can be roughly divided into three groups: carbohydrate-rich allergies, protein and lipid-rich legumes, soybean, seeds, nuts and vegetables rich in water-soluble vitamins and fruits. Although not listed here, algae are very good traditional foods rich in vitamins and minerals and can be included in groups such as vegetables and fruits. If you include three food groups in each diet, you are less likely to have nutritional deficiencies.*

of the calcium is stored in the bone and is broken down when necessary to control the concentration in the blood. The calcium concentration in the human body is about from 1/10,000 times to 1/100,000 times the concentration of the calcium in the blood, which is a very low concentration. When the calcium ion channel in the cell membrane is opened for any cell action, the calcium is transferred from the blood into the cell through the concentration gradients in the blood and the cell. From this point of view,the too high concentrations of the calcium can cause the inappropriate, adverse reactions to the metabolism of the human cells.

The second is that the beans, nuts, and seeds are rich in fat along with the high-quality proteins. Therefore, it is not necessary to divide the protein group and the fat group. In other words, the vegetarian protein and fat group becomes a protein/fat group. As shown in Table 11-1, the protein/fat group can be largely divided into three groups according to the ratio of the protein and the fat. The legumes are 18%~20% protein, while the lipids are 20%~30% protein. In the case of the soybean, the protein content is higher than 38%~40%, and the lipid had been somewhat decreased to 15%~17%. The seeds are 18%~20% protein but 40%~50% lipid. And the nuts have from 15 percent protein to 18 percent protein and from 50 percent to 60 percent fat.

Therefore, the vegetable foods should be composed of the three groups of the food groups. The first food group is the carbohydrate group, which includes the brown rice and the whole wheat. The second food group is the protein & fat group, which includesthe soybeans, the seeds, and the nuts. The third food group is the minerals & vitamins group, which are the fruits, the vegetables, and the seaweed. Therefore, when making a diet, if all three food groups are included as much as possible, there is no reason to lack any nutrient unless it is a special case.

This picture shows the Trinity vegetarian group as shown in Figure 11-2.

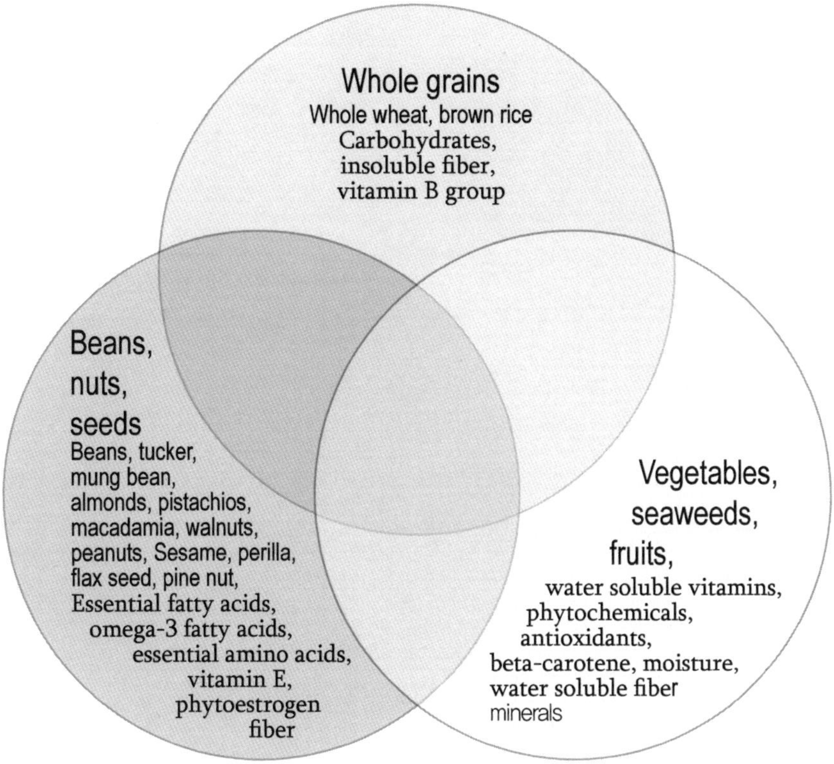

Figure 12-2. Triune vegetarian food group

When making a vegetarian diet, it is good to include three food groups. The first is the carbohydrate rich in fiber, the second is the high quality protein and lipid through the legumes, nuts and seeds, the third is the water soluble vitamins, phytochemicals and antioxidants through the vegetables, seaweeds and fruits, will be.

12.3. The reasons for, and the benefits of, vegetarianism

The reasons for, and the benefits of, the vegetarian diet can be divided into four broad categories−environmental protection, health promotion, hunger resolution, animal care, and may include the areas related to the religious tradition or spirituality. A research on the reasons for vegetarianism suggests that about 50% of the vegetarian motivations are due to the health reasons, and, more recently, the vegetarians have been increasingly involved in the environmental issues and the animal rights. Traditionally, Hinduism and Oriental Buddhism have encouraged vegetarianism in religion, while Christianity encourages vegetarianism in the Adventist schools. And many Indian yoga and meditation groups are encouraging vegetarianism.

The over−consumption of food is widespread not only in the advanced countries but also, in the developing countries. But, by the early 20th century,the humanity had suffered from the famines. This had been due to a limitation in the amount of the nitrogen introduced into the biosphere through the lightning or sprinkling bacteria in the natural world. The hunger situation has improved since Harbor and Bosch had used the chemical energy to fix the nitrogen industrially in the early 20th century. According to the Harbor−Bosch method, ammonia can be produced from the pressure of 200 atmospheres, 400° C ~ 500 ° C, and from the

<Box 1> Environmental and hunger problems related to sulfuric acid

Environmental issues

(1) Cow releases 20 times of human and 4 times of pig excrement. Most of them are released into animal wastewater and contaminate the environment. Due to the increase in costs, waste water treatment is often not performed.

(2) The amount of water required to produce 1 kg of food is as follows. 110 liters of tomatoes, 3,000 liters of rice, 1,000 liters of wheat, 100,000 liters of beef

(3) More than 60 percent of the world's pasture is over capacity and raising excess animals. As a result, grasslands are becoming increasingly deserted and tropical forests are being destroyed to create alternative land. Since 1900, more than 25% of the Central American forest has been harvested for grazing, and two–thirds of farmland is being used for livestock breeding.

Hunger problem

(1) Grains used as livestock feed are the amount that can feed 400 million people every year.

(2) 40 percent of the world's grain production is for livestock feed.

iron–catalyzed conditions. When this ammonia is mixed with the volcanic acid or the sulfuric acid, the ammonium fertilizer, such as the ammonium nitrate or the ammonium sulfate, is produced. After the Second World War, South Korea's chemical weapons factory had turned into a nitrogen fertilizer factory, which, in turn,had led to the Green Revolution [7].

In the 35 years since the 1960s, the world production of the grains had increased by a factor of 1.9, a change that had never occurred before in history. Now, the processing of the surplus grain has become an important issue. Because the Third World has not become an economical power to consume. The key solution for this was to convert to the livestock feed. Half of the livestock that had grazed the pastures had been converted into the factory livestock, and they had been fed and raised in the narrow wastes. 37 billion livestock are being cultivated globally, and the grain demand for them reached 40% of the world's grain production [8].

With the increase in meat consumption, the chronic diseases are increasing globally, and the medical expenses are starting to take up a considerable share of the national finances and resulting in the household bankruptcies. The list of the related diseases includes cancer, osteoporosis, gallstones, rheumatism, and the autoimmune diseases, as well as the metabolic syndrome, such as obesity, diabetes, hypertension, and the cardiovascular disease. It is, also,a time to report on the risks of the deficiencies in the nutritional science as well as the side–effects of overeating the calories and the over-toxicities of some nutrients.

12.4. The spread of the vegetarian books and vegetarianism.

The growing popularity of the popular vegetarian diet in the West since the 1970s has been fueled by the emergence of some popular books on vegetarian diet. Francis Moorephe emphasized the importance of the vegetarian diet related to the environment and the hunger through a small booklet "A meal for a small planet" [9].

And Peter Singer reminded the public of the ethical aspects of the harsh environment and the cruel slaughter of the livestock through "Animal liberation [10, 11]". The famous Baskin Robbins' heir John Robbins emphasized the health benefits of being vegetarian through "Diet for a New America [8, 12]".

Pimentel and Jeremy Rifkin are among the representatives regarding the importance of the vegetarian diet in relation to the environment. Pimentel had studied the various research papers through "Food, Energy, and Society" [13] and Rifkin, through "End of Meat" [14, 15], explains the meaning of the vegetarian diet for the sustainability.

The scientific and nutritional aspects of the book include John Savatte's "Vegetarian Nutrition" [16], Messina's "The Dietitian's Guide to the Vegetarian Diets" [17], and Lee's "Proof Positive" [18,

19].

The public, as written by the experts, has Colin Campbell's "What to Eat" and McDougall's "Confession of a Vegetarian Doctor". In Korea, the clinical cases related to the healing of the vegetarian diets have been reported by Song Sook-ja through the mass media [20, 21]. And the vegetarian books related to the various areas, including the vegetarian dishes, are being introduced constantly.

Although the contents of these books are somewhat different from each other due to the differences in the cited studies, they are generally related to the environment and the starvation, and they include the contents, such as Box 1.

Expanding the causal chain further widens the area associated with the dietary patterns. As you know, one of the main causes of the wars in the world is to secure the resources. The fossil fuels, especially those represented by the petroleum, are important, and a significant proportion of the demand for the fossil fuels is related to the livestock production. The need to include a series of the processes, such as the grain production, the transport, the packaging, and the sales, for the livestock is beyond our imagination.

In addition, as in the cases of China and India, an increase in the livestock consumption, which is accompanied by an increase in the economic power of the population, leads to an increase in the global grain prices [22]. Unlike the other commodities, the grain production is bound to be limited, so the food-related security

<Box 2> Decrease in medical expenses related to vegetarian [25]

40% of the cancer deaths occur because of eating meat.

The mortality rate for all cancers was 1.61 for the vegetarians.

Diabetes mellitus among vegetarians is 45%.

The diabetes diagnosis of the non–vegetarians is 1.9 times higher for men than the vegetarians and 1.6 times higher for women than the vegetarians.

When you look at the gall stones regarding the vegetarianism, the non–vegetarians are 1.9.

The incidence of cholelithiasis is 1.5% for vegetarians and 6.8% for non–vegetarians.

Compared to the non–vegetarians, the vegetarian men have the low systolic and diastolic pressures of 8mmHg and 6mmHg, respectively, and the vegetarian females are lower than 8mmHg for both.

The non–vegetarian hypertension is 1.74 times higher for women than for the vegetarians and 1.74 times higher for men than for the vegetarians. .

The mean body mass index (BMI) is 25.1 kg / m2 for the non–vegetarians, which is significantly higher than the 22.9 kg / m2 for the vegetarians

.

will become an increasingly important topic. Pimentel and Rifkin emphasized the fact that there is a very large energy gap between the direct consumption of the plants and the consumption of the animals. That is, more than half of the cereals that have been fed into the livestock feed are consumed by the heat energy of the livestock. And, except for the excrements and the non-digestible by-products, itsactual amount available is even smaller. What is interesting is that Socrates prophesied very precisely about the problems that would be derived from meat eating two thousand years ago.

"You will need the delicious dishes and the meat dishes. Besides, we will need the people for the farm pigs. These animals did not exist before because it had not been needed in our early city. (Syncopation)
And, if we live that way, we will need more doctors than ever before. And the land that had been sufficient to feed the population will now become smaller and insufficient. Should we then take away some of our neighbor's land if we want to have enough for the pasture and cultivation? And the next step will be a war. Now, we will not discuss the effects of war on the good or evil. But, we have now found the origin of war. It comes from these factors. It is the greatest source of evil for the individuals in the cities" [23].

According to Socrates, the source of war in the world is meat consumption. More land will be needed to raise the livestock. In the early stages of vegetarianism, land becomes scarce and a war has to take place. And more people are needed, and the slaves are needed to raise the livestock. As well as eating meat, many illnesses increase, which makes more doctors

12.5. Health and vegetarianism.

The health−related vegetarian studies can be divided into two main categories: First, the nutritionally sufficient; and, second, the prevention and healing of the vegetarian diets. The nutritional studies began in the 1970s, when the animal protection and the Oriental religions had spread to the Western countries and the vegetarians had increased. Until then, the nutrition−related topics had usually been associated with the deficiencies [16]. Thus, the view of the nutritional science regarding the vegetarian diet had been that a deficiency is possible. However, according to the results of a series of the close studies onthe suspicion, vegetarianism is nutritionally unproblematic and, rather, desirable in relation to the health. The final version of these studies was summarized in the official paper by the North American Dietetic Association, which includes the studies of the United States and Canada, on the position of the vegetarians [24].

"Considering the main stages of the life as the infancy, the childhood, the adolescence, the pregnancy, and the lactation, the various vegetarian diets can satisfy the nutrients needed for each cycle and allow for the normal growth. In childhood and adolescence, vegetarianism promotes the healthy eating habits in the long–term, and it has the advantage of lowering the cholesterol, the saturated fatty acid, and the total fat intake in the nutrition and increasing the dietary fiber intake through the fruits and the vegetables. The vegetarian children are, also, known to be thinner and to have the lower serum cholesterol than the non–vegetarian children [24]. "

The prevention and healing effects of the vegetarian diet include the relationships with a list of the various diseases–the cardiovascular disease, obesity, diabetes, rheumatoid arthritis, cancer, and gallstone. Although the difference between the degree of the prevention and the healing effect and the presence or absence of the statistical significance depend on the experimental methods and the conditions of the studies, the general tendency shows the healing effect of the vegetarian diet. A noteworthy article reported this more than 20 years ago.

However, in 1995, three researchers, including two medical doctors, reported an increase in the medical costs associated with meat [25]. Based on the results of the previous studies, they found that a considerable proportion of the medical costs regarding the various diseases could be reduced by having a vegetarian diet (Box

2). It is reminiscent of a research result that more than a third of the cancer causes are related to meat.

The beneficial effects of the vegetarianism on the disease prevention and the healing are compounded. As shown in Figure 2, the intakes of the calories, the cholesterol, and the triglycerides are reduced, and the fiber, the plant hormones, the phytochemicals, the antioxidants, the vitamins, and the water intake are increased. These nutrients are grouped together without moving individually, and they are very important for the health and the nutrition because they are closely related to the chronic diseases, such as the metabolic syndrome.

12.6. The decrease in the medical expenses by from 35 % to 78 % won when vegetarian.

Bernard of George Washington University in the United States reported that the medicial expenses of meat consumption is about from 35% to 78% of medical cost. Based on the comparative papers between vegetarian and non-vegetarians, he calculated the increased medical costs for meat consumption in 1992 dollars. First, the studies reported at the time were far more focused on lacto-ovo vegetarians not vegan. Rescently, many studies shows a more beneficial effect in the vegan diet than in the vegetarian diet. Several variables such as smoking, exercise, and alcohol consumption were statistically corrected. And they did not include costs such as reduced productivity of social other than direct medical expenses. At the time, 62.77 million Americans were diagnosed with hypertension with systolic blood pressure〉 140 / diastolic blood pressure〉 90 and medical expenses were $ 12.5 billion. Of these, doctors and nurses cost $ 5.1 billion, pharmaceuticals cost $ 3 billion, and hospital and nursing care centers cost $ 4.4 billion. We compared the Mormons who did not smoke, alcohol, and caffeine with the Sabbath. The difference here is that the Mormons do meat and the Sabbath do not. Compared to Mormons, the Sabbath men had a systolic 8mmHg/diastolic 6mmHg lower, and a female systolic 8mmHg / diastolic 8mmHg.

The body mass index was also lower at 22.9 for vegetarians

compared to 25.1 for non-vegetarians. Other studies have shown that if the diet was changed to vegetarian diet with other life patterns intact, systolic blood pressure decreased by 5 mmHg after 6 weeks, which was not related to weight changes.

In a study of 27,000 Sabbath church members, hypertension was 1.75 times higher for males and 1.74 times higher for females than for vegetarians. Body mass index (BMI) was 25.7 for males, 24.2 for vegetarians, and 25.2 for non-vegetarians and 23.6 for vegetarians. And the rate of diagnosis of hypertension by doctors was 37% for non-vegetarians, but only 14% for vegetarians. In the case of hypertension medication, non-vegetarians account for 22% and vegetarians account for 7%, while non-vegetarians account for 44% and vegetarians account for 18%.

Another study found that a 6-week vegetarian diet in hypertensive patients reduced systolic blood pressure to 140 mmHg in 30% of patients. However, if the diet contained meat as usual, only 8% had blood pressure dropping to 140 mmHg. There was also a study that conducted a vegan diet for one year, in which 20 of the 26 hypertensive patients participating in the study were able to terminate hypertension. The relief of blood pressure also has a beneficial effect on heart disease. For men aged 55~59 years, a 5 mmHg reduction in blood pressure reduces the risk of cardiovascular disease, including coronary vascular disease, by 7%. A reduction of 5 mmHg at age 35 and below is as effective as a reduction of 10 mmHg at age 65 and above. According to the above studies, the cost of hypertension due to meat consumption has increased by 59% to 68%. At that time, in the case of hypertension, if you pay $ 12.5 billion for medical expenses, about $ 2.8 billion to $ 8.5 billion is due to meat consumption. In the case of heart disease, 6.16 million Americans in 1992 had angina and myocardial infarction (heart attack)

1028,000 cardiac catheterization, 468,000 cardiovascular bypass, and 399,000 cardiovascular procedures were conducted. This resulted in a total of $ 40.4 billion in medical expenses for heart disease. Doctors/nurses cost $ 7.3 billion, drug costs $ 2 billion, and hospital/nursing center costs $ 31.1 billion.

In the 1990s, 1.2 million Americans were diagnosed with cancer each year. And every year 500,000 cancer resulted in the deaths of breast cancer, prostate cancer, lung cancer, rectal colon cancer. Lung cancer was diagnosed annually by 170,000 people and died of 149,000 people. According to a study of Sabbath people, vegetarians male were 0.67 times than non-vegetarians, and 0.47 times in female vegetarian. A 12-year study found that vegetarians had a cancer mortality rate of only 0.61, compared with non-vegetarians, after adjusting for smoking, BMI, and socioeconomic status as statistical variables.

In a study conducted in Germany for 11 years, the cancer mortality rate of vegetarians was 0.48 for males and 0.74 for females compared to non-vegetarians. Based on these studies, the cost of cancer deaths from meat consumption was estimated at $ 16.5 billion in 1992.

According to a study of the Sabbath churches surveyed in the 1960s,

Diabetes disease prevalence was 45% in vegetarian, less than half. Considering that not all Sabbath members are vegetarian, the prevalence of diabetes in real vegetarians will be even lower. According to a 21-year death study, the mortality rate from diabetes was 2.2 times higher for men and 1.4 times higher for women than for non-vegetarians comparing to vegetarians. Diabetic neuropathy and retinopathy were reduced by vegetarian diets centered on whole grains, legumes, vegetables, and fruits. According to these studies, increased diabetes care costs due to meat consumption were estimated at $ 14 billion to $ 17.1 billion.

According to a study conducted in the UK, 6.8% of non-vegetarians had gallbladder disease. But only in 1.5% of vegetarians. On ultrasonography, 17.8% of the non-vegetarians had no symptoms and 10% of the vegetarians had no symptoms. After adjustment for age and BMI, non-vegetarians had 1.9 times the rate of gallstones comparing to vegetarians. Based on a 1976 Sabbath study, $ 240 million is based on British research, and $ 2.4 billion is an additional cost of medical expenses due to meat consumption. Overweight is also a problem in metabolism, but it is also a burden on the musculoskeletal system. The cost of musculoskeletal disorders in 1980 was $ 1.31 billion, 10% of which was due to obesity. A study of 25,698 Sabbath church members found that over 30% of the standard body weight was 1.9 times higher for male non–vegetarians and 1.6 times higher for female non–vegetarian than for vegetarians. A study conducted in the UK found that 24% of non–vegetarians had a BMI greater than 24, while 14% were vegetarians. Thus, 10% of the $ 1.30 billion in musculoskeletal medical costs is $ 130 million, and $ 4.4 billion is a musculoskeletal disorder caused by obesity, based on a 31% increase in obesity rates from 1980 to 1992. Here, musculoskeletal medical costs of meat consumption were $ 1.9 billion.

59 to 69% of food poisoning is caused by fourfolded meat or poultry. The cost of medical expenses for five food poisoning bacteria, Salmonella, Campylobacter, O157, Listeria, and oxoplasma, was estimated to be between $ 230 million and $ 760 million in 1993. A study of 150 and 18 vegetarians and 41 non–vegetarians, respectively, found that 27 percent of non–vegetarians were admitted to hospital due to food poisoning, compared with only 12 percent of vegetarians. Drug prescribing experience was 22% for non–vegetarians, while only 11.3% for vegetarians.

There were also studies related to smoking and drinking, which showed that non–vegetarians were more likely than vegetarian. The percentage of non–vegetarians was 12%, but the percentage of non-vegetarians was 32% in smoking, while the rate of non-vegetarians was 16.2%, while the percentage of vegetarians was only 8.0% in alcohol drinking.

According to a study of 20,766 Sabbath church members who had been hospitalized for the past year. For males, 9.2% of non-vegetarians were vegetarians, while 7.2% were vegetarians, while 11.3% of vegetarians were vegetarians, compared to 13.3% of non-vegetarians. The percentage of non-vegetarians who answered that they did not use regular medication was 29.9% for men, but 70.3% for vegetarians. 21.3% of non-vegetarians were women non-vegetarian and 57.3% were vegetarians women. In the case of women, 11.8% of non-vegetarians had experience of emergency surgery, while 9.5% of vegetarians. The experience of x-rays. 12.9% of non-vegetarians and 11.2% of non-vegetarians of male.

To sum up, the rising cost of health care due to the consumption of meat is estimated to be between $ 28.8 and $ 8.5 billion. In the United States, $ 9.5 billion in heart disease, $ 16.5 billion in cancer, $ 14.1 to $ 17.1 billion in diabetes, $ 2 to $ 2.4 billion in gallbladder disease, $ 1.9 billion in obesity-induced musculoskeletal disorders, and $ 2 billion to $ 5.5 billion in food poisoning ~ $ 61.4 billion. There were no studies on the rise in medical costs due to the vegetarian diet until 1992. Nutrients, except for the whole vegan vitamin B12 was not a big problem. However, iron and calcium were the controversial nutrients. However, up to now, research has shown that excess iron intake through the heme iron of meat intake is associated with various diseases such as cardiovascular disease, cancer, diabetes, and dementia so on.

When this paper was published in 1992, there were a little studies on the benefits of vegetarianism. And most of it was a comparison between lacto-ovo vegetarian and non-vegetarian. Thus, the benefits of the vegetarian diet pattern for more diverse diseases may be added. This may include not only physical disorders, but also various neurological disorders, such as depression, autism, and schizophrenia ADHD, etc.

The bankruptcy of some European countries has increased due to medical costs. Medical expenses are involved in country bankruptcy. According to an American study in 2007, 70% of all individual bankruptcies were due to medical expenses, with half of these bankrupt families having homes and highly educated graduates.

Many countries that have increased social awareness about issues such as increased health care costs for meat consumption. The vegetarian population in Germany was only 2% in 2000, but 10% in 2010, 10 years later. In Korea, it is also necessary to implement a vegetarian selection system in day care centers and elementary and junior high schools. The National Health and Nutrition Survey should also include three variables vegetarian or not, vegetarian periods, vegetarian type or specturm. Big company with 300 or more employees will be required to choose the vegetarian menu.

References

1. Geiss HC, Otto C, Hund–Wissner E, Parhofer KG: Effects of ezetimibe on plasma lipoproteins in severely hypercholesterolemic patients treated with regular LDL–apheresis and statins. Atherosclerosis 2005, 180:107–112.

2. Lee KwangJo , Vegetarian in History. Seoul: Sallim Pub.; 2008.

3. Berry R: Famous Vegetarians and Their Favorite Recipes. N.Y. USA: Pythagorean Pub; 1993.

4. Union IV : What does 'vegetarian' mean? ; 2014.

5. Stepaniak J : Being Vegan. Lowell house anodyne; 2000.

6. Jin Sang–Hyun, Go Eun–Ju : The Difference of View Points of Dietitians and College Students on Vegetarian Diet: Openness of Decision Making Process in School Meal System. The Korean Association for Environmental Sociology, 2004, 7:115~139.

7. Jan Willem Erisman, Mark A. Sutton, James Galloway, Klimont Z, Winiwarter W: How a century of ammonia synthesis changed the world. Nature Geoscience 2008, 1:636 – 639.

8. Robbins J. Diet for a New America: How Your Food Choices Affect Your Health, Happiness, and the Future of Life on Earth: New World Library; 2011.

9. Lappe FM : Diet fo a Small Planet. Ballantine Books; 1985.

10. Singer P. Animal liberation: Random House; 1995.

11. Singer P: Animal Liberation. Ecco Press; 2001.

12. Robbins J: Diet for a New America. HJ Kramer; 1998.

13. Pimentel D, Pimentel MH: FOOD, ENERGY, AND SOCIETY. 3rd edn. FL, USA: CRC Press; 2008.

14. Rifkin J, Swanson T, Barbier E, Holmberg J, Wibe S, Jones T, Mcgehee W, Thayer P, Echenique Larrain J, Villavicencio Rivera M. Beyond beef: The rise and fall of the cattle culture: Banco Mundial, Washington, DC (EUA); 1992.

15. Rifkin J: Beyond Beef: The Rise and Fall of the Cattle Culture Plume; 1993.

16. Sabate J: Vegetarian Nutrition. CRC Press; 2001.

17. Messina V: The Dietitian's Guide to Vegetarian Diets: Issues and Applications. Jones & Bartlett Learning; 2004.

18. Nedley N: Proof Positive: How to Reliably Combat Disease and Achieve Optimal Health Through Nutrition and Lifestyle. Neil Nedley; 1999.

19. Nedley N, DeRose D. Proof Positive: How to Reliably Combat Disease and Achieve Optimal Health Through Nutrition and Lifestyle: The Author; 1999.

20. Song Sook-Ja : Miracle of natural remedy. SamYoung Pub.; 2011.

21. Song Sook-Ja : Natural remedi of diet therapy. Oblise; 2011.

22. Han SeokHo: The cause of international grain cost increasing and the effect on domestic product-value . Ori-Maeul, 92:50-59.

23. Plato: Republic. 3rd edn : Hackett Pbu Co; 2004.

24. American Dietetic A, Dietitians of C: Position of the American Dietetic Association and Dietitians of Canada: vegetarian diets. Can J Diet Pract Res 2003, 64:62-81.

25. Barnard ND, Nicholson A, Howard JL : The medical costs attributable to meat consumption. Prev Med 1995, 24:646-655.

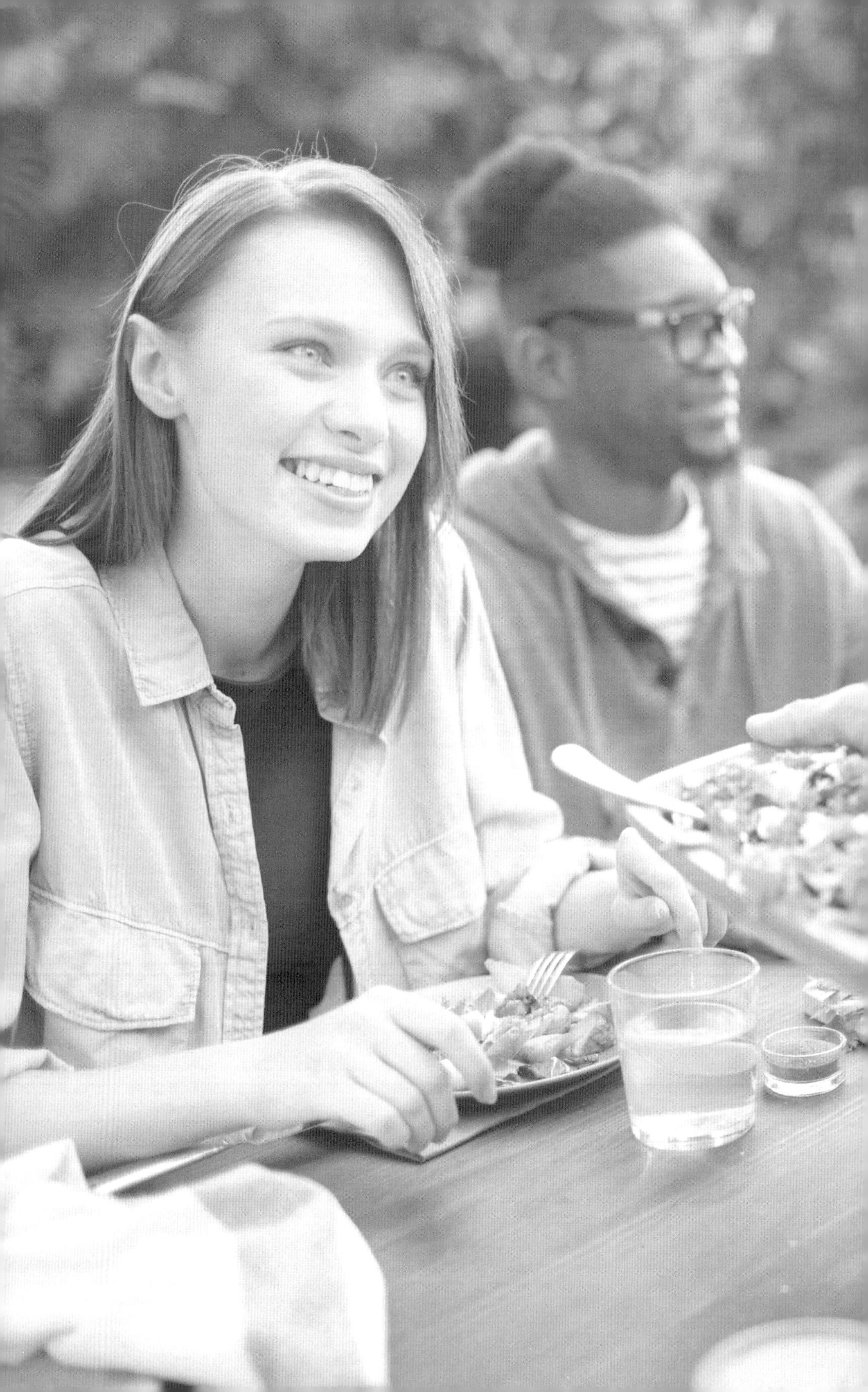

Epilogue

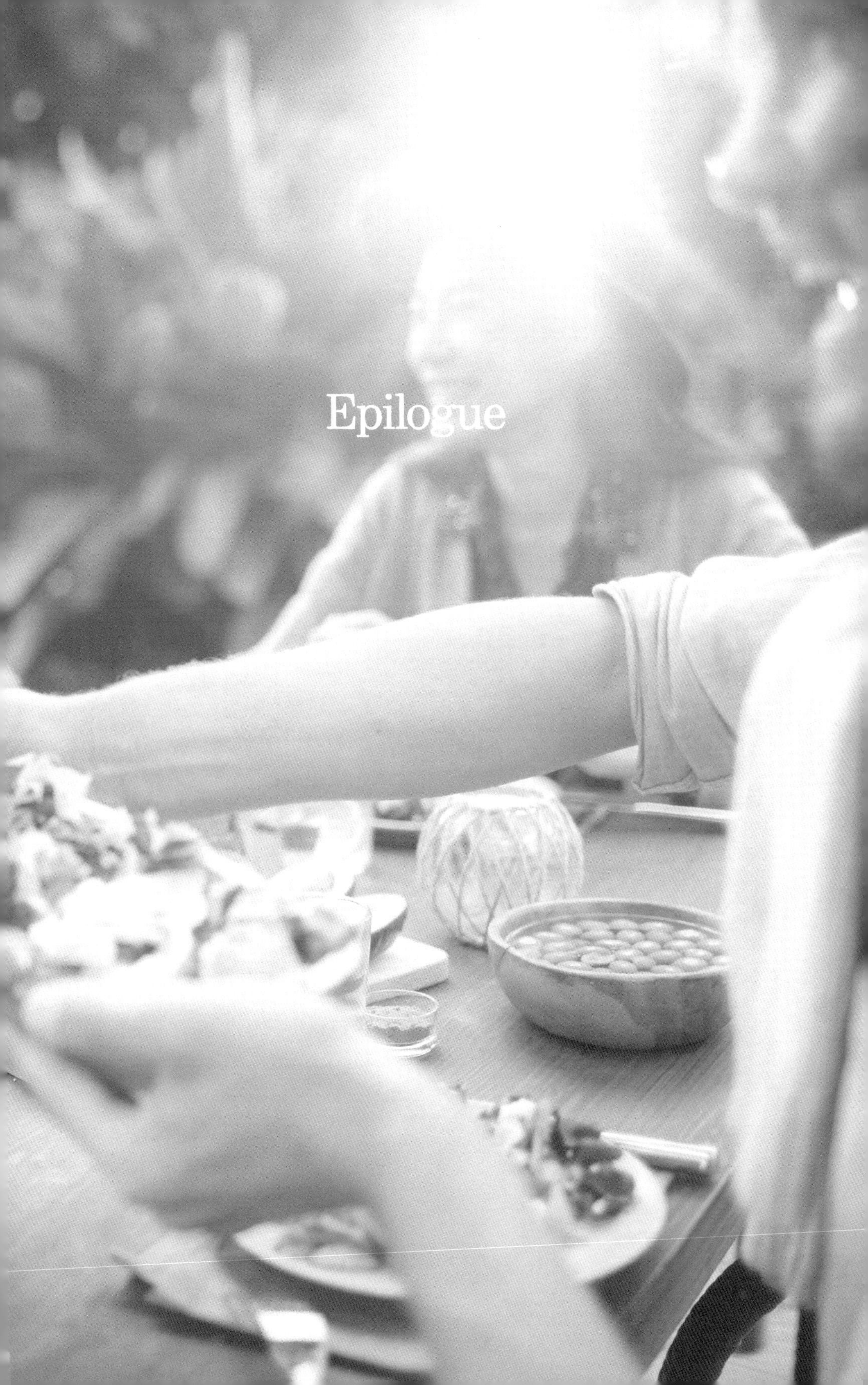

Vegetarianism and life.

People want a happy life. If we recognize that the world is based on causality, if we want a happy life, we can create the cause. One of the important conditions of a happy life is the health of the body. The health of the physical body is closely related to the health of the mind and, furthermore, to the spiritual health. Of these three factors, physical health is supported at the bottom by interacting with the other two. The title of 'the healing' in this article is to express that the vegetarian diet is related not only to the body but, also, to the healing of the mind and the spirituality.

A healthy body is possible through the healthy food and the healthy breathing. These two are the foundations of the existence of all living things. From an evolutionary point of view, humans have been eating the fruits for a long time, and it is, therefore, believed that the fruits are the most suitable for the human body and for the happiest state possible. In reality, we recommend a variety of the vegetable, dietary patterns for a happy life.

The human, vegetative evolution hypothesis.

The earth gave birth to the seed–bearing trees in the last period of the evolution, and the humans had evolved by eating the fruits while moving on the trees. Compared to the other animals, there is a strong grip (gripping force), the amalgamation of the molars, and the mouth of the herbivorous animals, and a frontal incarnate that is well–developed to eat the fruits.

As the humans came down to the prairie, the hand–gripping of the branches came to use the stones and the other natural objects as the tools. With the use of the tools, the language had been developed, and the human abstraction had been further expanded through the development of the language and the script.

The men who had been eating the fruits for a long time had been able to increase the population through the discovery of the grains 10,000 years ago and had been able to create a city. During the past 10,000 years, there has been an increase in the meat consumption in the harsh conditions of the various climates in the regions, but the main nutrient source for most humans has been the plants. Plants have provided the humans with the various nutrients, antioxidants, and vitamins that the humans have ingested for their growth and reproduction

Vegetarian and natural healing

For a long time, the human body has adapted to the global environment. To achieve the high energy production efficiency comparable to the other animals, a dozen systems of the digestive system, the respiratory system, the circulatory system, the nervous system, and the urinary system have elaborately developed their structures and functions. Indeed, the human body is supposed

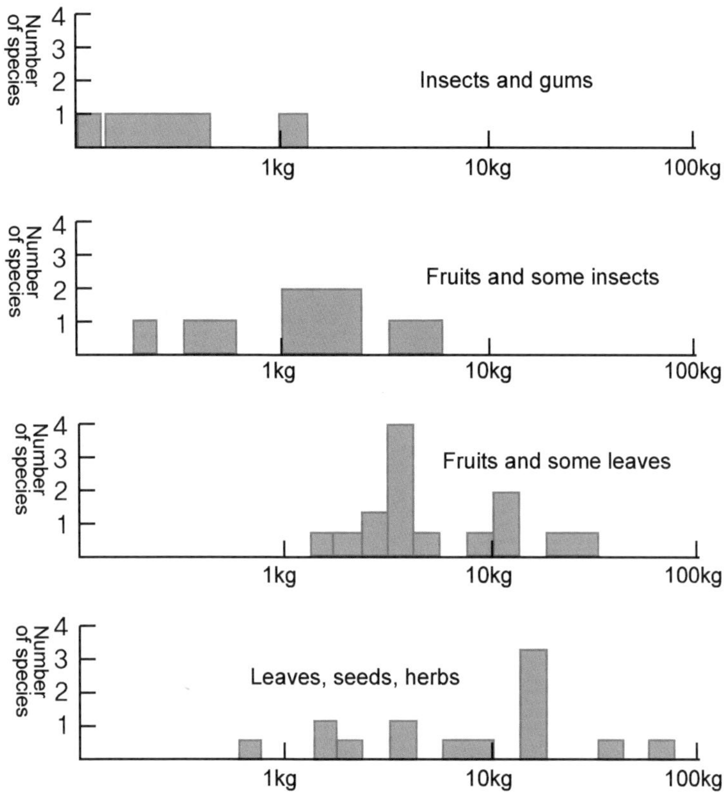

Figure 1. The weight of primates and the type of main food

Primates, the closest species to humans, almost all share vegetable food. Considering the type of food based on the weight of the primates, it is deduced that humans mainly eat fruits, leaves and herbs.

source: Boyd, R. and J.B. Silk, How Humans Evolved: Seventh Edition. 2014: W.W. Norton. p.127

to fulfill its function with a novel structure. The human body is originally healthy and having a disease is abnormal. If the oxygen supply, which is the most suitable material energy for the humans, is smooth through the vegetative diet and the abdominal respiration, the human body generates the energy through its high efficiency, thereby converting the human body into the health state and, in some cases, even more. Therefore, with only a few vegetables in the brown rice beans, people are healed from all kinds of the diseases.

On the other hand, if you supply an energy type, such as meat, that is not suitable for the human body, the human body gets stressed to make the maximum adaptation with the difficulty. All ten systems of the human body are stressed. What is commonly known is that the circulatory system fails due to the clogging of the blood vessels, and the urinary system fails because the waste is not caught properly. One of the mechanisms that has yet to be revealed is the neuroendocrine system and the immune system.

Vegetarianism,the mind, and the neuroendocrine system.

Cholesterol, by altering the levels of the five steroid hormones in the body, disturbs hundreds or thousands of the genes in the body. There are 48 nuclear receptors in the human body, which regulate

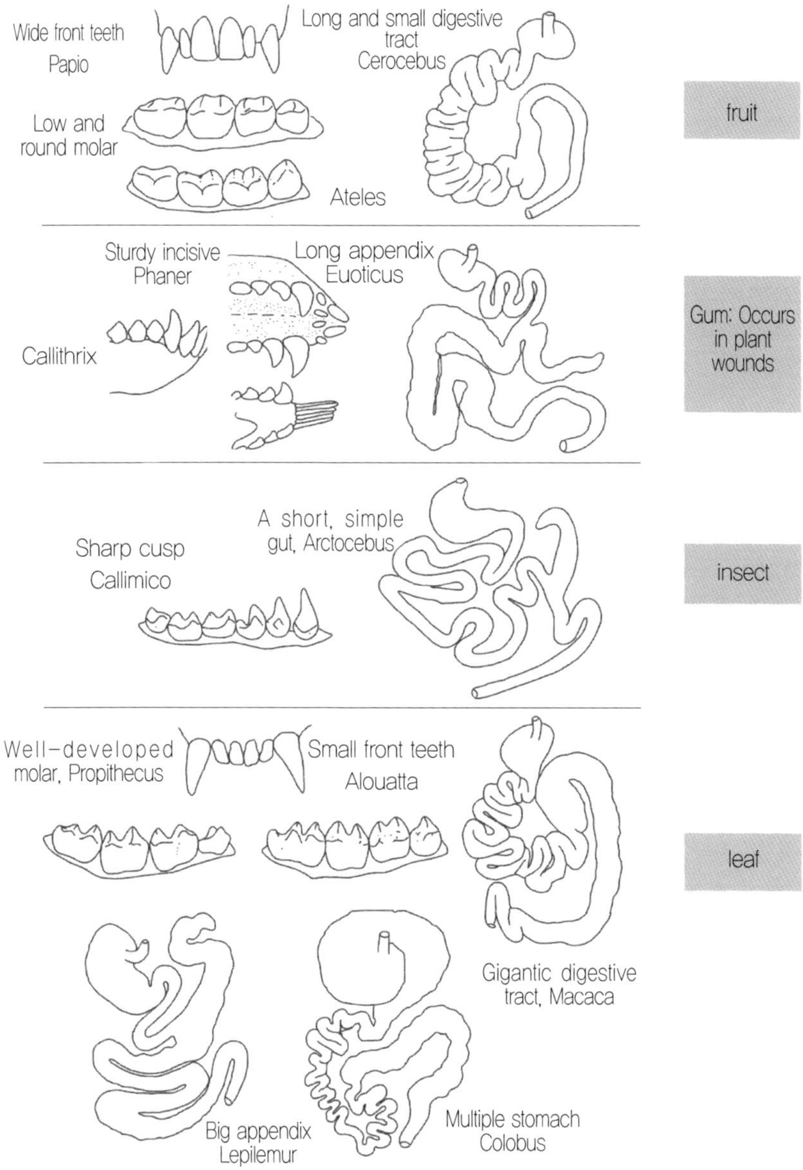

Figure 2. The structure of the digestive tract of primates and the type of main food
Primates, the closest species to humans, almost all share vegetable food. Considering the type of food based on the digestive tract of primates, it is deduced that humans mainly consumed fruits, leaves, herbs, and nuts.: Boyd, R. and J.B. Silk, How Humans Evolved: Seventh Edition. 2014: W.W. Norton. p.116

the genes in all the cells of the human body. A small molecule that signals these nuclear receptors is called a "ligand", and five steroid hormones play a role. In addition, I estimate that the various components of the plants will act as the ligands for the 48 nuclear receptors. An introduction to this was made briefly in Chapter 9.The endocrine system. The results are interesting if the studies of the vegetarian and endocrine systems are going to be carried out in the future.

The endocrine system and the nervous system are connected through the hypothalamus and the pituitary gland. Therefore, changes in the hormones soon lead to changes in the nervous system. The opposite is, also, true. From this point of view, the meat and the veggies produce a difference in the endocrine system, and the logic that it will, also, affect the nervous system is natural. One of these experiments was introduced at the end of Chapter 5 of this bookon the nervous system. Empathy is one of the human characteristics. The brain structures, such as the mirror neurons, which feel the pain of the others as their own, are a biological source of the human culture, civilization, and art. The dietary patterns of the vegetarians and the carnivorous make these brain responses different. This will be seen as a difference of the opinions on the socio-political, social security, and educational policies. Therefore, the sociology based on the diet becomes possible. I suppose that the future nutritional sociology, nutritional psychology, and nutritional neuroendocrinology will develop.

Vegetarianism, the medical expenses, and the sustainable nations.

Reports on the diverse benefits of vegetarianism continue. This is a very obvious fact that cannot be shaken, and the studies of the mechanism have been continuing. Since the 1950s, the production of the nitrogen fertilizer has increased after the Second World War, and the production of the grains has increased together. In order to solve the increased production of the grains in a short time, they had been converted to the grain feed, and, since then, the mankind has been consuming the meat at a very low price. Along with this, the various diseases, such as cancer, the cardiovascular disease, diabetes, obesity, osteoporosis, depression, atopy and the like, have increased rapidly. At the same time, each country experiences a financial crisis due to the medical expenses.

Along with the aging, the chronic spread of the diseases that require the chronic, lifelong treatment has become an important factor in reducing the vitality of the human civilization. We say that, in the next two to three years, one out of every four people in the country will become older than 65 and that the medical expenses will reach 400 trillion won. The national bankruptcy caused by the medical expenses is now only a matter of time. There is a surge in the meat consumption behind it. In the developed countries that recognize these linkages, the policy–based vegetarian dietary patterns are recommended. In this regard, I introduced the

'National Health Expenditure and Global Vegetarianism' (Seo-tae, 2015)'.

Bernard et al., who were introduced at the end of Chapter 11 on the medical costs that could be reduced due to the vegetarian diet, suggested from 35% to as much as 70% of the reduction of the medical costs. As of 2015, if the people pay a total of 100 trillion won for theannual, medical expenses in Korea, you can save from 35 trillion won to 70 trillion won annually through vegetarianism. These savings can be used more productively for the social health through the realizations of the old-age pension and the free education, regarding the high schools, for the university illiteracy, and for building the various social safety nets.

Vegetarianism and the sustainable nations.

In order to spread the vegetarian diet, Gwangju, Jeonbuk, and Jeonnam have already been providing the vegetarian meals once a week for the school lunches. This should be expanded to the day care centers. By 3 years of age, the brain cells are the most active in the lifetime. As introduced in Chapter 5, the average difference in the IQ's of the non-vegetarian and vegetarian children by 18 means how much the meat intake affects the brain development. This will affect not only the IQ, but, also, the various areas, such as the emotional intelligence, the art, and the physical education.

The second requirement is that the National Health and Nutrition

Survey requires a survey on the vegetarian and non-vegetarian levels. This will allow us to study the relationship between the dietary patterns and the health in a larger, more scientific, and empirical way.

The third is to provide a choice of the brown rice or the whole grains in the public food. In order to do this, it is possible to set the rice price higher than the brown rice in the grain policy. This makes it easier to supply the brown rice to the typical, small-sized restaurants.

This article introduces the diverse research literature related to the health benefits of the vegetarian diet to 10 human systems. We hope that we can continue to improve by supplementing the latest data in the future.

〈The Way Between Science and Transcendence〉

Ph.D. Aaron KJ Lee

The source of energy of all components of our body is food. Food can generate the energy by combining with the oxygen supplied through the breathing. The conversion of the energy through the breathing is the purpose of the human existence. This can be seen from the beginning of the universe through the understanding of the evolutionary process of the universe, the galaxy, the solar system, the earth, and the life. Though the names in, and the philosophical logic of, Buddhism, Christianity, Hinduism, Taoism, leading, Kabbalah, yoga, etc. are different, the fundamental core principle is the transcending through the transcendence. Who are you and what are you? The question about this can be answered through the breathing. This article is designed to link the reports of the scientific, philosophical, and mystical experiences to a consistent logic. Through this, we will be able to understand the original purpose of the human beings and find the ways to move toward it. Furthermore, our society will be able to make a system in a way that meets the purpose of life that was originally born with.

The Way Between Science and Transcendence

Contents

Chapter 9. Endocrine system

Chapter 10. Mind system

Part 3. Transcendence and science

Chapter 11. Mysticism and transcendental phenomena

Chapter 12. Meditation and Brain Science

Chapter 13. Light and Quantum Biology

Chapter 14. Quantum psychology and coherence of mind

Part 4. Transcendence and community

〈Cancer Healing and Cancer Prevention in Autophagy and Fasting〉

Aaron KJ Lee

Cancer gets better when you starve. Because cancer has damaged mitochondria and can not use lipids as an energy source. Mitochondria produce 90% of eukaryotic energy as a cell's power plant. In the human body, about 350 grams of glucose is stored in the glycogen format and becomes depleted in 12 hours. However, the lipid content of the human body is 13 kg, which can supply more than 78 days as an energy source. Therefore, when fasting, the human body uses lipid, not glucose, as a main energy source. Cancer cells die from starvation because the mitochondria are destroyed because they can not use lipids as an energy source, while normal cells are made healthier in the fasting process by using the modified ketone bodies as lipids and lipids as an energy source. This is because the mechanism of Autophagy works in the fasting process. Autophagy is the process of decomposing the damaged proteins and damaged mitochondria inside the cell to supply energy from inside the cell when it is not supplied with energy from outside the cell and recycling it as an energy source. This is also the theme of Nobel medical physiology in 2016. This paper explains the changing process of utilization of blood glucose and lipid ketone in the human body through the use of various figures, and explains how the fasting can cure cancer by a scientific principle.

Until now, tens of thousands of papers related to atopy have been published through specialized journals, but there have been almost no single studies on the human body. Modern medicine is trying to promote

Contents

the natural healing process of Autophagy by using drugs when fasting. Modern medicine, coupled with profits, makes it harder to promote the healing process through fasting. In this context, the authors propose that national and local governments should promote national health by running the national or public food service free of charge or at actual costs. By conducting the hunger joints together, healthcare providers will be able to conduct fasting more reliably and safely, and obtain more information in this process.

The autophagy process through fasting is effective not only for cancer, but also for the prevention and healing of diabetes, cardiovascular disease and dementia.